Dictionary of

COMPARATIVE PATHOLOGY and EXPERIMENTAL BIOLOGY

ROBERT W. LEADER, D.V.M.

Associate Professor and Head,
Laboratory of Comparative Pathology,
The Rockefeller University;
Clinical Professor of Pathology,
College of Physicians and Surgeons,
Columbia University

ISABEL LEADER, B.S.

Chief of Microbiology and Parasitology,
Beekman Downtown Hospital,
New York, New York

1971   W. B. SAUNDERS COMPANY

Philadelphia, London, Toronto

229840

W. B. Saunders Company: West Washington Square
Philadelphia, Pa. 19105

12 Dyott Street
London WC1A 1DB

1835 Yonge Street
Toronto 7, Ontario

Dictionary of Comparative Pathology and Experimental Biology   SBN 0-7216-5659-5

Print No.:   9   8   7   6   5   4   3   2   1

Foreword

Recognizing man when we encounter him in ancient documents or in remote places presents no problem. Yet, his biological characteristics cannot account for his uniqueness. He does not possess any noteworthy genetic or developmental singularity not already foreshadowed in lower forms. For example, the ability to walk erect, the liberation of the fore-limbs for manipulation, the crossing over of the optic tracts and binocular vision, the enlargement of the cerebral cortex, and the prolongation of childhood are fundamental human characteristics, but they are not bio-logical innovations of the human species; they are exaggerations or alterations of tendencies seen in all apes. Skills, biological drives, mental attributes, and social organizations considered typically human also appear in primitive forms among mammalian species.

Admittedly the idea of self, conscious reflection, and awareness of mortality are attributes which *seem* peculiar to man, but this is only an assumption and expression of our conceit, since we cannot rule out that other animals also possess these attributes. The only thing which is objectively certain is that man is characterized less by his biological and social endowments than by what he has created from them. He differs from the rest of the animal kingdom chiefly through his collective achievements over several thousands of generations, in other words through his cultural history.

In the preceding paragraphs, I have attempted to differentiate the two contrasting aspects of man's nature – his animal attributes and the humanness of his life – in order to define the scope of the Leaders' enterprise. In their dictionary, they focus attention on biological and behavioral characteristics which exist in a multiplicity of variant forms throughout the animal kingdom, and they leave out of consideration the cultural aspects of human life.

The Leaders have introduced in their text the word *anoman*, of their own making. *Anoman* is an acronym from the phrase "animal other than man" and refers to all species of animals other than *Homo sapiens*. It serves as a substitute for the vague expression "lower animals" and for the inaccurate phrase "man and animals." I have not yet become used to the sound of the word *anoman*, but I like very much the attitude it conveys, namely that man is an animal even though an extraordinary animal. This attitude is consistent with the fact that our unfortunate tendency to neglect our biological kinship to animals has delayed pro-gress toward the solution of biomedical problems and the understanding of behavior. In their dictionary, the Leaders have provided laboratory experimenters and students of human problems with a unique tool that will facilitate a more effective comparative approach to the study of biological, behavioral, and pathological phenomena. With factual exam-ples and lucid explanations, they document how these phenomena manifest themselves in multifarious but related forms throughout the animal kingdom, of which man is as much as ever a biological part, despite the sophistication of his cultural achievements.

RENÉ DUBOS
The Rockefeller University
New York, N.Y.
1971

Preface

Several medical dictionaries have useful entries on comparative and veterinary medicine but lack the range and specificity needed by the experimentalist or general biologist. Dictionaries of veterinary medicine for the most part lack depth in the comparative approach. This book has been written to bridge these gaps. It is intended primarily for use by persons who have considerable background in experimental biology and comparative pathology, and therefore omits general terms already adequately covered in standard medical dictionaries. We have been very selective. Some readers may be disappointed at the omission of favorite subjects, but will feel rewarded by our expanded definitions in many instances in which knowledge of comparative data is of special significance, e.g., *arteriosclerosis, leukemia,* and *zoonosis.*

As we weighed each entry we asked ourselves the question: "How important is this subject to readers in comparative pathobiology, including biologists, physicians, veterinarians, laboratory animal scientists, medical students, veterinary students, graduate students, and teachers of high school biology?"

Obviously a book this size cannot be all inclusive on a subject as broad as comparative pathology (see the definitions of pathology). Therefore a brief bibliography has been added to expand the scope of many entries. The reader will find that these bibliographic notations, while not extensive, will point the way to major segments of the literature and help the reader quickly gather knowledge about a subject unfamiliar to him. Most of the references are to books or symposia rather than individual journal articles. For example, the biologist who wishes to inquire further into immunologic diseases can find several references under *immunopathology, antibody, autoimmune disease,* and *immunoglobulin.* Even though the list is short, each citation leads to many additional sources of information.

In order to make the book more functional much information is presented in tabular form; see *acariasis, animal model,* and *immunoglobulin.* This not only saves space, but also allows the reader to scan complex subjects quickly. All the tables are included in the text, except two extensive ones, which are presented as addenda to avoid interrupting the continuity of the main entries.

Comparative medicine has emphasized infectious diseases since the time of Koch and Pasteur. Many of the greatest contributions to this science have come from studies in this field, and it is fitting that we have given them extensive coverage in our book.

Virtually no coverage has been given by other dictionaries to terms used by experimental behaviorists. The three hundred or so representatives of this vocabulary which we have included are a hopeful start in this direction.

Information about husbandry, breeds, genetic characteristics, and diseases of common laboratory animals is scattered in many books, and this is a major obstacle to teachers and students of biology and to scientists engaged in biological research. Recognizing this we have, with the invaluable assistance of Dr. Steven Weisbroth, included extensive information in this category, with special emphasis on the diseases of rats, mice, and rabbits. We have omitted much clinical information about the diseases of other species of domestic animals, such as cows, sheep, horses, and pigs, in deference to the need for more thorough treatment of the laboratory animals.

The coverage of invertebrates is limited, but the major diseases of these animals are included. The late Dr. Steinhaus, who along with Dr. Martignoni, assisted us with this material, spent his career proselytizing the scientific community to the cause of invertebrate pathology. Perhaps we can help his cause creep a small distance further forward.

The decades ahead will see pathology of the environment grow into an important area of study, and we must know more about the diseases of all animals, including invertebrates, in order to assess and control the environment. Arthropods, for instance, make up 82 per cent of the earth's species, and of these 92 per cent are insects. But insects have been studied principally for the diseases they carry to man and anomen. How do these diseases affect insects themselves? Can we control undesirable insects with biological methods? (See *Bacillus thuringiensis*.)

We found the vital area of genetics – especially as this science relates to disease – poorly covered in standard medical dictionaries. We have therefore devoted special effort to extracting what we considered the most significant data concerning this subject from textbooks and other sources. We believe that studies of disease by the use of animal models of genetic aberrations provide some of the most easily measured and readily interpreted study systems. If genetic modification is to become an important tool in correcting hereditary diseases, animal models will be indispensible.

The continuity of evolution and the stability of species are dependent in great measure upon two phenomena: the ability of the genome to pass along species information (see *gene*) and the ability of the individual member of a species to recognize and accept his own tissue components while rejecting those which are foreign (see *immunopathology*). Cancer, immunologic diseases, defense against infections, the capacity to conceive, and the ability to be born, all are bound up with the principles and mechanisms underlying genetics and immunology. Comparative pathology exists as a discipline and will grow as a science largely to the extent that it can unify and interpret these groups of phenomena. For these reasons we have given much space and emphasis to immunologic phenomena and heredity as they relate to disease.

R. W. LEADER
ISABEL LEADER
New York, N.Y.
1971

Acknowledgments

Help and advice were given often and generously to the authors by many colleagues, including Dr. John Gorham, Dr. George Padgett, and Dr. Keith Farrell of Washington State University; Dr. Carolyn Ripps, Dr. Caleb Finch, Dr. Arthur Hurvitz, Mr. William Bayless, Mr. Reynard Biemiller, and Dr. Lee Ehrman of The Rockefeller University; Dr. Bernard Wagner of The College of Physicians & Surgeons, Columbia University; and Dr. William Hardy of Sloan Kettering Institute.

Miss Ann Marie Quatela courageously and cheerfully endured many crises, short-notice deadlines, and revisions of material.

Mr. John P. Friel of W. B. Saunders Company helped immensely by exhibiting limitless patience and by supplying sound judgment and a precise sense of correctness.

Special credit is owed to Dr. Steven H. Weisbroth, formerly of The Rockefeller University, now at the State University of New York, Stony Brook, N.Y., who selected and prepared all drafts of material dealing with laboratory animals and transmissible tumors, as well as giving valuable consultation on many other subjects.

Consultants in other specific areas who aided us immensely are Dr. Gordon Ball, The Rockefeller University, in experimental behavior; Dr. Frank Fenner, The John Curtin School of Medicine, Canberra, Australia, in virology; and Dr. Mauro E. Martignoni, U.S. Department of Agriculture, and the late Dr. Edward A. Steinhaus, University of California, in invertebrate pathology.

R. W. LEADER
ISABEL LEADER

Contents

Page

VOCABULARY 1

ADDENDA

    Table of Animal Models 223
    Table of Zoonoses by Type of Etiologic Agent 229

BIBLIOGRAPHY 235

A

aardvark (earth hog; ant bear)   A mammal about 60 kg. in weight, native to Africa south of the Sahara Desert. Aardvark, an Afrikaans word meaning "earth-pig," is applied to these animals because of their burrowing habits.[110]

aardwolf (earth wolf)   A hyena-like mammal of southern and eastern Africa.[110]

ab-   A prefix signifying from, off, away from.

abiotic   In laboratory parlance, nonliving.

ablastin   An antibody that develops in response to invasion with certain parasitic protozoa and inhibits their reproduction. The development of ablastin in bacterial invasion has not been conclusively demonstrated.

Abolea   A genus of gerbil.

abomasitis   Inflammation of the abomasum. The most common causes are ingestion of unsuitable or spoiled fodder, acute infections, and consumption of irritant substances such as acids, lye, or newly slaked lime, or of certain poisonous plants or metallic poisons such as mercury, lead, or arsenic.

abomasum   The fourth or true stomach of the ruminant animal; it contains glands which secrete gastric enzymes. The other parts of the ruminant stomach are the rumen, reticulum, and omasum.

aboral   Situated away from or farthest from the mouth.

abort   1. To check the usual course of a disease. 2. To miscarry before the fetus is viable. 3. To become checked in development.

abortion   Expulsion of an embryo or nonviable fetus prior to the normal termination of gestation, as opposed to premature birth, which occurs after the stage of viability has been reached but before full term.

   a. from brucellosis, a variety caused by species of *Brucella: B. melitensis,* the agent of Mediterranean fever, gastric fever, or Malta fever causes abortion in goats and has been isolated from the milk of infected cattle and aborted fetuses of sheep; *B. abortus,* the agent of undulant fever, causes abortion in cattle (Bang's disease); *B. suis* causes abortion in swine and also infects horses, cattle, fowl, and dogs. All three species can infect man. *B. canis* causes abortion in dogs.

   contagious a., abortion caused by an infectious agent, particularly abortion in cattle caused by *Brucella abortus.*

   enzootic a. of ewes, abortion in ewes in California and Scotland for which an organism of the psittacosis-lymphogranuloma (*Chlamydia*) group has been found responsible. The abortion usually occurs during late gestation, the clinical symptoms closely resembling those of ovine vibriosis.

   equine viral a., an infection of the fetus with the virus of equine rhinopneumonitis; sometimes also caused by the virus of equine arteritis. See also *equine rhinopneumonitis.*

   Listeria a., abortion caused by *Listeria monocytogenes* during late pregnancy in cattle and sheep.

   mycotic a. of cattle, a form caused by several species of fungi of the genera *Mucor* and *Aspergillus.*

   paratyphoid a., a purulent hemorrhagic placentitis with necrosis of the chorionic villi, caused by *Salmonella abortus-equi.*

   Toxoplasma a., abortion caused by *T. gondii* and manifested as focal necrosis of placenta; most common in sheep.

   trichomonal a., abortion caused by *Trichomonas fetus* and transmitted by coitus.

   vibrionic a., abortion of cattle and sheep caused by *Vibrio fetus.*[16, 142]

ABR test (abortus-Bang-ring test)   A modified agglutination test used for detection of *Brucella* antibodies in milk. A suspension of *Brucella abortus* stained with hematoxylin is mixed with fresh milk, and a positive test is indicated by a decolorized milk column capped by a bluish violet layer of cream.

abrachia   A developmental anomaly characterized by complete absence of the arms.

abrachiocephalia   A developmental anomaly characterized by absence of the arms and head.

abscess   A circumscribed area of inflammation containing destroyed tissue, leukocytes, and miscellaneous debris (pus) which, in later stages, is frequently surrounded by a wall of fibrous tissue.

abscissa   One of two coordinates, the other of which is called the ordinate, used as a frame of reference. The abscissa is usually horizontal and the ordinate vertical, and when suitable values have been assigned to them the corresponding data can be plotted.

Absidia   A genus of pathogenic fungi of the family Mucoraceae capable of causing mycoses of the internal organs of animals. *A. lichtheimi* has been reported as the cause of mycosis in mink. *A. ramora* causes mucormycosis of swine and may also play a role in bovine mycotic abortions (see *mucormycosis*).

absolute zero   The hypothetical point in the temperature scale (−273.16° C. and 0° Kelvin) at which there is complete absence of heat.

absorbance   A measure of the loss of intensity of radiation passing through an absorbing medium.

abyssal   Living in the depths of the sea.

Acacia georgina   A tree of northern Austra-

1

lia; the fluoroacetate content of its leaves causes death in sheep and cattle.[13]

acantho- A combining form meaning thorny or spiny, or denoting a relationship to a sharp spine or thorn.

Acanthocephala (thorny-headed worm) A division (class) of nematodes which parasitize the digestive tract of fishes, amphibians, reptiles, and mammals (see table) and which possess a cylindrical body and a spiny proboscis, by which they attach themselves to the host.

ACANTHOCEPHALIDS AND THEIR
HOSTS[11, 21, 99, 116]

SPECIES	HOST
Acanthocephalus anthuris	Amphibians
A. lucii	Fish
A. ranae	Amphibians (mainly frogs)
Corynosoma inerme	Seal
C. strumosum	Lamprey
C. semerme	Lamprey
Echinorhynchus salmonis	Lamprey
Macracanthorhynchus hirudinaceus	Swine, occasionally cattle
Moniliformis moniliformis	Man, rat, mouse
Neoechinorhynchus spp. N. vutili	Reptiles (chiefly Chelonia, the long-necked turtle)
Oncicola canis	Dog, immature forms in turkey, swine
Plagiorhynchus formosus	Chicken, flicker, crow, robin
Polymorphus boschadis	Duck
Pomphorhynchus laevis	Fish
Immature forms of other acanthocephalids	Snakes

acanthocephaliasis Infestation with any species of the class Acanthocephala.

acanthosis A thickening of the epidermis characterized by proliferation and downgrowth of the stratum germinativum (prickle cell layer).

a. nigricans, in anomen, this condition is seen most commonly in Dachshund dogs as lesions of the axillae and inner side of the thighs, probably caused by endocrine imbalance.[78]

acardia A developmental anomaly characterized by absence of the heart.

acardius An imperfectly formed free twin fetus lacking a heart and invariably lacking other body parts as well.

acariasis (mange) Infestation with mites (see table).

acarid A mite or tick. See table.

acarine disease A disease of adult bees caused by the parasitic mite *Acarapis woodi*. The mite mainly infests the tracheae leading from the first pair of thoracic spiracles. Bees so affected become incapable of flight and the life of overwintered infested bees is shortened. See also *Isle of Wight disease* and *acariasis*.

acclimatization The physiological and behavioral adjustment of a species to a new environment over several generations.

accomplice A bacterium that accompanies the chief infecting agent in a mixed infection and that influences the virulence of the chief organism.

acenaphthene A chemical agent that induces polyploidy.

acentric Lacking a centromere, so that the chromosome will not survive subsequent cell divisions.

acephalia A developmental anomaly characterized by absence of the head.

acephalobrachia A developmental anomaly characterized by absence of the head and arms.

acephalocardia A developmental anomaly characterized by absence of the head and heart.

acephalocyst A headless, baglike hydatid filled with liquid; it is one of the stages in the existence of a sterile cestoid worm (Laennec, 1804).

acephalopodia A developmental anomaly characterized by absence of the head and feet.

acetaldehydase An enzyme that catalyzes the oxidation of acetic aldehyde to acetic acid.

acetic thiokinase An enzyme of the Embden-Meyerhof pathway that converts acetate to acetyladenylate and acetyladenylate to acetyl coenzyme A, using ATP and Mg^{++} as co-factors.

acetoacetate decarboxylase An enzyme of the lipogenic-lipolytic pathway that converts acetoacetate to acetone.

acetoacetyl-succinic thiophorase An enzyme of the lipogenic-lipolytic pathway that catalyzes the conversion of acetoacetate to acetoacetyl coenzyme A.

acetolase An enzyme that catalyzes the conversion of alcohol into acetic acid.

acetonemia (ketosis) The presence in the blood of ketone (acetone) bodies in abnormally large quantities, commonly seen in diabetes mellitus. The ketone substances comprise three chemical compounds—beta-hydroxybutyric acid, acetoacetic acid, and acetone—which represent successive stages in the catabolic oxidation and utilization of fatty acids.

bovine a., an abnormal rise in the level of ketone bodies related to impaired gluconeogenesis, seen frequently in dairy cattle during the postparturient period. See also *toxemia of pregnancy*.

ovine a. (pregnancy disease of ewes), ketosis of ewes which occurs during the last few weeks of pregnancy and is accompanied by severe hypoglycemia. See also *toxemia of pregnancy*.

aceto-orcein A dye consisting of orcein dissolved in acetic acid; used to stain squash preparations of chromosomes.

acetylation The introduction of an acetyl group into an organic molecule.

acetylcholine A reversible acetic acid

ACARIDS PARASITIC ON MAN AND ANOMEN[21, 116]

SPECIES	SITE	HOST
Acarapis woodi	Trachea	Adult bees (see also *Isle of Wight disease* and *acarine disease.*)
Chyletiella parasitivorax	Skin	Cat, rabbit, dog
Chorioptes spp.	Skin, feet, base of tail	Sheep, horse, goat, cow, rabbit (ear)
Cytodites nudus	Air sacs	Bird
Demodex folliculorum	Hair follicles, sebaceous glands	Dog, cat, man, pig, sheep, cow
D. phylloides	Hair follicles, sebaceous glands	Pig
Dermanyssus gallinae	Skin	Poultry
Entonyssus spp.	Trachea, lungs	Snake
Hannemania spp.	Skin	Amphibian
Cnemidocoptes gallinae	Feather follicles	Chicken
C. mutans	Skin of legs	Chicken
Linguatula serrata	Nasal respiratory passages	Man, dog, fox, wolf, horse, goat, sheep
Notoedres cati	Skin	Cat, rabbit, others
Ophionyssus natricis	Skin	Snakes
Ornithonyssus spp.	Feathers, skin	Chicken
Pneumonyssus caninum	Paranasal sinuses	Dog
P. simicola	Bronchioles, alveoli	Rhesus monkey
Psorergates ovis	Skin (forms cysts)	Sheep
P. simplex	Skin (forms cysts)	Mouse
Psoroptes communis	Ears	Rabbit, sheep, cow, horse
Sarcoptes spp.	Skin	Cow, dog, man, sheep, pig, horse, rabbit
Trombicula spp. (chiggers)	Skin	Birds, mammals, including man
Tyroglyphus	Urinary, intestinal tract	Man, dog

ester of choline, $CH_3 \cdot CO \cdot O \cdot CH_2 \cdot CH_2 \cdot N-(CH_3)3 \cdot OH$, normally present in many parts of the body and having important physiological functions, such as the transmission of a nerve impulse across a synapse; used as a parasympathomimetic agent.

acetylcholinesterase An enzyme that catalyzes the cleavage of acetylcholine to form choline and acetate. High concentrations are found in neuronal synapses.

acetylphosphatase An enzyme in muscle that catalyzes the splitting of acetylphosphate.

acheilia A developmental anomaly characterized by absence of one or both lips.

acheiria A developmental anomaly characterized by absence of one or both hands.

acheiropodia A developmental anomaly characterized by absence of hands and feet.

achondroplasia (chondrodystrophy) An abnormality in the conversion of cartilage into bone, resulting in asymmetrical dwarfism. This anomaly has been preserved by selective breeding in certain breeds of dogs such as the Dachshund.

  bovine a., an autosomal recessive trait, seen in "bull-dog" calves of the Dexter breed.

  a. of domestic fowl, an autosomal dominant trait affecting Scots, Dumpies, and Japanese bantams. Homozygous birds usually die during the first week of incubation.[67]

achordate Without a notochord; used with reference to animals below the chordates.

Achorion See *Trichophyton.*

acid 1. Any compound of an electronegative element with one or more hydrogen atoms that are replaceable by electropositive atoms. 2. A colloquialism referring to lysergic acid diethylamide (LSD).

acid-fast bacteria Organisms which, after being stained with warm solutions of fuchsin, resist the decolorizing action of strong acids. This reaction is characteristic of *Mycobacterium* species and certain other higher bacteria.[16]

  atypical acid-fast b., a group of microorganisms capable of producing disease in man; some may have originally infected anomen. They are classified as follows: group I or photochromogens, which produce no pigment in the dark, and yellow pigment in the light (*Mycobacterium ulcerans, M. marinum, and M. kansasii,* the last having been derived from the cow); group II or scotochromogens, which produce yellow-orange-red pigment (*M. scrofilaceum*); group III or nonphotochromogens (the "Battey" group), which are pleomorphic and produce *Nocardia*-like filaments and seem to be closely related to the avian types; group IV or rapid growers (*M. fortuitum*), which are pathogenic for man and lower animals.

acid fuchsin A mixture of sulfonated fuchsins used in complex stains and in Andrade's indicator.[153]

aconitase An enzyme of the Krebs cycle that converts citrate to *cis*-aconitate, and *cis*-aconitate to isocitrate.

aconite (monkshood; wolfsbane) An extremely poisonous plant, *Aconitum napellus,* found in all parts of the world.[36]

acorn calf A calf affected with congenital achondroplasia.[13, 67]

acorn poisoning Oak leaf poisoning.[13]

acquisition A term used in behavioral science to indicate progressive increments in response strength observed over a series of occasions on which the response is measured.

acrania   A developmental anomaly characterized by partial or complete absence of the cranium or skull.

acridine orange   A basic dye of the acridine group soluble in water, alcohol, and glycerol and used in fluorescence microscopy for staining bacteria and other cells, for differentiating living from dead cells in soil, for the differential staining of DNA from RNA, for the cytodiagnosis of cancer, and as an indicator of the viability of cells after thermal and radiation damage.[37, 57]

acriflavine   A basic dye of the acridine group. Solubility at 15° C.: water 5 per cent, absolute alcohol, 0.5 per cent; and glycerol 4 per cent. Originally used by Benda to stain trypanosomes, it is now used to demonstrate infectious microorganisms, as a vital stain for nuclei, and to label transfused leukocytes to determine their life-span in the circulation.[37, 57, 153]

acro-   A combining form denoting relation to an extremity, top, or summit, or to an extreme.

acrobrachycephaly   A condition resulting from fusion of the coronal suture, causing abnormal shortening of the anteroposterior diameter of the skull.

acrocentric   Having the centromere near one end of the replicating chromosome, so that one arm is much longer than the other.

acronym   A word formed by the initial letters of the principal components of a compound term, as laser (light amplification by stimulated emission of radiation) or anoman (animal other than man).

acrophobia   Fear of high places.

acrosome   A caplike organelle of the anterior sperm head which contains hydrolytic enzymes that are thought to digest the egg coat to facilitate fertilization.

actin   A muscle protein discovered by Szent-Györgyi. It occurs in filaments, which, acting along with myosin particles, are responsible for the contraction and relaxation of muscle. See also actomyosin.

actinic   Pertaining to those rays of light beyond the violet end of the spectrum that produce chemical effects.

actino-   A combining form denoting relation to a ray, as ray-shaped, or pertaining to some form of radiation.

actinobacillosis (wooden tongue)   A bacterial infection caused by gram-negative bacilli of the genus Actinobacillus, seen mainly in cattle but also in other species (see Actinobacillus). It may affect the jaw but is more frequently seen in soft tissue such as the tongue, cervical lymph nodes, and occasionally other organs. The lesions consist of heavily encapsulated granulomata with focal areas or streaks of suppuration. Colonies of organisms found in the pus are visible as tiny granules less than 1 mm. in diameter, which are referred to as sulfur granules.[16]

Actinobacillus   A genus of rod-shaped microorganisms which form small cheeselike granules similar to the sulfur granules of actinomycosis. There are five species: A. lig-nieresi causes actinobacillosis in cattle, A. actinomycetemcomitans infects man, A. equuli infects foals, A. actinoides causes chronic pneumonia in calves, and A. mallei (formerly Malleomyces mallei) causes glanders in solipeds.[16]

Actinomyces   A genus of microorganisms which grow in the form of branched mycelium that breaks up into segments. They are anaerobic or microaerophilic, gram-positive, nonacid-fast saprophytes which occasionally cause disease in man and anomen. A. bovis infects cattle, A. israeli infects man and occasionally cattle, and A. baudetii infects dogs and cats.[16, 36]

actinomycetin   A poorly characterized substance produced by most species of Streptomyces, which can cause lysis, especially of gram-positive bacteria.[49]

actinomycin   Any of a family of antibiotics isolated from species of Streptomyces, which are active against gram-positive organisms and are potent immunosuppressants that inhibit DNA-dependent RNA synthesis by formation of complexes with DNA.[36, 49]

actinomycosis (lumpy jaw)   A disease of cattle, swine, and sometimes man caused by species of Actinomyces. Most commonly it affects the jaw but may invade the brain, lungs, or abdominal organs, the lesions consisting of granulomata which may eventually discharge viscid pus containing minute yellowish granules. The organism is a common inhabitant of soil and the oral cavity and enters a wound to establish infection. In dogs, it may invade the abdominal organs from bite wounds.

actithiazic acid   An antibiotic produced by species of Streptomyces that is active against mycobacteria because of its antagonism against biotin.[49]

actomyosin   The system of actin filaments and myosin particles constituting muscle fibers and responsible for the contraction and relaxation of muscle. See also actin and myosin.

acu-   A combining form denoting relationship to a needle.

acupuncture   The insertion of needles into a part for the production of counterirritation.

acute   Denoting a disease process having a short course, usually less than one week. It is frequently misused to denote a disease process of severe nature but should be used only in relation to time, as contrasted to its antonym, chronic.

acute bee paralysis   See acute paralysis under paralysis.

ad-   A prefix expressing to or toward, addition to, nearness, or intensification.

-ad   A suffix expressing direction toward, as in cephalad, caudad.

adactylia   A developmental anomaly characterized by the absence of digits on the hand or foot.

adamantanamine   A tricyclic amine that inhibits cell infection by myxoviruses. The mechanism is not known but has its effect before the virus enters the cell.

adaptability The capacity of an organism or a population to change in response to environmental demands, so that continued survival is favored. This may be phenotypic adaptability (as in acclimatization) or genotypic. Cf. *adaptedness.*

adaptable enzyme Inducible enzyme; see under *enzyme.*

adaptation 1. The fitness of an organism for its environment, or the process by which it becomes fit. Such adaptation may be structural, physiological, behavioral, or color adaptation. See *adaptedness.* 2. A condition in reflex activity marked by a decline in the frequency of responses when sensory stimuli are repeated several times. See *habituation.*

    sensory a., in behavioral science, an incremental or decremental change in response or response strength that has been demonstrated to depend solely upon changes in the state of a receptor organ exposed to protracted or repetitive stimulation.

adaptedness The state of a population with respect to its environment, as the ability of a species to survive and reproduce in a given environment. Cf. *adaptability.*

adaptive coloration Adjustment of color patterns of animals either to make them more conspicuous or to conceal them.

adaptive convergence Superficial similarities of behavior, structure, and physiology in widely different groups that inhabit the same environment.

adaptive enzyme Inducible enzyme; see under *enzyme.*

adaptive peak A figurative estimate of the greatest possible degree of adaptability of an organism to its environment; any deviation from the tip of the peak indicates a lesser degree of adaptation.

adaptive radiation Evolutionary changes of a single phyletic line that affect the physiology, structure, and behavior of a single species to make it better adapted to different environmental conditions.

addax An antelope, *Addax nasomaculatus,* that inhabits the Sahara Desert.

adder A poisonous snake, *Vipera berus,* of the family Viperidae. See table accompanying *snake.*

Addison's disease (bronzed skin; melasma suprarenale) A disease characterized by a bronzelike pigmentation of the skin, severe prostration, progressive anemia, low blood pressure, diarrhea, and digestive disturbance. It is due to disease (hypofunction) of the adrenal glands and is usually fatal.

addled A term used in apiculture to describe eggs that fail to hatch, larvae that fail to pupate, and pupae of honeybees that die without any apparent infection. Addled eggs and addled brood are the results of genetic anomalies. Highly inbred queen bees have been shown to produce addled progeny.

adenase A deaminizing enzyme that catalyzes the conversion of adenine to hypoxanthine and ammonia.

adeno-, aden- A combining form denoting relationship to a gland or glands.

adenoacanthoma An adenocarcinoma in which some of the constituent elements exhibit malignant metaplasia to cells of a squamous type.

adenoameloblastoma Ameloblastoma characterized by the formation of ductlike structures in place of or in addition to the typical odontogenic pattern.

adenocarcinoma Carcinoma in which the cells are arranged in the form of glands.

    enzootic intestinal a., terminal ileitis of hamsters; see under *ileitis.*

    gastric a. 303, a tumor first induced by the injection of 20-methylcholanthrene into the wall of the glandular stomach of the C3H mouse, in the laboratory of H. L. Stewart at the National Cancer Institute in 1948. It has since been carried in C3H or C3H$_f$ inbred mice, in which it grows in nearly 100 per cent of cases, killing the most approximately 100 days after subcutaneous transplantation.[150]

    gastric a. 328, a tumor first induced in a strain C57B1 mouse by the injection of 20-methylcholanthrene into the wall of the glandular stomach, in the laboratory of H. L. Stewart at the National Cancer Institute in 1949. From the outset subcutaneous transplants grew progressively in 100 per cent of C57B1 hosts. It has a transplant interval of four weeks. An interesting feature of this tumor is the hypervolemia that accompanies tumor growth in most hosts.[150]

    mammary a. C3HBA, a spontaneous tumor found at necropsy in a nine-month-old C3H mouse in the laboratory of H. B. Andervont at the National Cancer Institute in 1946. When transplanted subcutaneously, it becomes palpable in seven to nine days and kills the host in ten to twenty-eight days, only rarely metastasizing. The tumor has been shown to contain the mammary tumor milk agent.[150]

    mammary a. R2426, a spontaneously arising adenocarcinoma of the mammary gland observed in a female rat of the August strain in the laboratory of M. R. Curtis and W. F. Dunning at the Institute of Cancer Research, Columbia University, in 1939. The tumor may be transplanted by a variety of routes, with 100 per cent successful growths in the August strain of inbred rats. It is not adaptable to rats of other strains. Pulmonary metastases occur frequently.[150]

    pulmonary a. C4661, an alveologenic carcinoma of the lung induced in strain A inbred mice by subcutaneous injections of 20-methylcholanthrene. The tumor was developed in Heston's laboratory at the National Cancer Institute in 1943. From the outset the tumor grew progressively, without regression, in 100 per cent of strain A mice. A subcutaneous transplant becomes palpable seven days after inoculation, measures 2 cm. in diameter by the twenty-first day, and kills the host within six weeks. It is continued by serial passage in strain A mice with transplant intervals of 14 to 21 days.[150]

    renal a. (Lucke frog tumor; Lucke renal adenocarcinoma), a spontaneous renal ad-

enocarcinoma first observed by B. Lucke in
1932 in about 2 per cent of leopard frogs
(*Rana pipiens*) used in student laboratories
at the University of Pennsylvania. The spontaneous tumor is twice as common in males
as females and varies in size from a pinpoint
to those that entirely replace the kidney. The
propensity for metastasis is found to be influenced by the nutritional plane and body
temperature of the poikilothermic host.
Lucke argued, and produced experiments
consistent with, an etiology based on viral
induction, but this view is not accepted by
all. The tumor may be maintained by transplantation to the subcutis, eye, or kidney of
frogs or tadpoles. Virus particles have been
observed in electron photomicrographs.[150]

adenofibroma   A tumor composed of connective tissue containing glandular structures.

adenoma   A glandular benign tumor.

adenomatosis   A condition characterized by
multiple glandular growths.

   pulmonary a., an ovine disease of unknown origin characterized by the proliferation of bronchiolar, alveolar, or septal cells
in the lungs in progressive pneumonia, so
severe that it resembles neoplasia. Metastases to lymph nodes have been reported.[142]
See also *jaagsiekte* and *maedimaedi*.

adenosine diphosphate (ADP)   A product,
along with organic phosphate, of the hydrolysis of adenosine triphosphate.

adenosine triphosphate (ATP)   A nucleotide compound occurring in all cells; it represents energy storage.

adenosinetriphosphatase   An enzyme that
catalyzes the splitting of adenosine triphosphate into adenosine diphosphate, with liberation of inorganic phosphate. Abbreviated
ATPase.

adenovirus   Any of a group of DNA-containing viruses which cause disease in man
and anomen (see table). They replicate in
the nucleus of cells and are characterized by
a structure of 252 capsomeres. Certain
strains are capable of causing tumors when
inoculated into newborn hamsters and are
able to transform cultured cells into malignant variants. These oncogenic properties
have made them valuable tools in the search
for greater knowledge about the nature of
virus-induced neoplasms. The best known
adenovirus of anomen is the virus of canine
hepatitis (fox encephalitis).[39] See also classification, under *virus*, and see *oncogenic
viruses.*

adjuvant   In immunology, a substance or
substances which, when added to injected
antigen, enhance antibody production; they
are particularly useful when only small
amounts of antigen are available. Several
substances have been used, including alum,
aluminum hydroxide, lanolin, various oils,
bacteria, and tapioca.

   Freund's a., a water-in-oil emulsion of sa-
line and a mixture of an emulsifier such as
Aquaphor in mineral oil. *Complete Freund's
a.* contains, in addition, heat-killed acid-fast
mycobacteria.

adjuvant arthritis   See under *arthritis.*

ad lib.   Abbreviation of L. *ad lib'itum,* at
pleasure.

Adonis   A genus of poisonous ranuncula-
ceous plants, native to Europe, Asia, and Africa. *A. aestiva'lis* and *A. verna'lis* are valuable cardiac stimulants.

adoral   Near or toward the mouth.

ADP   Adenosine diphosphate.

adrenal cortical carcinoma WK1546   A tumor of the adrenal cortex that arose spontaneously in a spayed 18-month-old (DBA × -
CE)F₁ hybrid mouse, observed at necropsy in
the laboratory of M. Dickie at the Jackson
Memorial Laboratory in 1950. The tumor is
maintained by subcutaneous transplantation
in (DBA × CE)F₁ hybrids, either intact or
castrated, with an interval of six to nine
months.[150]

Aedes   A genus of culicine mosquitoes responsible for the transmission of many arbo-
viruses. See *mosquito.*

Aegyptianella   Protozoan blood parasites
closely related to the *Babesia* group, differing in that the forms in erythrocytes divide
several times. Cf. *Babesia.*

Aelurostrongylus abstrusus   The lungworm of cats. Adults inhabit branches of
the pulmonary artery, where they produce
ova which enter the alveoli to develop into
larvae, which are then coughed up, swallowed, and passed in the feces. The life cycle
outside the definitive host is unknown.[100]

aerobe   A microorganism that can live and
grow in the presence of free oxygen.

aerobic   Growing only in the presence of molecular oxygen.

aerobiology   That branch of biology which
deals with the distribution of living organisms by the air, either the exterior or out-

ADENOVIRUS INFECTIONS[2, 39, 114]

ADENOVIRUS	DISEASE
Avian	None
Bovine	Probably viral diarrhea
Canine	Viral hepatitis, fox encephalitis
Human: 28 antigenic types, of which types 7, 12, and 18 have shown oncogenic properties	Conjunctivitis, diarrhea, respiratory infections
Murine	None except by injection of suckling mice
Simian	Rhinitis, conjunctivitis; some strains are oncogenic for newborn hamsters

door air (extramural a.) or the indoor air (intramural a.).

aerosol A suspension of liquid or solid particles in a gas. In biology, usually an air-suspended population of microorganisms. In animals exposed to aerosol clouds, particles larger than 5μ are probably trapped before reaching the lung alveoli.

aerosol apparatus A machine that produces aerosol clouds for the exposure of animals.

aerosol infection One due to exposure to an aerosol cloud. Some organisms that may be used to produce infection by the aerosol method are *Bacillus anthracis, Brucella, Coccidioides immitis, Diplococcus pneumoniae, Mycobacterium tuberculosis, Pasteurella pestis, P. tularensis,* and monkey B virus.

aerosol vaccination Vaccination by exposure to an aerosol cloud. This method has been used to produce immunity against Newcastle disease of chickens and canine distemper and, in Russia, against plague, anthrax, tularemia, and brucellosis in man and anomen.[29]

Aerospace Medical Association Washington National Airport, Washington, D.C. 20001.

AFIP Armed Forces Institute of Pathology.

aflatoxicosis Aflatoxin poisoning; see *aflatoxin.*

aflatoxin A toxin produced by *Aspergillus flavus* in moldy peanuts (ground nuts). One outbreak of aflatoxicosis from contaminated feed killed more than 100,000 turkeys in England. The toxin may be excreted in the milk of cows fed toxic material. Consumption of aflatoxin may be linked to hepatoma of Bantu natives in Africa and to hepatoma of rainbow trout.

African horse sickness (equine plague; pestis equorum) An acute, subacute, or chronic infectious disease of solipeds, horses being most susceptible. It is caused by a virus that is stable at pH 6 and survives for years in the cold in an oxalate-phenolglycerol mixture. There are nine immunologic types. The disease, which is transmitted by several species of mosquitoes and possibly by flies, was originally limited to South Africa, but has spread in recent years to Egypt, Lebanon, Turkey, Afghanistan, India, and Cypress. It spreads rapidly and is potentially a serious threat to horses of other countries.[16, 142]

African swine fever (East African swine fever; wart hog disease; Montgomery's disease) An acute, highly fatal disease of domesticated swine, in which the primary lesions are in the lymphatic tissues and in the walls of arterioles and capillaries. Although it has many features in common with hog cholera, it is caused by a different virus, which has been cultivated in chick embryos. Originally the infection occurred only in Africa, where it is carried as a latent infection by wild swine (wart hogs). The wild swine can transmit it to domesticated swine, in which the mortality rate is nearly 100 per cent. Recently it has spread from Africa to Spain and Portugal, where it has caused the death of thousands of swine.[2]

African white-tailed rat See under *rat.*

after image (ocular spectrum) A visual impression persisting briefly after cessation of the stimuli causing the original image.

aftosa Foot-and-mouth disease.

agammaglobulinemia Deficiency or absence of gamma globulin in the blood, which may be idiopathic or occur secondarily to a disease of the lymphatic or reticuloendothelial system.

agar A dried extract of certain red algae, used principally as a nutrient medium and to give solid form to media used for the culture of bacteria and other microorganisms.

agastria Absence of the stomach.

age (estimation of) In many species of animals, age can be judged from a careful examination of the teeth.[29] In young animals, eruption and shedding of teeth follow fairly regular time patterns; in adults, the amount of wear visible can be used to estimate age. The wear depends on several factors, such as nutritional state, exposure to toxic materials, experience with infectious disease, metabolic state, and degree of abrasiveness of food. Typical dentition can be expressed by a basic dental formula of the primitive mammal, as deduced from examination of fossil remains: $I\frac{3}{3}\,C\frac{1}{1}\,Pm\frac{4}{4}\,M\frac{3}{3}$ = 44 teeth, where I means incisors, which are named central, middle, and corner and are cutting teeth; C indicates canines, which are used for tearing flesh and are most highly developed in carnivores; Pm means premolars and M means molars, both types being grinding teeth, which reach the greatest state of complexity in herbivores. The premolars and molars are designated numerically as Pm 1, 2, 3 and M 1, 2, and 3. The upper and lower figures in the formula represent the teeth on one side of the jaw in the maxilla and mandible, respectively. The number of each type is therefore multiplied by 2 to get the total number.

The horse:

Deciduous formula: $I\frac{3}{3}\,C\frac{0}{0}\,Pm\frac{3}{3} = 24$ teeth

Adult formula: $I\frac{3}{3}\,C\frac{1}{1}\,Pm\frac{3\ or\ 4}{3}\,M\frac{3}{3}$

or 42 teeth

The lower teeth, because they can be more easily observed, are most commonly used for age estimation. The timetable of eruption in the horse is as follows:

Status	Age
Central I just visible	Birth
Pm1, 2, 3 may be visible	
Pm1, 2, 3 erupted	1 month
Middle I visible	
Central and middle I well developed	6 months
M1 erupted but not in apposition	
Corner I visible but not in apposition	1 year
I show wear	2 years

M2 erupted but not in apposition
Total of five pM and M present

Permanent central I appear	2 years 6 months
Central I fully out; deep infundibula	3 years
Pm1 and 2 shed; permanent Pm appear	
Permanent middle I fully erupted	4 years
Full permanent set of Pm and M	
Canines may appear	
Corner I in apposition	5 years
Permanent dentition present	

From this time on, age must be estimated by a combination of characteristics such as depth and shape of the infundibula, shape of table surfaces, and grooving of the labial surfaces.

The cow:

Deciduous formula: $I\frac{0}{4} \, C\frac{0}{0} \, Pm\frac{3}{3} = 20$ teeth

Adult formula: $I\frac{0}{4} \, C\frac{0}{0} \, Pm\frac{3}{3} \, M\frac{3}{3} = 32$ teeth

The fourth I is probably a modified C. The timetable of eruption is as follows:

STATUS	AGE
I and Pm just visible	Birth
All deciduous teeth erupted	1 month
M1 erupted and developed	6 months to 1 year
I worn level	
M2 erupted	1 year to 1 year 6 months
Central permanent I fully erupted	2 years
Second intermediate (lateral) I cut	3 years
Permanent corner I in apposition	4 years
Permanent dentition complete	

The dog:

Deciduous formula: $I\frac{3}{3} \, C\frac{1}{1} \, Pm\frac{3}{3} = 28$ teeth

Adult formula: $I\frac{3}{3} \, C\frac{1}{1} \, 4\frac{Pm}{Pm} \, M\frac{2}{2} = 42$ teeth

The number of molars may be reduced in breeds with shorter heads, and the teeth may erupt more rapidly in larger breeds. There are no teeth present at birth, but the full deciduous formula is present by six weeks. The timetable of eruption of permanent teeth is as follows:

STATUS	AGE
Central and middle I, Pm1	4 months
Corner I, C, M1 erupted	5 months
Pm2, 3, 4 and M2 erupted	5 to 6 months
M3 erupted	
Full permanent dentition present	6 to 8 months

From this time until 18 months, it is not possible to estimate age accurately. After this period, approximate age can be estimated by the degree of wear of the three cusps of the incisors; however, diet (e.g., whether bones are chewed) causes great variability in this criterion. For this reason these are very loose estimates.

STATUS	AGE
Lower central I worn	1 year 6 months
Lower middle I worn	2 years plus
Upper central I worn	3 years plus
Upper middle I worn	4 years plus
Lower corner I worn; canines show wear	5 years
Cusps worn off lower corner I; canines blunt	6 years
Central lower I worn flat; table elliptical	7 years
Table of lower I slanted forward	8 years
Table of lower middle I and I elliptical upper central	10 years
I start to shed	12 years

The cat:

Deciduous formula: $I\frac{3}{3} \, C\frac{1}{1} \, M\frac{3}{2} = 26$ teeth

Adult formula: $I\frac{3}{3} \, C\frac{1}{1} \, Pm\frac{3}{2} \, M\frac{1}{1} = 30$ teeth

Eruption begins at two to three weeks and is completed by four weeks. The permanent teeth erupt during fourth to sixth month of life. Considerable variations in number occur.

The rabbit:

$$I\frac{2}{1} \, C\frac{0}{0} \, Pm\frac{2 \text{ or } 3}{2} \, M\frac{2 \text{ or } 3}{2 \text{ or } 3} = 22 \text{ to } 28 \text{ teeth}$$

The rat, mouse, and hamster:

$$I\frac{1}{1} \, C\frac{0}{0} \, Pm\frac{0}{0} \, M\frac{3}{3} = 16 \text{ teeth}$$

The guinea pig:

$$I\frac{1}{1} \, C\frac{0}{0} \, Pm\frac{1}{1} \, M\frac{3}{3} = 20 \text{ teeth}$$

agenesis   The absence of an organ due to failure of the organ to develop embryologically.

agenosomia   A developmental anomaly characterized by absence or rudimentary development of the genitals and eventration of the lower part of the abdomen.

agerasia   An unusually youthful appearance in a person of advanced years.

agglutination   The clumping that occurs when cells are suspended in serum containing specific antibodies. In this reaction, the antigen is present in the structure of an organized cell such as bacteria, red blood cells (hemagglutinin), or spermatozoa.

agglutinin   Antibody that aggregates a specific antigen, e.g., bacteria, following combination with the homologous antibody.

aggressive See under *behavior.*

aglossia 1. Congenital absence of the tongue. 2. Absence of the power of speech.

aglyphous Without venomous fangs.

agnathia A developmental anomaly characterized by total or virtual absence of the lower jaw.

agnotobiotic Xenic, or bearing one or more organisms not known to the investigator. This condition differs from that in the conventional animal in the sense that one may reasonably be expected to determine all the living species in the association.[86]

-agogue A word termination meaning an agent that leads to or induces.

agonadal 1. Having no sex glands. 2. Due to the absence of sex glands.

agonal 1. Pertaining to the death agony; occurring at the moment of or just before death. 2. Pertaining to terminal infection.

agonistic See under *behavior.*

agoraphobia A feeling of fear at being, or at the thought of being, alone in a large open space.

agouti 1. A rodent of the genus *Dasyprocta,* which is represented by two dozen species that extend from Southern Mexico to Central America, Southern Brazil, and the Lesser Antilles. Agoutis may reach the size of a large rabbit and have an elongate body, small ears, a vestigial tail, and slender feet with three toes with hooflike claws on the hind foot. The fur is reddish brown and multibanded in agouti (see def. 2) pattern. It is a terrestrial herbivore, is active at night, and eats roots, leaves, and fruits. 2. A grizzled color of the fur resulting from alternate light and dark bands on individual hairs.

-agra A word termination meaning a seizure of acute pain.

agranulocytosis A disease characterized by a marked drop in the number of circulating granulocytes. See *cyclic neutropenia.*

    infectious feline a., see *panleukopenia.*

Agricultural Research Institute 2101 Constitution Ave., N.W., Washington, D.C. 20418.

agromania Intense passion for solitude or for wandering in fields.

agrypnia Sleeplessness or insomnia.

agyria A malformation in which the normal convolutions of the cerebral cortex are not developed.

ahypnosis Morbid wakefulness or insomnia.

aichmophobia Abnormal fear of sharp-pointed objects.

ailurophilia A morbid or inordinate fondness for cats.

Ailurus (red panda; red catbear) The lesser panda, *Ailurus fulgens,* which inhabits bamboo forests of Yunnan and Szechwan in China and of northern Burma, Sikkim, and Nepal.[110]

air sac Air-containing extensions of the primary and secondary bronchi of birds which connect with bone cavities. The principal sacs are the thoracocervical, connecting with the vertebrae; the anterior thoracic, connecting with cavities in the bones of the shoulder girdle and humerus; the sternal, connecting with the ribs and sternum; the posterior thoracic (paired); and the lesser abdominal (paired). The air sacs are apparently weight-saving devices.

-al In chemistry, a suffix used in forming the names of compounds indicating the presence of the aldehyde group.

alar Pertaining to the wing.

albatross See *procellariiform birds.*

albinism Congenital leukoderma, or absence of pigment in the eyes and the skin and its appendages, which may be partial or complete. See also *Chediak-Higashi syndrome* and *cyclic neutropenia.*

    partial a. (localized a.; naevus anaemicus), absence of pigment in local areas only. See also *Chediak-Higashi syndrome.*

    total a., complete absence of pigment in the eyes and in the skin and its appendages, often attended with astigmatism, photophobia, and nystagmus.

albomycin An antibiotic produced by species of Streptomyces. It is a cyclic iron-containing peptide which inhibits the growth of gram positive cocci, chiefly pneumococci and staphylococci but which is also active against some gram-negative bacteria. Its mode of activity is not well understood, but it probably interferes with the transport of metabolic precursors through bacterial membranes.[36, 49] See also *sideromycin.*

alcian blue A stable dye derived from copper phthalocyanin; used to demonstrate acid mucopolysaccharides in tissue sections.[153]

alcoholase An enzyme that converts lactic acid to alcohol.

Aleutian disease A disease of mink caused by a filterable agent, probably a virus, and characterized by hypergammaglobulinemia, plasmacytosis, nephritis, arteritis, and bile duct proliferation.[82]

Aleutian mink A mutation of ranch mink which occurred in Oregon in 1941 as an autosomal recessive trait characterized by diluted pigmentation of the fur and eyes. See also *mink* and *Chediak-Higashi syndrome.*

alexin See *complement.*

algae A group of cryptogamous unicellular plants, being the simplest plants that contain chlorophyll and are thus capable of photosynthesis.

algal poisoning (water brood) Poisoning of livestock from drinking water contaminated by certain species of blue-green algae, including *Microcystis aeruginosa.* It occurs when algae become concentrated in one area of a body of water because of prevailing wind.

-algia A word termination indicating a painful condition.

alizarin red A coal tar dye of the anthraquinone group. Solubility at 15° C.: water 6.5 per cent, absolute alcohol 0.1 per cent, and glycerol 8 per cent. It is used as a pH indicator and to identify calcium in tissue sections and hemoglobin in erythrocytes.[57, 153]

alkali disease Chronic poisoning of livestock from consumption of selenium-concentrating plants such as *Astragalus* and *Oxytropis*.[13]

allelo- A combining form denoting relationship to another.

allergen (atopen) A substance or substances capable of causing allergic reactions. Some common allergens are plant pollens, bacteria, foods and drugs, and cutaneous debris from animals. See table.

allergic granuloma A condition characterized by proliferation of epithelioid, lymphoid, and giant cells produced by an allergic reaction, as in fungal infections and tuberculosis.[142]

allergy An altered or hypersensitive state of reactivity toward specific substances after previous exposure to the same substance or antigen. Allergic responses are divided into two broad categories: (1) The immediate type, which occurs quickly after injection of antigen into a sensitized animal and is characterized by circulating or "humoral" antibody. Included in this group are hay fever, asthma, serum sickness, anaphylaxis (q.v.), and glomerulonephritis. (2) The delayed type, in which the reaction may require one or two days to develop after exposure of a sensitized individual to antigen. In this group are tuberculosis, tularemia, brucellosis, mycotic infections, contact dermatitis, and graft rejection. Circulating antibodies are not found.[36] A number of pharmacologically active substances have been associated with various allergic reactions (see table).

allo- A combining form denoting a condition differing from the normal, or a reversal, or referring to another.

alloantigen See *isoantigen*.

allochromacy The formation of a stain from an unstable material such as Nile blue.

allochthonous See under *behavior*.

allogeneic Of disparate or foreign origin or genotype within a given species. The term homologous has also been used in this sense.

allograft A graft of tissue in which the donor and recipient are of the same species, but genetically dissimilar. Formerly called *homograft*.

  first-set a., the original tissue or tissue constituents transplanted from a given donor (or inbred strain) to a specified recipient of the same species. This original graft usually heals in place and becomes vascularized. Rejection usually occurs 10 to 14 days after transplantation and is caused by immunologic reactivity of the recipient against isoantigens in the transplanted tissue. The latter process is often termed "first-set rejection."

  second-set a., the second tissue constituent transplanted from a given individual (or inbred strain) to the original recipient. This tissue does not ordinarily heal in place and does not become vascularized. By the second or third day it is invaded by leukocytes, and rejection usually occurs by the fourth or fifth day. The latter process is referred to as "second set rejection" and, although accelerated, is histologically identical to the first set rejection. It implies an anamnestic response by the recipient. The *third-set allograft* is rejected no faster than the second set and there is no further acceleration with the fourth, fifth, or sixth set.

allotrio- A combining form meaning strange or foreign.

MEDIATORS OF ALLERGIC REACTIONS*

SUBSTANCE	SOURCE	ACTIVITY
Acetylcholine	Freed from the protein complex by nerve impulse	Parasympathomimetic contraction of bronchial tone, increased glandular secretion, and intestinal motility
Bradykinin	Produced by the activation of proenzyme in plasma, which is induced by the action of enzymes in the pancreas and salivary glands	Bronchoconstriction, dilatation of coronary vessels and skin vessels, increased capillary permeability
Complement	Serum	Reaction with globulin or antigen-antibody complex to cause cell lysis
Heparin	Mast cells	Inhibition of blood coagulation
Histamine	Mast cells, rabbit platelets, human white blood cells	Bronchoconstriction, capillary relaxation
Kallidin	Produced by the action of kallikreins on plasma alpha-2-globulin	Vasodilatation, increased capillary permeability, pain. See *kinin*.
Serotonin	Chromaffin cells of intestine, nervous tissue, platelets, mast cells of rodents	Constriction of smooth muscle of intestine and uterus, especially in the rodent
Slow-reacting substance (SRS-A)	Sensitized guinea pig lung	Constriction of guinea pig ileum, rabbit jejunum, and human bronchioles

*Adapted from M. W. Chase: The Allergic State. *In* R. J. Dubos and J. G. Hirsch (Eds.): Bacterial and Mycotic Infections of Man. 4th ed. J. B. Lippincott Co., Philadelphia, 1965.

allotriophagia See *pica.*

allotype A genetic unit factor or mendelian character demonstrable because of its immunologic properties. This term is borrowed from immunochemistry, where it is applied to variant forms of the serum proteins, but it is equally applicable to the histocompatibility isoantigens.

allotypic Of different genetic origin. In experimental biology, it means not inbred.

alopecia Loss of hair or wool, seen in a variety of infections and in metabolic, toxic, or nutritional disorders.

   a. areata, localized loss of hair without any definite cause.

   a. of canines (Cushing's syndrome; adrenal cortical hyperplasia), alopecia occurring on the surface of the abdomen, where the affected skin may also be hyperpigmented.

   endocrine a., hair loss due to various endocrine disorders. All types exhibit thinning of the epidermis and inspissated keratinous debris in the hair follicles.[142]

   a. of hyperestrogenism, hair loss seen most commonly in Sertoli cell tumors of male dogs.

   hypothyroid a., hair loss due to hypothyroidism. More commonly than myxedema, thyroid deficiency in the dog is apt to cause hair loss accompanied by atrophy and pigmentation of the skin. Lesions are usually bilaterally symmetrical, with the neck and the backs of thighs affected first.

   pattern a. (common baldness), nonpathologic loss of pelage occurring as a consequence of maturation in several species in the mammalian Order Primates, notably man, stumptail macaques (*Macaca speciosa*), red uacaris (*Cacajao rubicundus*), and to a lesser extent, orangutans (*Hylobates*) and chimpanzees (*Pan*). Especially in stumptails the pattern of hair loss – from the forehead dorsally toward the parietal scalp and the greater extent of balding in males than females – closely mimics the development of balding in man. The types of hair follicles and their histologic and biochemical characterization have been intensively examined.

   sexual a., alopecia due to decreased sex gland activity in dogs over five years of age. In castrated cats, it may occur in either the male or the female, beginning on the inner aspect of the thighs.

alpaca A ruminant native to southern and western South America in semidesert habitats from sea level to elevations of 5000 meters. The alpaca is important for its valuable wool.

ALS antilymphocyte serum.

alsike clover A legume, *Trifolium hybridum*, which on ingestion causes photosensitization related to liver damage, and accumulation of phylloerythrin. It is also a molybdenum converter and may cause molybdenosis when eaten by livestock in areas where the soil is high in this element.[13]

altitude sickness (brisket disease; mountain sickness) A sporadic disease of cattle kept at high altitudes, characterized by pulmonary hypertension, congestive heart failure, and subcutaneous edema. Its cause is not fully understood but may be related to a combination of anoxia and ingestion of certain kinds of plants.[13]

altricial Having young which when hatched or born are very immature and helpless.

alveld A typical hepatogenous photosensitization syndrome that causes death in lambs, and occasionally older sheep, in the southwest coastal areas of Norway. The photodynamic agent is phylloerythrin. The disease has long been associated with grazing on *Narthrecium ossifragum*, also known as the bog asphodel. See also *photosensitization.*

alveolo- A combining form denoting relationship to an alveolus, probably most often used in reference to dental and pulmonary alveoli.

alveolus A general term used in anatomical nomenclature to designate a small saclike dilatation.

Amanita A genus of mushrooms some species of which produce a highly toxic substance known as amanitine, including *A muscaria, A. phalloides* (the white or deadly mushroom), *A. rubescens* (a species considered edible but which contains a powerful hemolysin), and *A. verna.*

Amaranthus reflexus (red root) A plant that can cause nitrate poisoning in livestock.

amathophobia Morbid dread of dust.

amaurosis Blindness, especially blindness occurring without apparent lesion of the eye, as from disease of the optic nerve, spine, or brain, seen in familial lipodystrophy of the brain of dogs, which resembles Tay-Sachs disease of man.

Amazona aestiva A variety of Amazon parrot that may be a source of human psittacosis.

Ambystoma mexicanum Axolotl.

ameba disease 1. A disease of adult honeybees caused by *Malpighamoeba mellificae.* The ameba develops and ultimately encysts in the lumen of the malpighian tubules. 2. A disease of grasshoppers in which an ameba, *Malameba locustae*, infects primarily the malpighian tubules, has also been called ameba disease (or *amebic disease*).

amebiasis Infection with *Entamoeba histolytica*, the cause of severe dysentery in man. Cats can be used as experimental hosts. Dogs may become infected but pass few if any cysts and probably do not constitute a hazard as a source of human disease. Several species of amebae infect birds as well as the rat and guinea pig.[142]

ameloblastoma A true neoplasm of tissue of the type characteristic of the enamel organ, but which does not undergo differentiation to the point of enamel formation.

   pituitary a., craniopharyngioma.

American Academy for Cerebral Palsy 1520 Louisiana Avenue, New Orleans, La. 70115.

American Academy of Allergy 756 N. Milwaukee Street, Milwaukee, Wisc. 53202.

American Academy of Dermatology, Inc. 636 Chruch Street, Evanston, Ill. 60201.

American Academy of Forensic Sciences 700 Fleet Street, Baltimore, Md. 21202.

American Academy of Microbiology, Inc. 900 Market Street, Wilmington, Del. 19801.

American Academy of Oral Pathology National Institutes of Health, Institute for Dental Research, Building 102B07, Bethesda, Md. 21214.

American Anthropological Association 1530 P Street, N.W., Washington, D.C. 20005.

American Association for Accreditation of Laboratory Animal Care 4 E. Clinton Street, P.O. Box 13, Joliet, Ill. 60434.

American Association for the Advancement of Science 1515 Massachusetts Avenue, N.W., Washington, D.C. 20005.

American Association for Cancer Research, Inc. 7701 Burholme Avenue, Fox Chase, Philadelphia, Pa. 19111.

American Association for Laboratory Animal Science P.O. Box 10, Joliet, Ill. 60434.

American Association for the Study of Neoplastic Diseases 10607 Miles Avenue, Cleveland, Ohio 44105.

American Association of Avian Pathologists, Inc. 1626 E. First Street, Long Beach, Calif. 90802.

American Association of Immunologists 9650 Rockville Pike, Bethesda, Md. 20014.

American Association of Medical Record Librarians 211 E. Chicago Avenue, Chicago, Ill. 60611.

American Association of Physical Anthropologists Fels Research Institute, Antioch College, Yellow Springs, Ohio 45387.

American Association of Physicists in Medicine International Atomic Energy Agency, Karntnerring, Vienna, Austria A-1010.

American Association of Veterinary Anatomists Department of Anatomy, School of Veterinary Science and Medicine, Purdue University, Lafayette, Ind. 47907.

American Association of Veterinary Nutritionists New York State Veterinary College, Cornell University, Ithaca, N.Y. 14850.

American Association of Veterinary Parasitologists School of Veterinary Medicine, University of Missouri, Columbia, Mo. 65201.

American Board of Oral Pathology 3601 Greenway, Baltimore, Md. 21218.

American Board of Pathology, Inc. Department of Pathology, University of Michigan, 1335 E. Catherine Street, Ann Arbor, Mich. 48104.

American Cancer Society, Inc. 219 E. 42nd Street, New York, N.Y. 10017.

American Chemical Society 1155 16th Street, N.W., Washington, D.C. 20036.

American College of Laboratory Animal Medicine 2101 Constitution Avenue, N.W., Washington, D.C. 20418.

American College of Medical Technologists 5608 Lane, Raytown, Mo. 64133.

American College of Veterinary Pathologists Armed Forces Institute of Pathology, Washington, D.C.

American Dairy Science Association 903 Fairview Avenue, Urbana, Ill. 61801.

American Entomological Society Academy of Natural Sciences of Philadelphia, 1900 Race Street, Philadelphia, Pa. 19103.

American Genetic Association 1507 M Street, N.W., Washington, D.C. 20005.

American Heart Association, Inc. 44 E. 23rd Street, New York, N.Y. 10010.

American Institute of Biological Sciences 3900 Wisconsin Avenue, N.W., Washington, D.C. 20016.

American Institute of Chemical Engineers 345 E. 47th Street, New York, N.Y. 10017.

American Institute of Fishery Research Biologists College of Fisheries, University of Washington, Seattle, Wash. 98105.

American Institute of Ultrasonics in Medicine University of Illinois, Urbana, Ill. 61801.

American Medical Association 535 N. Dearborn Street, Chicago, Ill. 60610.

American Medical Technologists, Inc. 710 Haggins Road, Park Ridge, Ill. 60068.

American Medical Writers Association 3150 Wilson Boulevard, Arlington, Va. 22210.

American Microchemical Society Department of Chemistry, Fordham University, Bronx, N.Y. 10458.

American Philosophical Society 104 S. 5th Street, Philadelphia, Pa. 19106.

American Physiological Society 9650 Rockville Pike, Bethesda, Md. 20014.

American Phytopathological Society Department of Plant Pathology, University of Wisconsin, Madison, Wisc. 53706.

American Psychological Association 1200 17th Street, N.W., Washington, D.C. 20036.

American Registry of Pathology A registry of pathological material maintained at the Armed Forces Institute of Pathology in Washington, D.C.

American Rheumatism Association Section of the Arthritis Foundation, 1212 Avenue of the Americas, New York, N.Y. 10036.

American Society for Cell Biology The Rockefeller University, York Avenue at 66th Street, New York, N.Y. 10021.

American Society for Experimental Pathology 9650 Rockville Pike, Bethesda, Md. 20014.

American Society for Microbiology 115 Huron View Boulevard, Ann Arbor, Mich. 48103.

American Society of Animal Science Oregon State University, Corvallis, Ore. 97331.

American Society of Biological Chemists, Inc. 9650 Rockville Pike, Bethesda, Md. 20014.

American Society of Clinical Pathologists 445 N. Lake Shore Drive, Chicago, Ill. 60611.

American Soceity of Human Genetics State University of New York, Stony Brook, N.Y. 11790.

American Society of Ichthyologists and Herpetologists Division of Reptiles and Amphibians, United States National Museum, Washington, D.C. 20560.

American Society of Laboratory Animal Practitioners 505 King Avenue, Columbus, Ohio 43201.

American Society of Mammalogists Zoology Department, Oklahoma State University, Stillwater, Okla. 74074.

American Society of Medical Technologists Suite 1600, Hermann Professional Building, Houston, Tex. 77025.

American Society of Naturalists Biology Department, Princeton University, Princeton, N.J. 08540.

American Society of Parasitologists Suite 1711, 333 N. Michigan Avenue, Chicago, Ill. 60601.

American Society of Pharmacognosy Eli Lilly and Company, 740 S. Alabama Street, Indianapolis, Ind. 16225.

American Society of Zoologists Department of Zoology, University of California, Berkeley, Calif.

American Veterinary Medical Association 600 S. Michigan Avenue, Chicago, Ill. 60605.

aminoaciduria The presence of abnormal quantities of one or more amino acids in the urine resulting from a defect in the metabolism or transport of the amino acid(s). The resultant syndrome usually affects many organ systems and frequently involves abnormalities of the central nervous system, such as mental retardation, convulsions, or psychosis.[144, 147]

aminopeptidase An enzyme that cleaves the peptide bond of terminal amino acids that contain free amino acid groups. It occurs in lysosomes and is used to indicate their presence[90, 118]

aminopherase An enzyme by which transamination is effected; transaminase.

aminoprotease An enzyme that hydrolyzes a protein by reacting with the free amino group of its substrate.

aminopterin A folic acid antagonist, one of the early antimetabolites used as an oncolytic drug.

aminotransferase Transaminase.

ammonia burn See *hutch burn.*

Amoebataenia sphenoides A tapeworm of the chicken and turkey.

Ampertas (crested-tailed marsupial "mice") A genus of highly intelligent marsupials of central Australia.

amphi- A prefix signifying on both sides, around or about, double.

amphioxus A primitive marine animal of the chordate class Leptocardii, which is of special biological interest because it possesses the three distinctive characteristics of the phylum Chordata in simple form—(1) single dorsal nerve cord, (2) notochord, (3) gill slits in the pharynx—and is believed to resemble some ancient ancestor of the phylum. Examples of amphioxus include *Branchiostoma virginiae* in the Atlantic and *B.*

californiense in the Pacific. They are used as food by the Chinese.

amphixenosis A disease, such as staphylococcosis, the cycle of which is perpetuated in nature by both man and anomen.[136]

ampho- A prefix signifying both.

amphophilic Stainable with either acid or basic dyes.

amphotericin B An antifungal antibiotic.[36, 49] See *polyene antibiotics.*

amplexus The embrace during mating, as by anuran amphibians.

Amsinckia intermedia (tarweed) A plant the seeds of which cause severe chronic hepatic degeneration, especially in the horse. Ingestion may result in photosensitization and hepatogenic encephalopathy.[13]

amusia Inability to produce or comprehend musical sounds.

amyelia A developmental anomaly characterized by absence of the spinal cord.

amylase An enzyme that catalyzes the hydrolysis of starch.

    pancreatic a., amylopsin.

    salivary a., ptyalin.

amyloidosis Deposition of hyaline glycoprotein material in the tissues, especially in the walls of arterioles, renal glomeruli, liver, spleen, and myocardium. It is most frequently seen in animals that have been repeatedly injected with antigenic substances (as in antitoxin production), but it also occurs in long-standing chronic infections. Certain strains of mice show a very high incidence, and it also occurs as deposits in the spermathecal epithelium of mated queen honeybees, where it may cause premature drone laying.

    primary a., that which occurs with no known exposure to the above conditions.

ana- A prefix indicating upward, backward, excessive, or again.

anabiotic Able to return to life after apparent death.

anadromous Denoting fishes which spend most of their adult life in the sea but which enter and ascend rivers in order to spawn.

anaerobe A microorganism that lives and grows only in the complete or almost complete absence of molecular oxygen.

    facultative a., a microorganism that is able to live under either anaerobic or aerobic conditions.

    obligate a., a microorganism that can live only in the complete absence of molecular oxygen, oxygen being toxic to it.

anaerobic Growing only in the absence of molecular oxygen.

analog, analogue 1. A part or organ having the same function as another, but of different evolutionary origin. 2. A chemical substance with a structure similar to that of another but differing from it in respect to a certain component; it may have a similar or opposite action metabolically.

analogous Denoting structures or organs that have the same function but are of different phylogenetic origin.

anal sac Either of the paired sacs in the dog, one on each side of the anal canal between the internal and external anal sphincter muscles, each sac emptying into a duct on the lateral aspect of the anus. The sacs are formed by pockets of skin into which apocrine and sebaceous glands open. They are frequently confused in the literature with the perianal or circumanal glands.[96] Cf. *perianal gland.*

anamnestic reaction A rapid immunologic reaction that occurs when a previously sensitized animal is reinjected with the original antigen, and thus constitutes evidence of immunologic memory.

anaphase That stage in mitosis, following the metaphase, in which the halves of the divided chromosomes move apart toward the poles of the spindle to form the diaster. See *mitosis.*

anaphylaxis An acute systemic reaction of the immediate type resulting from injection of a specific antigen into a previously sensitized animal (see *allergy*). The name was coined by Richet in 1902. The resultant symptoms vary among species and have been studied extensively to elucidate the mechanisms of immunologic phenomena. In the *guinea pig,* sensitivity is readily produced by a single injection of soluble protein such as ovalbumin or horse serum; less potent antigens may require several injections. Within three to five minutes after intravenous injection of the specific antigen in sensitized animals, convulsions, cyanosis, and death ensue. The process is characterized by constriction of smooth muscles, especially of the bronchioles, resulting in death from suffocation.

In the *dog,* several injections of protein are required for sensitization. Intravenous injection of antigen into sensitized animals leads to restlessness, vomiting, diarrhea, and collapse. There is a profound drop of blood pressure, and leukopenia results from entrapment of leukocytes in the lungs.

In the *rabbit,* less is known of the mechanisms. Some show shock with irregular respiration, but bronchospasm is absent.

The actively sensitized *rat* or *mouse* is less susceptible to shock. The chief site of increased capillary permeability is the intestine, where serotonin is released by enterochromaffin cells.

Anaphylaxis can also occur in the horse, cow, monkey, and birds, especially the pigeon.[36] For mediators of anaphylaxis, see table accompanying *allergy.*

anaplasia A condition in tumor cells in which there is loss of normal differentiation, organization, and specific function.

Anaplasma A genus of small coccoid organisms that parasitize the red blood cells of cattle, sheep, and goats. Formerly classified as *Sporozoa,* they are now considered to be closer to the *Rickettsia* and are placed in the family Anaplasmataceae, order Rickettsiales. *A. centrale* is observed in the central portion of the red blood cells. *A. marginale* develops on the periphery of red blood cells. *A. ovis* infects red blood cells of sheep and goats, but not cattle. See *anaplasmosis.*[159]

anaplasmosis An important disease of cattle and sheep resembling piroplasmosis, and caused by *Anaplasma marginale* and *A. centrale,* which parasitize and destroy red cells. Overt disease occurs only in adult animals; most calves undergo an inapparent infection unless splenectomized prior to exposure. Anemia is the essential effect produced by the organism and is manifested by weakness, pallor of the mucosae, accelerated respiration, and sometimes icterus. The organism, a spherical body 0.3 to 0.8 μ in diameter, is found within erythrocytes and is best demonstrated in blood smears with Giemsa stain. It reproduces by binary fission, passing through four stages. The disease is transmitted by ticks, biting flies, and mosquitoes, although it can be passed from infected to noninfected animals by careless use of surgical instruments.[13]

Anatidae See *anseriform birds.*

Ancylostoma (hookworm) A genus of nematodes that parasitize the duodenum. They are bloodsuckers that cause chronic blood loss in the host, resulting in severe microcytic hypochromic anemia (see *anemia*). Their eggs are passed in the feces and, after the larvae develop in moist soil, the larvae of the infective stage enter the body by burrowing through the skin, from which they reach the intestine and there grow to adulthood. *A. caninum* infests the dog and cat, *A. duodenale* infests man, and *A. (Uncinaria) braziliense* infests man and the dog and cat. Related genera include *Necator, Bunostomum,* and *Globocephalus.*[21]

andrase A hypothetical enzyme-like substance regarded as the material basis of maleness in heredity.

anemia A condition in which the number of red blood cells or their hemoglobin content is reduced below normal. When only the number of red blood cells falls below normal, the term oligocythemia may be used. Since anemia is rarely a primary disease, the term should be qualified by indicating its cause (see table).[73, 76, 79, 91, 133, 142]

autoimmune a., anemia in which serum antibodies react with red blood cells and the Coombs test is positive. It is seen in several so-called autoimmune diseases, including lupus erythematosus, idiopathic thrombocytic purpura, and chronic thyroiditis. In animals, the most striking examples occur in canine lupus erythematosus and autoimmune hemolytic anemia. It is also a prominent feature of NZB mouse disease.

congenital a., see *hemophilia.*

a. in congenital porphyria, see *porphyria.*

equine infectious a. (swamp fever; Vallee's disease; EIA), a disease of members of the genus *Equus* probably caused by a virus and transmitted by bloodsucking insects or by contaminated needles or tattooing instruments. The virus has been isolated from blood, feces, urine, and milk. Since the disease is usually transmitted by mosquitoes and biting flies, it is seasonal in occurrence and most common in swampy

A CLASSIFICATION OF ANEMIAS

ETIOLOGY	MORPHOLOGY OF RED BLOOD CELLS
I. Blood Loss	
A. Acute posthemorrhagic anemia	Normocytic normochromic (macrocytic if regeneration is active)
B. Chronic hemorrhagic anemia	Microcytic hypochromic
1. Blood-sucking or blood-destroying parasites	If there is adequate protein and iron, same as in acute. If prolonged, animals
2. Blood donors (excessive)	usually develop iron deficiency and
3. Bleeding ulcers	the cells become microcytic hypo-
4. Neoplasms	chromic.
5. Impaired coagulation	
II. Decreased Blood Formation	
A. Deficiency of factors necessary for hematopoiesis	
1. Iron deficiency (nutritional and/or defective absorption)	Microcytic hypochromic (also cobalt copper deficiency)
2. Protein deficiency	Normocytic or microcytic
3. Deficiency of various B vitamins and/or erythrocyte maturing factor in liver	
a. Pyridoxine deficiency	Microcytic, slightly hypochromic (experimental anemia in dogs and swine)
b. Pterolyglutamic (folic) acid (vitamin B_{12}) deficiency (pernicious anemia; also seen in gastric disorders, diarrhea, and hepatitis)	Macrocytic normochromic with megaloblastic bone marrow.
c. Erythrocyte maturing factor deficiency	Same as above
B. Injury, displacement, or obscure dysfunction of bone marrow	
1. Injury due to chemicals	Normocytic normochromic
2. Injury from irradiation	Normocytic normochromic
3. Displacement of bone marrow; myelophthisic (neoplasm metastasis) leukemia	Normocytic normochromic
4. Obscure dysfunction of bone marrow	Microcytic or normocytic normochromic
Acute and chronic infections; nephritis with high nitrogen retention	Same as above
III. Increased Destruction of Blood	
A. Congenital defects	
1. Sickle cell anemia of man	Great variability depending on response of bone marrow
B. Acquired Anemias	
1. Poisonous plants: mushrooms, bracken, fern	
2. Chemical agents: naphthalene, gasoline, saponin, Aniline dyes, coal tar, sodium or potassium chlorate	
3. Infectious agents: equine anemia virus, hemobartonella, streptococci, epeyrythrozoon, Leptospira, Babesia, Clostridium, hookworm	
4. Drugs: sulfonamides, antipyretics	
5. Miscellaneous: certain neoplasms, burns, hemolytic anemia of newborn in horses, anti-A factor in dogs, autoimmune diseases such as canine lupus erythematosus	
6. Snake venom	

areas. Equine infectious anemia is usually a chronic disease with periods of exacerbation, especially following stress. Animals have been known to carry active virus in their blood for as long as 18 years, but the disease does not seem to be contagious through contact. Some aspects, including arteritis, glomerulonephritis, and plasma cell proliferation, indicate that immunologic mechanisms may be involved.

hemolytic a. of newborn animals, a disease of foals and piglets. The pregnant female develops antibodies against the red blood cells of the fetus, the antibodies are secreted in the colostrum, and, shortly after the young animals begin to nurse, hemolysis of red blood cells begins. Hemolytic icterus, edema, and evidence of red blood cell regen-

eration are characteristic. Death may ensue from the resultant anemia. If female dogs that possess type A⁻ blood have been sensitized by type A⁺ blood, a similar disease may develop in pups possessing type A positive blood.

infectious a., a form caused by members of the family Bartonellaceae and seen in several species. These organisms are tiny intracellular parasites of red blood cells which may be rod-shaped, ring-shaped, coccoid, or filamentous. They can be seen with Giemsa stain and fall in a classification intermediate between bacteria and rickettsiae. *Bartonella bacilliformis* causes human bartonellosis (Carrion's disease; Oroyo fever).

iron deficiency a. of piglets, microcytic hypochromic anemia caused by inadequate iron in food. Piglets are vulnerable because their liver reserves are small and sow's milk contains very little iron.

leptospiral hemolytic a., hemolytic anemia in dogs and cattle caused by infection with *Leptospira*. In the dog, this is more commonly seen in infections with *Leptospira icterohaemorrhagiae* than in those with *L. canicola*. Hemolytic crisis may be accompanied by hemoglobinemia and hemoglobinuria.

sickle cell a., see *sickling*.

anemo- A combining form denoting relationship to the wind.

anemophobia Morbid fear of wind or drafts.

anencephaly A developmental anomaly characterized by absence of the cranial vault and by cerebral hemispheres that are completely absent or reduced to small masses attached to the base of the skull.

anergy Originally, a lack of ability to react to tuberculin, even though the individual being tested may be infected. The term has taken on broader meaning and may indicate a lack of ability to react to an allergic stimulus, because of desensitization (specific), depressed immunologic mechanisms of unknown cause (nonspecific), or tolerance (nonspecific). See also *hyperergy* and *hypoergy*.[36]

anesthesia 1. Loss of sensation, especially touch and pain, in the skin or mucous membranes as a result of some nervous lesion or other abnormality. 2. Loss of sensation in a part of the body (local anesthesia) or the entire body (general anesthesia) induced by a drug.

Achievement of functional anesthesia in experimental animals is of concern to scientists who must satisfy themselves and legal requirements that the agent used is effective, both for the outcome of the experiment and as a preventive of pain and suffering for the animal. The agents used include those which induce sleep or depress the central nervous system, such as hypnotics, narcotics, or tranquilizers, and those which specifically produce insensibility to pain, either regionally or locally, i.e., the analgesics. Many other types of agents, such as muscle relaxants, may be used in occasion as supplements to anesthesia. References should be consulted for details of technic.[45, 87, 95] See Bibliography.

Anesthetic agents can be classified as local (or regional) and general. Local anesthetics are used for operations of brief duration in which body relaxation is not a necessary factor. Procaine and lidocaine are commonly used when injection is the method of application. Ethyl chloride may be applied topically.

General anesthetics are used when unconsciousness and relaxation are desirable. These may be given by inhalation, as with ether, nitrous oxide, trichloroethylene, halothane, methoxyflurane, cyclopropane, or chloroform. Of the nonvolatile anesthetics, barbiturates are the most common; the intravenous route is most desirable but the

intraperitoneal, intrapleural, oral, or rectal route may also be used. Dosages are based on the body weight of the animal, but levels of tolerance vary for different species and caution is necessary. Some examples of anesthesia procedures, including those for preanesthesia, follow:

The dog: Preanesthesia—(a) Subcutaneous injection of 1–2 mg. per kg. morphine sulfate and 0.05–10 mg. atropine sulfate per kg. of body weight one-half hour prior to anesthesia; (b) intravenous injection of chlorpromazine 1.0 mg. per kg. of body weight 10 minutes before anesthesia. Anesthesia—Volatile: preferably administered with an anesthesia machine so that oxygen can be mixed with it and in order to achieve maximum control of depth. Methoxyflurane or halothane (with or without N_2O), ether, or cyclopropane may be used. Nonvolatile: for short-acting anesthesia, thiopental sodium 12 to 16 mg. per kg. of body weight or 4.0% thiamylal sodium 17.6 mg. per kg. For intermediate period of action, pentobarbital sodium 30 mg. per kg. given intravenously.

The rabbit: Preanesthesia—Intramuscular injection of chlorpromazine 25 to 100 mg. per kg. of body weight.

Anesthesia—Volatile: ether or halothane. Use restraint box or wrap in towel for administration. Nonvolatile: drugs similar to those used in the dog. There is a wide variation of response to barbiturates and a narrow margin of safety. Dosage: short-acting barbiturates such as pentobarbital 30–50 mg. per kg. of body weight. Routes of administration: anterior marginal ear vein or intraperitoneal route. For nonrecovery experiments in which prolonged anesthesia is desired, Urethan at a dosage of 1.69 gm. per kg. is widely used. Paraldehyde at a dosage of 1.0 and 1.5 ml. per kg. for intramuscular injection and gastric intubation respectively is also a satisfactory anesthetic for rabbits.[95]

The guinea pig: Preanesthesia—After a 12-hour fast prior to induction, a subcutaneous injection of 2.5 mg. of atropine sulfate 30 minutes prior to anesthesia.

Anesthesia—Volatile: methoxyflurane. ether, N_2O, or halothane. Nonvolatile: pentobarbital sodium 3.0 mg. per 100 gm. of body weight injected intraperitoneally. Use sixfold dilution of stock solution. Routes of administration: cephalic vein, recurrent tarsal vein on lower lateral third of tibia, sublingual veins (to augment anesthesia after induction), jugular vein, marginal auricular vein, or intraperitoneal. Barbiturates are extremely damaging to tissues and should never be given subcutaneously. For short procedures CO_2 derived from dry ice under a platform-supported guinea pig is an excellent method.[95]

The cat: Preanesthesia—(a) Subcutaneous or intramuscular injection of meperidine hydrochloride not to exceed 5 to 10 mg. per kg. of body weight, 45 minutes prior to induction. The dosage is very critical in Felidae. (b) Intramuscular injection of chlorpromazine hydrochloride 1.5 mg. per kg. 30 minutes prior to anesthesia.

Anesthesia — Volatile: methoxyflurane, halothane, or ether. Nonvolatile: drugs and procedures similar to those for the dog, except that the use of morphine is strictly contraindicated in Felidae.

Primates (*Rhesus monkey*): Restraint is a serious problem, but sedation combined with preanesthesia can be achieved by intramuscular injection of promazine at a dosage of 2 mg. per kg. or phencyclidine at a dosage of 0.5 mg. per kg. Anesthesia—Volatile: methoxyflurane, halothane, or ether. Nonvolatile: drugs and procedures similar to those for the dog.

The rat: Anesthesia—Volatile: methoxyflurane, halothane, or ether in bell jar or with nose cone. Nonvolatile: intraperitoneal injection of pentobarbital sodium 1.0 mg. per 100 gm. of body weight in dilute (10 mg. per ml.) solution. Young rats require lower dosage per gram of weight than adults.[95]

The mouse. Anesthesia—Volatile: methoxyflurane, halothane, or ether. Nonvolatile: intraperitoneal injection of pentobarbital sodium 5.0 (3–7) mg. per 100 gm. of body weight in dilute (10 mg. per ml.) solution. Mice of both sexes, but especially males, are extremely sensitive to the hepatotoxicity of chloroform.[95]

The hamster: Anesthesia—Volatile: methoxyflurane, halothane, or ether. Nonvolatile: intraperitoneal injection of pentobarbital sodium 6.0 mg. per 100 mg. of body weight in dilute solution.

Birds: Anesthesia—Volatile anesthetics must be used with caution because the material may saturate the air sacs, resulting in overdosage. It can be controlled by careful intermittent administration; methoxyflurane is advocated for this purpose. Nonvolatile—intramuscular injection of Equithesin (mixture of pentobarbital, chloral hydrate, and magnesium sulfate) in a dosage of 2.5 ml. per kg. of body weight. The limits of tolerance are narrow and the dose must be carefully calculated. Procaine is quite toxic and contraindicated in parakeets, but is widely used as an anesthetic in pigeons, chickens, and ducks with no untoward effects.

Fishes: Several agents have been used, including ether, sodium amytal, carbon dioxide, and cresol. Tricaine methanesulfonate is probably the currently most popular and efficacious. The fish is placed in water containing 50 to 100 mg. of this agent per liter; when the fish has become immobilized it can be removed and manipulated.

Amphibians and reptiles: Tricaine methanesulfonate can be used in ambient water concentrations of 1:1000 to 1:10,000 depending on the requirements of the experimenter. Hexobarbital is widely used by injection into the dorsal lymph sac at dosages of 120 mg. per kg. of body weight, and pentobarbital sodium, by the same route, at a dosage of 60 mg. per kg.

aneuploid   Having more or less than the nor-mal number of chromosomes. See *chromosomal aberration.*

aneurysm   Localized dilatation of an artery. The most common type in anomen is the verminous aneurysm of horses involving principally the anterior mesenteric artery near its origin in the aorta. It is caused by irritation due to the presence of the larvae of *Strongylus*, which attach themselves to the endothelial surface of the vessel. Because thrombi which form in the arterial lumen may embolize into smaller branches and interfere with blood supply to the intestine, intermittent colic (thromboembolic colic) may result. The aneurysms seldom rupture.

   dissecting a. of turkeys, this form occurs in the aorta, principally in males but occasionally in females. It may rupture, resulting in death from intra-abdominal hemorrhage. The cause is unknown, although similar lesions appear in birds made lathyritic by the administration of beta-aminoproprionitrile, a chemical found in the sweet pea, *Lathyrus odoratus.*

angio-, angi-   A combining form denoting relationship to a vessel, usually a blood vessel.

angioma   A tumor whose cells tend to form blood vessels (*hemangioma*) or lymph vessels (*lymphangioma*); a tumor made up of blood vessels or lymph vessels.

angiomatosis   A diseased state of the vessels, with formation of multiple angiomas.

Angiostrongylus   A genus of nematodes of the family Metastrongylidae.

   A. cantonensis (Rattostrongylus cantonensis), a species known as the rat lungworm. It is also the cause of human meningoencephalitis in Hawaii and Tahiti.[21] See *helminth parasites,* under *rat.*

   A. vasorum, a species occurring in the pulmonary artery of the dog and fox.

angolamycin   See *macrolide.*

Angstrom unit   The unit of wavelength of electromagnetic and corpuscular radiations, equal to 10^{-7} mm. Called also *angstrom.*

angustmycin   An antibiotic produced by a species of *Streptomyces* that is active against gram-positive bacteria and against Walker 256 tumor. Its activity is directed against purine metabolism in a fashion similar to that of psicofuranine.[36, 49]

anhydrase   An enzyme that catalyzes the removal of water from a compound.[90, 118]

   carbonic a., an enzyme that catalyzes the decomposition of carbonic acid into carbon dioxide and water, and thus facilitates the transfer of carbon dioxide from tissues to blood and to alveolar air.

aniline blue   A basic coal tar dye of the triphenylmethane group. Solubility at 15° C.: water, absolute alcohol, 1.5 per cent; and glycerol, 5 per cent. It is used for staining spermatozoa, and is especially suitable for canine and human semen. It is also incorporated in stains to demonstrate muscle fibers, glial fibrils, collagen, reticulum, glomerular stroma, erythrocytes, and nuclear chromatin.[57, 153]

animal A living organism requiring oxygen and organic food and capable of motion and sensation, as distinguished from a vegetable. Sometimes incorrectly used to refer to the lower animals as distinguished from man (see *anoman*). This inclination of man to separate himself from the apes and other animals is an outgrowth of ego, a delusion which has impeded progress in the understanding of social behavior and the solution of biomedical problems.[101]

    specific pathogen-free a., see *SPF.*

Animal Behavior Society 333 N. Michigan Avenue, Chicago, Ill. 60601.

animal disease See *animal model* and *zoonosis.*

animal model In its broadest sense, any condition found in anomen which is of value in studying a biological phenomenon. In the limited scope of this book, models for study of human diseases will be emphasized. The following references cite several recent symposia on this subject and publications of tabulated lists which contain extensive bibliographies: 7, 25, 28, 35, 42, 43, 47, 72, 76, 81, 105, 132, 149, 164. See addenda, table of Animal Models and Bibliography.

Animal Nutrition Research Council Department of Poultry Science, Rutgers University, New Brunswick, N.J. 08903.

aniso- A combining form denoting unequal or dissimilar.

anisotropic Substances composed of fibers or crystals with a high degree of molecular orientation. When a ray of plane-polarized light passes through anisotropic material, it is split into two rays polarized in perpendicular planes, which property is called birefringence.

anneal In biochemistry, to cool slowly a denatured nucleic acid so that the double strand may reform. See *melting out temperature.*[90]

annelid Any member of the phylum Annelida, the segmented worms. As a group they are characterized by elongated, segmented bodies with fine bristle-like structures (setae) for locomotion. The cuticle is thin, the digestive tract is complete and tubular, the coelom is large, the blood vascular system is closed with a chambered heart, and the nervous system comprises a dorsal brain and ventral nerve cord with ganglia and lateral nerves in each somite. Most forms are marine, but some members inhabit fresh water, some are terrestrial. Four classes are recognized: Archiannelida, including *Polygordius*; Polychaeta, including the blood worm, *Glycera*, the clamworm, *Nereis*, and the parchment worm, *Chaetopterus*; Oligo-

chaeta, including the earthworms (e.g., *Lumbricus*); and Hirudenea, including the leeches (e.g., the medical leech, *Hirudo medicinalis*).

anodontia Congenital absence of the teeth. It may involve all or only some of the teeth, and both the deciduous and the permanent dentition or only teeth of the permanent dentition.

anomaly Marked deviation from the normal standard; applied especially to congenital defects.

anoman (plural *anomen*) An acronym from the phrase "*animal other than man*," indicating all species of animals other than *Homo sapiens.* Pronounced *ah'no-man* (pl. *ah'nomen*). This term is offered as a concise substitute for the unsatisfactory "lower animals" and as an alternative to the inaccurate phrase "man and animals."

Anopheles See *mosquito.*

anophthalmia A developmental defect characterized by absence of the eyes, which has been reported in calves, puppies, and foals.

Anoplocephala magna The tapeworm of the horse.

anorchism, anorchidism Congenital absence of the testis, which may occur unilaterally or bilaterally.

ansa A general term used in anatomical nomenclature to designate a looplike structure.

anseriform birds Any member of the avian order Anseriformes. The largest family (Anatidae) in this order contains the ducks, geese, and swans. A number of common terms are used to distinguish the sexes and young of these birds (see table). Groups of ducks or swans are called flocks; geese may be called flocks or gaggles. In flight, groups of these birds may be referred to as a flight or skein. All members of the Anatidae are essentially aquatic, and are characterized by long necks and spatulate bills, with three toes being linked by webs. Many species are agriculturally important, all are of concern to conservationists, and several are important in research (see table).

ant- See *anti-.*

ant bear See *aardvark.*

ante- A prefix signifying "before" in time or place.

anteater (spiny anteater; echidna) A monotreme, *Tachyglorsus aculeatus*, inhabiting Tasmania, Australia, and New Guinea, which has a body covering of fur intermixed with dorsal and lateral barbless spines; it feeds on termites, ants, insects, and worms, which it traps with its long sticky tongue.

antechinus (speckled marsupial mouse) A

COMMON NAMES OF ANSERIFORM BIRDS

SUBSTANTIVE NAME	MALE	FEMALE	YOUNG
Duck	Drake	Hen	Duckling
Goose	Gander	Goose	Gosling
Swan	— — —	— — —	Cygnet

IMPORTANT SPECIES OF ANSERIFORM BIRDS

DOMESTIC OR BREED NAME	SCIENTIFIC NAME	WILD DERIVATION
Indian runner duck	*Anas platyrhynchos*	Mallard
Khaki Campbell duck	*A. platyrhynchos*	Mallard
Muscovy duck	*Cairina moschata*	Muscovy duck
Peking duck	*Anas platyrhynchos*	Mallard
Chinese goose	*Anser cygnoides*	Swan goose
Domestic goose	*A. anser*	Greylag goose

marsupial, *Paranthenus apicalis*, inhabiting the southwestern corner of Australia.

antelope   Any of the slender ruminants of the Old World having hollow horns; their size varies considerably according to species.

    American a. (pronghorn antelope; prong buck), an artiodactyl, *Antilocapra americana*, inhabiting the desert and grasslands in southwestern Canada, western United States, and northern Mexico. It is not a true antelope, but rather the only living representative of a group of ungulates that arose and developed in North America.

anthracosis   A condition caused by the inhalation of carbonaceous pigment, which becomes deposited in macrophages of the lungs. The pigment may be carbon or other material. The disease is very common in city horses, dogs, and cats.

anthrax   A bacterial infection caused by *Bacillus anthracis*. Principally a disease of herbivores, it may affect other species, including man. In man the infection is usually acquired by contact with animals or their products such as hides, wool (woolsorter's disease), or shaving brushes. The disease is important historically, for Pasteur and his colleagues first demonstrated active immunization by using attenuated anthrax cultures in their famous public experiment in 1881. Spores of the organism are extremely resistant and remain dormant but viable in the soil for many years.

anthropo-   A combining form denoting a relationship to man.

anthropoid   Resembling man. The anthropoid apes are the tailless apes of the family Pongidae, including the chimpanzee, gibbon, gorilla, and orangutan. See *ape* and *primate*.

anthropology   The science that treats of man, his origins, historical and cultural development, and races.

anthropomorphism   The attribution of human form or character to nonhuman objects.

anthropopathy   The ascription of human emotions to nonhuman subjects.

anthropophilic   Preferring human beings to other animals; said of certain mosquitoes. Cf. *zoophilic*. See also *dermatomycosis*.

anthropophobia   Morbid dread of human society.

anthropozoonois   A disease that can be transmitted to man from anomen or the reverse, e.g., rabies, brucellosis, and anthrax.[136] See also *zoonosis*.

anthropozoophilic   Attracted to both human beings and animals; said of certain mosquitoes. Cf. *anthropophilic* and *zoophilic*.

anti-, ant-   A prefix signifying against or over against.

antibiotic   1. Destructive of life. 2. A chemical substance that has the capacity, in dilute solutions, to inhibit the growth of or to destroy bacteria and other microorganisms. Antibiotics are used in the treatment of infectious disease of man, anomen, and plants, and are also valuable in biochemical dissection of cellular metabolic functions because of the specificity of their effect on cells.[1, 32, 36, 49] See table for list of antibiotics. See also entries of individual antibiotics for summary of the characteristics of each.

ANTIBIOTICS ACCORDING TO THEIR SITE OF ACTION*

CELL WALL SYNTHESIS
Bacitracin
Cephalosporin
D-Cycloserine
O-Carbamyl-D-serine
Penicillin
Ristocetin
Vancomycin

MEMBRANE FUNCTION
Albomycin
Amphotericins
Antimycoin
Ascosin
Bacitracin
Candicidin
Candidin
Circulin
Colicin E1, K
Colistin
Endomycin
Etruscomycin
Filipin
Flavicid
Fungichromin
Gramicidin S, J1, J2, A
Gramicidin B, C, D
Hamycin
Lagosin
Nystatin
Pentamycin
Perimycin
Pimaricin
Polyenes
Polymyxins
Rimocidin
Streptomycin
Trichomycin

Tyrocidines
Valinomycin

RIBONUCLEIC ACID METABOLISM
Aurantin
Chromomycin
Cinerubin
Colicin E1, K, E2, 1a, 1b
Daunomycin
Griseofulvin
Kanamycin
Minomycin
Mithramycin
Neomycin
Nogalamycin
Novobiocin
Olivomycin
Phytoactin
Pluramycin
Streptomycin
Streptonigrin

DEOXYRIBONUCLEIC ACID METABOLISM
Actidione
Actinomycin
Bruneomycin
Cinerubin
Colicin E1, K, E2, 1a, 1b, E2, CA-42
Cycloheximides
Daunomycin
Edeine
Griseofulvin
Mitomycin A, B, C
Novobiocin
Phleomycin
Pluramycin
Porfiromycin
Sarkomycin
Streptonigrin
Xanthomycin

PURINE AND PYRIMIDINE SYNTHESIS
Angustmycin A
Azaserine
Cordycepin
Decoyinine
DON (6-diazo-5-oxo-L-norleucine)
Hadacidin
Psicofuranine
Sangivamycin
Sarkomycin
Toyocamycin
Tubercidin

PROTEIN SYNTHESIS
Acetoxycycloheximide
Actinospectacin
Actiphenol
Amicetin
Angolamycin
Bacitracin
Blasticidin S
Bluensomycin
Carbomycin
Catenulin
Chalcomycin
Chloramphenicol
Chlortetracycline
Cohcin E2, E3, 1a, 1b
Cycloheximide
Demethylchlortetracycline
Dihydrostreptomycin
Edeine
Erythromycin
Fermicidin

Framycetin
Fusidic Acid
Fusidin
Gentamycin
Glutarimides
Gougerotin
Hygromycin B
Hydroxystreptomycin
Inactone
Kanamycin
Kasugamycin
Lancamycin
Lincomycin
Mannosidostreptomycin
Methymycin
Mikamycin
Minomycin
Naramycin B
Neomycin
Niromycin
Nucleocidin
Ostreogrycins
Oxytetracycline
Pactomycin
Paromomycin
Protomycin
Pristinamycins
Puromycin
Rifamycin
Sarkomycin
Sparsomycin
Spectinomycin
Spiramycin
Staphylomycins
Streptimidone
Streptogramins A, B
Streptomycin
Streptonigrin
Streptoviticins
Synergistins
Tenuazonic Acid
Tetracycline
Vernamycins
Viomycin
Viridogrisein

RESPIRATION
Antimycin A1, A2, A3, A4, A35, A102
Aurovertin
Flavensomycin
Nigericin
Oligomycins
Patulin
Pyocyanine
Rutamycin
Usnic Acid

OXIDATIVE PHOSPHORYLATION
Aurovertin
Colicin E1, K
Dinactin
Gramicidin S, J1, J2, A, B, C, D
Monactin
Nonactin
Oligomycin
Rutamycin
Trinactin
Tyrocidine
Usnic Acid
Valinomycin

OTHER SITES
Bacitracin
Novobiocin
Sideromycin

*From D. Gottlieb and P. D. Shaw: Antibiotics. Vol. I. Mechanisms of Action. Springer-Verlag, New York, 1967.

antibody A modified type of serum globulin synthesized by lymphoid tissue in response to antigenic stimulus, each different haptenic structure of one antigen molecule being capable of inciting a distinct response. By virtue of two specific combining sites, each of which is complementary in structure to the inciting haptenic group, antibody molecules combine with antigen in vivo and in vitro. Antibodies are classified according to their behavior on electrophoresis, ultracentrifugation, and immunoelectrophoresis. They are also classified according to the mode of their observed action, as agglutinins, amboceptors, antienzymes, antitoxins, bacteriolysins, blood group antibodies, cytoxins, hemolysins, opsonins, and precipitins.[32, 36, 93] See *immunoglobulin*.

    cytophilic a., a globulin formed by lymphoid tissue that has a strong affinity for macrophages and may be related to delayed hypersensitivity by enhancing antibody formation through the removal of antigen that may interfere with the function of the lymphocyte.

    cytotropic a., a subclass of IgG antibodies that bind to target cells and sensitize for anaphylaxis.[32]

    evolution of a., see *immunoglobulin*.

    natural a., an immunoglobulin that does not require administration of an antigen for its elicitation, but occurs as a response to naturally occurring antigens such as food or undetected infections.

    synthesis of a., the means by which antigens stimulate certain cells to manufacture specific antibodies has remained a subject of controversy since Ehrlich proposed the first reasonable theory. Recently the clonal selection (q.v.) theory has received considerable support. Proponents of this theory hold that there are clones of cells available in every individual that are able to produce antibodies against any conceivable antigen. The general pattern of maturation of these cells is shown in the accompanying diagram.[108] See *immunoglobulin,* and see *monoclonal gammopathy,* under *gammopathy.*

anticipatory See under *error.*

anticodon The triplet of nucleotides in transfer RNA which matches, by complementary base pairing, with the specific codon (q.v.) in messenger RNA during translation in the ribosome.

antigen A substance capable of inducing the formation of an antibody and reacting specifically with the same antibody.

    Forssman a., a heterogenetic antigen from various animals which will produce antisheep hemolysin; originally isolated from the guinea pig kidney.

    heterophile a., an antigen common to more than one species, such as Forssman antigen.

antigen-antibody complex A combination of antigen with its specific antibody and complement. This reaction may neutralize the antigen (toxin, infectious agent, etc.), but may also be damaging to tissues.[93, 129] See *glomerulonephritis* and *arteritis.*

antigen-free The state of an organism or material, which has had no contact with haptens or any biologically distinct products of another species that will elicit antibody response.[86]

antigenic determinant That portion of the antigen molecule which determines the specificity of antigen-antibody reactions.

antigenostic Free from antigens other than those known to be present.[86]

antigen unit The least quantity of antigen that will fix one unit of complement so as to prevent hemolysis.

antilymphocyte serum (ALS) (antilymphocyte globulin [ALG]) Antiserum produced by the injection of lymphocytes into horses or other animals. It possesses immunosuppressive activity. Its mode of action, although not thoroughly understood, probably involves reactivity with surface antigens of lymphocytes. It appears to have con-

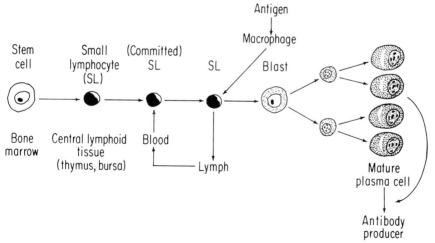

Figure 1. Synthesis of antibodies: clonal selection.

siderable value in delaying the rejection of transplanted organs.[163]

antimetabolite A substance that interferes with the function of living cells by blocking one or more metabolic processes. Many of these are analogs of vital substances, known as competitive antagonists. Some have greater effect on neoplastic than on normal cells and are used in cancer chemotherapy. Some act to suppress immune reactions and are used to aid transplantation experiments. Some have value as antiviral agents. Some affect bacteria and/or fungi more severely than vertebrate cells and are used as antibiotics. Their greatest value, however, may lie in the increased knowledge gained about cell metabolism by studying the specific effects of their activity on the biochemical machinery of cells.[1, 32, 36, 49, 64, 94, 130, 144] See table.

antimycin A complex of antibiotics produced by species of *Streptomyces* which were first studied because of their inhibition of pathogenic fungi. Included in the group

ANTIMETABOLITES
(See also entries under individual names)

SUBSTANCE	BASIS FOR ACTIVITY	APPLICATION
Actinomycin	Blocks messenger RNA synthesis (see *antibiotic*)	Immunosuppressant, antibiotic
Adamantanamine	Interferes with cell-virus interaction	Myxovirus inhibitor
Amethopterin	Folic acid analog	Immunosuppressant
Amniopterin (methotrexate)	Folic acid analog	Immunosuppressant
Asparaginase	Destroys asparagine	Oncolytic
Azaserine	Unknown	Oncolytic
Azathioprine (Imuran)	Purine analog	Immunosuppressant, oncolytic
6-Azathymine	Pyrimidine analog	Immunosuppressant
6-Azauridine	Pyrimidine analog	Immunosuppressant
5-Bromo-2'-deoxyuridine (BUDR)	Pyrimidine analog	Immunosuppressant, anti-DNA virus
Busulfan (Myleran)	Alkylating agent	Immunosuppressant
Buthioprine	Purine analog	Immunosuppressant, oncolytic
Colchicine	Inhibits mitosis by interference with formation of spindle	Immunosuppressant, oncolytic; gout treatment
Cyclophosphamide (Cytoxan)	Alkylating agent	Immunosuppressant
Cytosine arabinoside	Affects nucleic acid metabolism	Oncolytic and antiviral; experimental lesions of central nervous system
5-Fluoro-2'-deoxyuridine (FUDR)	Pyrimidine analog	Immunosuppressant, anti-DNA virus
p-Fluorophenylalanine (FPA)	Amino acid analog	– – –
5-Fluorouracil	Pyrimidine analog	Immunosuppressant, anti-DNA virus
Griseofulvin	Inhibits mitosis (see *antibiotic*)	Antifungal, oncolytic
Guanidine HCl	Inhibits viral RNA polymerase	Picornavirus inhibitor
2-α-(Hydroxybenzyl)-benzimidazol (HBB)	Inhibits viral RNA polymerase	Picornavirus inhibitor
Hydroxyurea	Interferes with DNA formation	Oncolytic
5-Iodo-2'-deoxyuridine (IUDR)	Pyrimidine analog	Immunosuppressant, anti-DNA virus
Isatin-beta-semicarbazone	Inhibits synthesis of virus-specific proteins	Poxvirus inhibitor
N-Isopropyl-α-(2-methyl-hydrazino)-P-toluamide (MIH)	Unknown	Oncolytic
Kethoxal bis (thiosemi-carbazone) (KTS)	Interferes with DNA formation	Oncolytic
6-Mercaptopurine (6MP)	Purine analog	Immunosuppressant, oncolytic
6-Methylthiopurine ribonucleoside (6MMPR)	Purine analog	Immunosuppressant, oncolytic
Nitrogen mustard	Alkylating agent	Immunosuppressant
Nogalamycin	Interferes with RNA synthesis	Oncolytic in Hodgkin's disease
6-Thioguanine	Purine analog	Immunosuppressant, oncolytic
Trichloroethylamine	Alkylating agent	Immunosuppressant
Vinblastine (Vinca alkaloid)	Inhibits mitosis	Oncolytic
Vincristine	Inhibits mitosis	Antifungal, oncolytic

are antimycin A (used as a fish poison), virosin, blastmycin, and phyllomycin. Their activity has not been well characterized but consists of interference with oxidative metabolism.[36, 49]

antiserum A serum that contains antibody or antibodies. It may be obtained from an animal that has been subjected to the action of antigen either by injection into the tissues or blood, or by infection.

antiviral substance Any of a number of chemicals that can interfere with replication of viruses. These have been studied extensively in cell cultures and have aided experimenters in understanding the mechanisms of virus synthesis, but they have been of relatively little value as therapeutic agents. See *antimetabolite.*

antivivisection Opposition to the use of living animals for purposes of experimentation or demonstration of life processes to students of physiology, zoology, and other biological sciences.

ANTU Alpha-naphthyl thiourea, a derivative of thiourea that is antithyroid in activity, but also highly toxic, especially to small mammals. It acts specifically to increase the permeability of lung capillaries, with resultant severe pulmonary edema and hydrothorax. It is popular as a rat poison, usually being mixed with meat or grain for that purpose. Accidental or purposeful poisoning of dogs with ANTU is common, the dog usually dying in the sternal recumbent position with frothy fluid bubbling from the mouth and nose.

anxiety 1. A feeling of apprehension, uncertainty, and fear. 2. A secondary drive established as the development of a discriminated avoidance-conditioned response (see *avoidance conditioning,* under *conditioning*). It may be manifested either as a negative reinforcing stimulus for other responses, or in the form of behavior unusual under the circumstances, for instance, defecation, urination, huddling, vocalization, flight, or excessive general activity. Some theories now tend to consider all drives as instances of the expression of anxiety.

apandria Morbid aversion to the male sex.

apanthropia 1. Morbid fear of human companionship. 2. Apandria.

ape A member of the family Pongidae, the anthropoid apes, which comprises five genera and about ten species that inhabit forests in equatorial Africa, southeastern Asia, Sumatra, Mentawi Islands, Java, and Borneo. The members of this family, the closest living relatives of man, may be divided into two groups: (1) the "great apes," such as the orangutan, chimpanzee, and gorilla, and (2) the gibbons, which are smaller and have longer arms and slenderer bodies. The best developed senses of the apes are hearing and vision, including color perception. They have vocalization and a variety of facial expressions. The chimpanzee is an intelligent manlike ape extensively used in laboratory research. See *primate.*

aphilopony Fear of or disinclination to work.

aphtha A small ulcer.

aphthous fever See *foot-and-mouth disease.*

apiculture The breeding and culture of bees.

apimyiasis Myiasis of the adult honeybee caused by the larvae of *Senotainia tricuspis* Meigen, *Rondanioestrus apivorus* de Villers, and certain other fly species. See also *myiasis.*

apisination Bee sting.

aplasia Lack of development of an organ; frequently used to designate complete suppression or failure of development of a structure from the embryonic primordium.

apo-, ap- A prefix signifying separation or derivation from.

apodiform birds Any member of the avian order Apodiformes, including the swifts and hummingbirds, which are birds having long, narrow wings.

apoenzyme The protein portion of an

A Brief Classification of Arachnids

Order	Suborder	Representative Forms
Scorpionida		Scorpions; many forms poisonous and allergenic
Pedipalpi		Whip scorpions
Palpigrada		— — —
Araneae		Spiders, many forms poisonous and allergenic
Solpugida		Sun spiders
Pseudoscorpionida		False scorpions
Podogona		
Phalangida		Harvestmen, daddy longlegs
Acarina	Mesostigmata	Mites, including *Laelaps, Halarchne, Liponyssus, Dermanyssus,* and *Allodermanyssus*
	Ixodides	Ticks, including argasine ticks (no dorsal shield), e.g., *Argas* and *Ornithodorus;* and ixodine ticks (with dorsal shield) e.g., *Dermacentor* and *Boophilus*
	Trombidiformes	Mites, including *Demodex,* and chiggers, e.g., *Trombicula.*
	Sarcoptiformes	Mites, including *Sarcoptes, Psoroptes, Chorioptes,* and *Knemidocoptes.*

enzyme, which requires the presence of coenzyme to become a complete enzyme (holoenzyme).[90, 118]

Aporina delafondi A tapeworm of the pigeon.

aposymbiotic Symbiont-free; usually used in reference to mutualistic symbionts.

appeasement See under *behavior.*

appendix A diverticulum of the tip of the cecum. The wall of the cecum or appendix contains areas of lymphoid tissue similar to that seen in the bursa of Fabricius (q.v.). Its purpose is not well understood, but studies in the rabbit indicate that it may function as one unit of central lymphoid tissue (q.v.).

appetitive See under *behavior.*

approach A drawing near, as in response to a stimulus.

    gradient of a., see *goal-gradient.*

approach-approach See under *conflict.*

approach-avoidance See under *conflict.*

apterium An area of the skin of birds, from which no feathers grow (except down in the young). Plural *apteria.*

apterygiform birds Members of the avian order Apterygiformes, flightless birds with vestigial wings, typified by the kiwi.

apterygote Belonging to the group of insects which are primitively wingless. See also *insect.*

aquarium A container of fresh or salt water for growth of fish, amphibians, reptiles, or plants. Careful attention must be given to establishment of the proper habitat and maintenance of the environment within the correct range of salinity, temperature, oxygenation, pH, etc.[50]

arachnid Any member of the phylum Arthropoda, subphylum Chelicerata, class Arachnida. This large group includes the spiders, ticks, scorpions, and mites. In general they are terrestrial with two pairs of mouth parts, pedipalps and chelicerae, and four pairs of legs. The abdomen lacks locomotor appendages, the eyes are simple, the cuticle has sensory hairs or scales, and gills are absent. Most forms are oviparous, and do not metamorphose (except *Acarina*). They are chiefly terrestrial. (See table on page 23.)

arbovirus Arthropod-borne virus, i.e., a virus transferred by a biting arthropod. These viruses undergo replication both in the arthropod and in the vertebrate host (see also *zoonosis*). The host range of most species is known only superficially (see table).[2, 66] See also *classification*, under *virus.*

ARCP American Registry of Comparative Pathology. Armed Forces Institute of Pathology, Washington, D.C. 20305.

arcus A general term used in anatomical nomenclature to designate any structure having a curved or bowlike outline.

Argas persicus The chicken tick, which also infests geese, ducks, turkeys, guinea

Vectors and Hosts of Certain Arboviruses

Virus or Disease	Vector	Vertebrate Host
The Mosquito-borne Viruses		
California encephalitis	*Culex* and *Aedes*	Man and anomen
Chikungunya	Mosquito	Man
Dengue	*Aedes*	Man
Eastern equine encephalomyelitis	Mosquito	Bird, man, horse
Ilheus	Mosquito	Man
Japanese B encephalitis	*Culex*	Bird, pig, horse, man
Murray Valley encephalitis	*Culex*	Man, horse
O'Nyong-Nyong virus	*Anopheles*	Man
St. Louis encephalitis	*Culex*	Man, bird
Semliki Forest virus	*Aedes*	Man, wild primates
Sindbis virus	*Culex*	Man, bird
Turkey meningoencephalitis	Mosquito	Turkey
Venezuelan equine encephalomyelitis	Mosquito	Man, horse
Wesselsbron disease	*Aedes*	Sheep, cow, man
Western equine encephalomyelitis	*Culex tarsalis*	Bird, man, horse
West Nile fever	*Culex*	Man
Yellow fever	*Aedes*	Wild primates, hedgehog, man
The Tickborne Viruses		
Central European tickborne fever	*Ixodes ricinus*	Man, goat
Colorado tick fever	*Dermacentor andersoni*	Man
Kyasanur forest disease	*Hemaphysalis spihigera*	Wild primates, man
Louping ill	*Ixodes ricinus*	Sheep, cow
Nairobi sheep disease	*Rhipicephalus*	Sheep, goat
Omsk hemorrhagic fever	*Dermacentor*	Man
Russian Far East encephalitis	*Ixodes ricinus*	Man
Other Arboviruses		
Blue tongue	*Culicoides*	Sheep
Lagos bat virus	Unknown	Bat
Phlebotomus fever	*Phlebotomus papatasi*	Man
Rift Valley fever	Mosquito	Sheep, goat, cow, man, forest rat
Vesicular stomatitis	Unknown	Cow, horse, pig, man

fowl, pigeons, canaries, and various wild species of fowl.

argentaffinoma A tumor of the gastroenteric tract (carcinoid) formed from the argentaffine cells (Kultschitsky's cells) of the enteric canal.

arginase An enzyme of the liver that splits arginine into urea and ornithine.

argyrophil Staining or easily impregnated with silver.

arhinia A developmental anomaly characterized by absence of the nose.

arithmomania A morbid impulse to count, with worriment about numbers.

Arizona Academy of Science Room D-203, Physical Science Center, Arizona State University, Tempe, Ariz. 85281.

Arkansas Academy of Science University of Arkansas, Fayetteville, Ark. 72701.

armadillo A small member of the genus *Dasypus*, order Edentata. There are several species in South America. The nine-banded armadillo, *D. novemcinctus*, which ranges into North America, is useful for embryological and immunological studies because it always produces monozygotic quadruplets, each with a separate blood supply to the placenta.

Armed Forces Institute of Pathology Washington, D.C. 20305.

Arnhart's black-egg disease See *melanosis*.

ARP American Registry of Pathology.

arrheno- A combining form meaning male.

arrhenoblastoma A malignant tumor of the ovary consisting of immature gonadal elements with male hormonal secretion, and producing masculine secondary sex characteristics.

arrhythmia Irregularity or loss of rhythm, especially an irregularity of the heart beat. The heart beat of the dog normally exhibits sinus arrhythmia, particularly when at rest. This arrhythmia may disappear in fever or cardiac disease, because of tachycardia or an increased work load on the heart.

arsenic A heavy metal that is a common cause of poisoning in animals, especially from insecticides or smelter fumes. Since it is secreted in milk, suckling animals can be poisoned if the dam has ingested arsenic.

arteriosclerosis Thickening and hardening of the arteries. There are three different types, which are probably separate etiologic entities: (1) atherosclerosis, in which a mushy substance of nondescript nature is deposited in the intimal layer (see *atherosclerosis*); (2) medial sclerosis of Mönckeberg, which affects the medium-sized muscular arteries and consists of hyaline and fatty degenerative changes in the muscular tissue of the media, eventually leading to necrosis and calcification; (3) diffuse arteriolar sclerosis (*arteriolosclerosis*) of the smaller arteries, or arterioles. The term "hyperplastic sclerosis" has also been used and is descriptive of some of the changes that occur in the small peripheral arteries, especially in those of the lung, kidney, spleen, and pancreas. The hyperplasia consists of proliferation of the cells of the intima and media, which form concentric lamellations that may nearly fill the lumen. (This is especially common in cats.) The intima may be replaced with connective-tissue hyaline or there may be swelling and necrosis of the medial layers, with marked compression of lumen. An interesting form of coronary arteriosclerosis occurs in Pacific salmon (*Salmo gairdneri*) and steelhead trout during upstream migration for spawning. In the steelhead, the process appears to be reversible upon return to ocean waters.

Medial arteriosclerosis is an important spontaneous disease of female multiparous rats and laboratory rabbits. In both species, the lesion consists of medial arteriosclerosis of the Mönckeberg type. The earliest lesions arise as sclerotic plaques at the base of the ascending aorta. As the disease progresses, the plaques become more extensive, eventually confluent, and the entire arterial tree becomes sclerotic and pipelike. Microscopically, the events begin as degeneration of the medial layer of the artery with fragmentation of collagenous bundles. These lesions mineralize, and with advancement may become cartilaginous and bony, and even contain islets of bone marrow. In rabbits, there is a well delineated syndrome of cachexia, hypertension, and terminal congestive heart failure as consequences of the arterial disease. The pathogenesis is unknown. In multiparous breeder rats, the disease is clearly exacerbated by calcium depletion as a consequence of bearing young and lactation, but again, the mechanism of aberrant metabolism is not well understood.

In both rats and rabbits, the spontaneous lesions have been confused with those induced experimentally by cholesterol. It is most important to recognize that spontaneous atheromas have never been observed in laboratory rats or rabbits, that the spontaneous lesions are medial and not subintimal, and that they stain (both grossly and microscopically) with Von Kossa's stain, and not Sudan IV, as they do not contain lipids.[122] See also *atherosclerosis* and *periarteritis nodosa*.

arteritis Inflammation of an artery. Polyarteritis (involvement of several arteries) similar to that seen in man has been reported in several species. See table on page 26.

equine infectious a. (epizootic cellulitis; pink eye syndrome), a viral infection of horses, characterized by fever, stiffness of gait, edema of the limbs, and swelling around the eyes. It also causes abortion. In fatal cases it produces conjunctivitis, edema of the palpebra and nictitating membrane, and excessive lacrimation. The nasal membranes become congested and a serous nasal discharge is present. One strain of virus has been grown in horse and hamster kidney cells. Attenuated virus has been used for immunization.

arthritis Inflammation of a joint (*polyarthritis* when several joints are involved).

SUMMARY OF ANIMAL ARTERITIDES*

ANIMAL	DISEASE	ASSOCIATED FEATURES	CAUSE
Cow	Malignant catarrhal fever, encephalitis, ophthalmitis	Nonsuppurative encephalitis	Virus
Cow	Sporadic encephalitis	Encephalitis	Virus(?)
Cow, sheep	Listeriosis-vasculitis	Microabscesses of brain	Bacterium
Horse	Equine viral arteritis, necrosis, thrombosis; arteries of all organs involved	Leukopenia, edema, abortion, nephritis, myocarditis; may be antigen-antibody complexes	Virus
Horse	Equine anemia, periarteritis, fibrinoid degeneration	Hypergammaglobulinemia, glomerulonephritis, plasmacytosis, anemia	Virus
Aleutian mink	Aleutian disease; necrosis and inflammation in 25% of cases	Hypergammaglobulinemia, glomerulonephritis, infarction, plasmacytosis; antigen-antibody complexes	Virus
Mouse	Segmental pulmonary arteritis; lymphocytes, but some polymorphonuclear leukocytes; no necrosis or thrombosis	Myocarditis; bodies in polymorphonuclear leukocytes	Rickettsia-like organism; transmissible
Mouse	NZB mouse disease	Glomerulonephritis arteritis	Virus(?)
Mouse	Lymphocytic choriomeningitis	Nephritis, periarteritis; antigen-antibody complexes; persistent viral infection	Virus
Pig	Periarteritis, African swine fever, hog cholera, Teschen disease, baby pig encephalitis	– – –	Virus
Pig	Salt poisoning, eosinophilic periarteritis	Cerebral edema	Excessive salt ingestion
Rat	Necrosis of arteries; lymphocytes and polymorphonuclear leukocytes, thrombosis	Hypertrophic osteoarthropathy, leukemia	Transmitted by cells
Rat	Arteritis, especially of lungs and kidneys; necrosis, polymorphonuclear leukocytes	Glomerulonephritis	Benzanthracene, single dose
Rat	Necrosis; affects mesenteric and renal arteries	Nephropathy	Unknown
Sheep	Necrosis; lymphocyte and macrophage infiltration; affects arteries in kidneys and muscles	– – –	Unknown
Chicken	Chronic respiratory disease	Pneumonia, periarteritis	*Mycoplasma*
Dog	Lupus erythematosus	Nephritis; antigen-antibody complexes	Unknown
Dog, cat	Polymorphonuclear infiltration; necrosis; affects coronary, pulmonary, and gastric arteries	– – –	Unknown, perhaps hypersensitivity

*From R. W. Leader, J. R. Gorham, and B. M. Wagner: Connective tissue diseases of animals other than man. *In* B. M. Wagner (Ed.): The Connective Tissue. The Williams & Wilkins Co., Baltimore, Md. 21202, U.S.A. © 1967.

Acute inflammation of a joint is commonly serous, fibrinous, or purulent. The serous form is equivalent to an excessive formation of synovial fluid, which distends the joint capsule. When infection is present, the exudate is fibrinous or, in the presence of pyogenic organisms, purulent. The articular surfaces may be eroded, and the surrounding tissues may become edematous.

adjuvant a., an experimentally induced arthritis that has been produced in rats by injection of Freund's adjuvant. It resembles human rheumatoid arthritis.[36]

avian a., a form caused by several bacteria, including *Bacterium arthropyogenes, Escherichia venezuelensis, Salmonella pullovum,* and the staphylococci.

bacterial a., inflammation of synovia and articular surfaces. The most common known agents are *Escherichia coli,* streptococci, staphylococci, *Erysipelothrix,* and *Corynebacterium pyogenes.*

Chlamydia a., polyarthritis of the serous type in sheep and cattle. See *osteoarthritis* and *osteoarthropathy.*

degenerative a., inflammation of the

weight-bearing joints and the spine (spondyloarthritis) of older animals.

neonatal a., bacterial polyarthritis of newborn animals resulting from invasion through the umbilical vein, most commonly seen in foals. The agents are many and include *Corynebacterium, Escherichia, Shigella,* streptococci, and staphylococci. See *omphalophlebitis.*

rheumatoid a., a form occasionally diagnosed in old dogs and old cows. Its manifestations are variable and obscure. The condition as it occurs in man is not seen in anomen, although *Erysipelothrix* arthritis of swine and adjuvant arthritis of rats are somewhat similar.

arthro-, arthr- Combining form denoting relationship to a joint or joints.

arthropod Any member of the phylum Arthropoda (joint-footed animals). Typically the body is composed of a head, thorax, and abdomen formed of segments (somites) like or unlike, variously separate or fused, and four or more pairs of jointed appendages. A chitinous exoskeleton covers all parts and is molted at intervals to permit growth. The digestive tract is complete, the coelom is reduced, the blood vascular system consists of heart, vessels, and body spaces (hemocoel), and respiration is performed by gills, tracheae, or book lungs. The brain is dorsal; the paired nerve cord is ventral with ganglia to each somite or concentrated anteriorly. The sexes usually separate. Various forms may be terrestrial or aquatic (marine and fresh water), and free-living, commensal, or parasitic. See also under *guinea pig, primate, rabbit,* and *rat.*

arthrospore A fungal spore or segment produced by fragmentation of hyphae.

Arthus reaction (local anaphylaxis) A condition resulting from repeated injections of antigen into the skin, in which the antigen reacts with antibody in the tissue fluids, resulting in antigen-antibody complex formation and tissue damage. The presence of complement and polymorphonuclear leukocytes is necessary for the reaction to take place. The reverse reaction occurs when antibody is injected into the dermis and antigen is given intravenously. This reaction requires very small amounts of antibody (24 to 225 μg. of antibody nitrogen).

Artiodactyla An order of ungulates or hoofed animals that have an even number of toes such as cattle, goats, swine, and deer.

Ascaridia galli A large intestinal nematode of chickens.[21]

Ascaris A genus of extremely common nematodes (phylum Nemathelminthes, family Ascaridae), adult forms of which are found in abundance in the gastrointestinal tract of birds and mammals throughout the world. The adults, usually large robust worms, are found in the small intestine. Their eggs are thick-shelled and unsegmented when laid, and a period of incubation and two molts within the shell are required before the embryo becomes infective. The eggs are resistant to desiccation, low temperatures, and many chemical agents. Young animals are particularly susceptible to infection with ascarids, whereas many adults shed their ascarid parasites spontaneously.[21]

A. suum A nematode of the family Ascaridae, commonly found in pigs.[21]

ascidian (sea squirt) A tunicate of the class Ascidiacea, one of the lower chordates. Larval forms possess chordate characteristics, which may be absent in sessile adult forms. Ascidians are marine animals with a tunic composed of cellulose, a material rare in animals. They are commonly known as "sea squirts" because of their habit of suddenly squirting water from body openings when touched. Examples include the clear sea squirt, *Clavelina gigantea,* the sea squirt, *Mogula manhattensis,* and the leathery sea squirt, *Styelia plicata.*

ascigerous Productive of ascospores and associated structures of the perfect state of the *Ascomycetes.*

ascites tumor See *Ehrlich tumor.*

Ascoli test A thermoprecipitation test used for the detection of anthrax-infected hides.

Ascomycetes Fungi in which the perfect state is manifest by production of asci and (within them) ascospores.

ascorbiasis See *scurvy.*

ascorbic acid (vitamin C) An organic compound in citrus and other fruit, deficiency of which causes scurvy in primates and the guinea pig.

ascorbic acid deficiency A metabolic error in the metabolism of glucose in the glucuronic acid pathway (q.v.) which is characterized by the absence of the enzyme that catalyzes the conversion of L-gulonolactone to 2-keto-L-gulonolactase. Man, other primates, and the guinea pig lack the enzyme completely, and are vulnerable to ascorbic acid deficiency unless the vitamin is present in the diet. See *scurvy.*

ascospore Genetically segregated spores of the perfect (sexual) state in *Ascomycetes.*

-ase A word termination used in forming names of enzymes, ordinarily affixed to a stem indicating the general nature of the substrate, the actual name of the substrate, the type of reaction catalyzed, or a combination of these factors.

Asiatic pit vipers See table accompanying *snake.*

asoma A fetal monster with an imperfect head and the merest rudiments of a trunk.

asparaginase An enzyme that catalyzes the hydrolysis of asparagine to aspartic acid and ammonia. Found by Kidd to be present in rather large amounts in guinea pig serum. His early studies have led to extensive exploration of the enzyme as a tool in cancer chemotherapy because of its ability to inhibit the growth of certain neoplastic cells which require asparagine in their metabolism or which lack asparagine synthetase. The cells of acute leukemia appear to be especially vulnerable.[130]

aspartase An enzyme that splits aspartic acid into fumaric acid and ammonia.

aspergillosis Infection with mycotic organisms of the genus *Aspergillus*, particularly *A. fumigatus*. It is most prevalent in birds but may occur in mammals. The organisms are extremely common in nature, occurring on food stuffs and plants. Young birds are believed to become infected from contaminated bedding, usually while they are in the brooder stage of growth, hence the term "brooder pneumonia." Infection in man has been called pigeon-feeder's disease. Infections in horses, cats, and, rarely, sheep and cattle have been reported. Predisposing factors include debilitating conditions, administration of adrenal cortical hormones, irradiation, diabetes, and disturbance of normal flora by long continued treatment with antibiotics. Aspergillosis sometimes takes the form of placentitis, a frequent cause of abortion in cattle.[11, 112]

Aspicularis tetraptera An intestinal nematode parasite of the family Oxyuridae (pinworm) which infests the rat and mouse.[21] See *helminth parasites,* under *rat.*

ass (burro; donkey) An ungulate, *Equus asinus,* of the family Equidae native to Asia and Africa, most frequently in desert plains.

assassin bug A biting insect of the family Reduviidae.

Association for Gnotobiotics c/o Oak Ridge National Laboratory, Biology Division P.O. Box Y, Oak Ridge, Tenn. 37830.

assortative mating Nonrandom mating; sexual reproduction in which pairing is controlled by the tendency of certain males to select a female of a particular genotype. The tendency to select a mate of the same genotype is positive assortative mating; of a different genotype, negative assortative mating.

asternia A developmental anomaly characterized by absence of the sternum.

Asterococcus Obsolescent name for *Mycoplasma.*

asthma Dyspnea characterized by recurrent attacks of bronchial spasms, often caused by allergy. Asthma as seen in man is virtually unknown in anomen, although there have been rare reports of it.

bovine a. (fog fever), atypical interstitial pneumonia of uncertain etiology in cattle characterized by pulmonary edema, emphysema, and proliferation of the bronchiolar-alveolar epithelium.

Astragalus (loco weed) A genus of plants capable of extracting selenium from the soil in sufficient concentration to cause poisoning in cattle, horses, or sheep that consume the plant in grazing. It also contains an alkaloid toxin that affects the nervous system.

astro- A combining form indicating some relation to a star, as star-shaped.

astrocytoma C3H(18) A tumor developed by selection from an originally mixed cell glioma induced by intracranial injection of methylcholanthrene in a C3H/St mouse in the laboratory of H. M. Zimmerman at Montefiore Hospital, New York City, in 1948. Transplantation is successful in nearly 100 per cent of C3H hosts. The tumor may be implanted by a variety of routes; it kills the host about 14 days after inoculation by invasion without metastasis.[150]

astrophobia Fear of the stars and celestial space.

atavism Reappearance of a recessive character unexpressed during several generations.

ataxia Loss of muscular coordination with impaired balance.

a. of calves, a specific cerebellar disease in Jersey calves that is thought to be inherited as a simple mendelian recessive trait.

cerebellar a., a form seen frequently in cats. The signs are not detectable in kittens until they are able to walk, at about one month of age. The cerebellum is much smaller than normal, a defect long presumed to be inherited. Recent findings indicate that certain viruses (panleukopenia viruses) attack the germinal layer of the cerebellum of the fetus or newborn animal (i.e., rats, hamsters, ferrets, and kittens), destroying cells of the molecular and granular cell layers and resulting in apparent hypoplasia of the cerebellum.

a. of foals (wobbles), a disease of young horses and mules in which nonparalytic disturbances of gait are present. Degeneration is seen in the spinal cord, particularly in the cervical region.[142]

a. of lambs (swayback), failure of myelination of the brain and spinal cord, seen in lambs born to mothers fed a copper-deficient diet.

-ate A word termination forming a participial noun, as the object of the process indicated by the root to which it is affixed, e.g., *hemolysate,* something hemolyzed; *homogenate,* something homogenized.

atelencephalia A developmental anomaly characterized by imperfect development of the brain.

atelo- A combining form meaning imperfect or incomplete.

atelocardia A developmental anomaly characterized by incomplete development of the heart.

atelocheilia A developmental anomaly characterized by incomplete development of a lip.

ateloencephalia Atelencephalia.

ateloglossia A developmental anomaly characterized by incomplete development of the tongue.

atelognathia A developmental anomaly characterized by incomplete development of the jaw.

atelomyelia A developmental anomaly characterized by incomplete development of the spinal cord.

atelopodia A developmental anomaly characterized by incomplete development of the foot.

ateloprosopia A developmental anomaly

characterized by incomplete development of the face.

atelorachidia   A developmental anomaly characterized by incomplete development of the spinal column.

atelostomia   A developmental anomaly characterized by incomplete development of the mouth.

atherosclerosis   A form of arteriosclerosis in which the primary lesion consists of lipid infiltration of the tunica intima of the aorta and other arteries. There may or may not be reduced functional capacity. The symptoms of atherosclerosis as seen in man (angina, cerebrovascular insufficiency, intermittent claudication) are the results of reduced function. While not common in anomen in the natural state, atherosclerosis can be artificially induced in rabbits, dogs, primates, and other species. Some forms of naturally occurring atherosclerosis of anomen are as follows.

Swine: Old animals exhibit lesions quite similar to those seen in man, involving the aorta, coronary arteries, and cerebral arteries. Little is known about the state of arteries in very old swine, because most swine are slaughtered for meat while young. They are not known to suffer myocardial infarction from coronary artery thrombosis.

Fowl: Chickens, turkeys, and pigeons are affected, white carneau pigeons showing a very high incidence. Lesions are most common at the bifurcation of the thoracic aorta into the abdominal aorta and celiac axis, but also occur in the coronary arteries. Myocardial infarction occurs occasionally. Other birds, including the parrot and cockatoo, may be affected by atherosclerosis.

The rat: Old animals are affected, especially female breeders. The lesions, however, differ considerably from those in man.

Wild animals: Most cases have been reported in captive animals and are thought by some to be related to environmental stress. Wild canines and edentates appear to be moderately susceptible.

The dog: These animals seldom develop atherosclerotic changes, even in old age. Occasionally coronary artery disease occurs in concert with extreme elevation of serum cholesterol levels.

Nonhuman primates: Baboons, chimpanzees, and squirrel monkeys develop lesions similar to those in man, but much less severe. Atherosclerosis is rare in *Rhesus* and *Cebus* monkeys.

The rabbit: Rabbits seldom, if ever, develop spontaneous atherosclerosis. Degeneration and calcification of the tunica media, however, is quite common.[23, 122]

ATP   Adenosine triphosphate.

atresia   Congenital absence or pathologic closure of a normal opening, passage, or cavity.

    a. ani (imperforate anus), a failure of development of the anal opening. Often there is little more than the skin and subcutis remaining imperforate, and it may be possible to establish a satisfactory opening by surgery. The muscular sphincter and the rectum are also inadequately developed. Frequently seen in young pigs.[142]

atrophic rhinitis (porcine rhinitis)   A disease of swine that commences in young pigs with slight catarrhal rhinitis and sneezing. The lesions consist of erosion and disappearance of the nasal turbinate bones and mild inflammation. The cause of atrophic rhinitis has never been determined. Some workers maintain that the disease can be transmitted to young pigs and occasionally to older swine by local instillation of nasal exudate from affected animals. Others believe that the sole cause is related to high phosphorus and low calcium levels in the diet.[73]

atrophy   A defect or failure of nutrition manifested as a wasting away or diminution in the size of a cell, tissue, organ, or part.

attack   See under *behavior.*

attend   In behavioral science, to give any type of response to a stimulus.

attenuation   Alteration of a microorganism to diminish its virulence. Several methods of attenuation are available: cultivation at an unfavorable temperature, the heating of cultures or infective material for a short time; cultivation on an unfavorable medium; plating on a suitable medium and selecting a nonvirulent colony; adaptation of the organism in other than the native host by serial inoculations (a method frequently used for attenuation of viruses); and serial passage in tissue culture.

audiogenic seizure   A seizure induced by sound. Laboratory animals of several species, especially certain strains of mice, rats, and rabbits, exhibit convulsions when subjected to intense sound stimulation. Typically mice first appear startled, may freeze briefly, become agitated, and then go into a clonic phase, falling on their sides and kicking rhythmically. Many mice also go into tonic extension with fixation of the trunk muscles in the inspiratory position, which, unless reversed by artificial respiration, will result in death.[51]

Aujeszky's disease (pseudorabies; infectious bulbar paralysis; mad itch)   A lethal disease of the nervous system that affects cattle, dogs, cats, rats, and swine. Sheep are susceptible to experimental exposure. Shope demonstrated that the disease is transmitted to cattle by contact with swine that harbor the virus. Adult swine suffer only mild clinical disease, but death occurs in young pigs as a result of pharyngeal paralysis and indications of bulbar involvement.[16] See also *herpesvirus B.*

auramine O   A basic diphenyl methane dye used in fluorescence microscopy for staining tubercle bacilli, *Treponema pallidum*, and other bacteria, and for staining trypanosomes in dried blood films.[37, 153]

aurantia   An acid coal tar of the nitro group, used for staining mitochondria. Solubility at 15° C.: in water, 0.1 per cent; in absolute alcohol, 0.55 per cent, and in glycerol, 1 per cent. It is a highly explosive chemical which may cause severe dermatitis.[37, 57]

aurovertin See *oligomycin*.

australopithecine A member of an extinct group of manlike apes that lived in South Africa during the early Pleistocene era, about 700,000 years ago.

auto-, aut- A prefix denoting relationship to oneself.

autoagglutination Clumping or agglutination of an individual's cells by his own serum; autohemagglutination.

autoantibody An antibody directed against the tissues of the individual in which it is produced, by the stimulus of either exogenous or endogenous antigen.[93, 129] Autoantibodies can combine with antigens as complexes together with complement, and may be deposited in the renal glomeruli or arterial walls, where they cause lesions. See *autoimmune disease*. Some of the body organs or substances which are the origin of such antigens and/or the targets of such antibodies are the following: adrenal gland, red blood cell, liver, glomerular basement membrane, brush border of renal tubule, connective tissue, nucleoprotein, cytoplasm (ribosomes), thyroid gland, arterial wall, gamma globulin, brain, skeletal muscle, myocardium, insulin, sperm, testis, uveal tissue, thyroglobulin, platelets and leukocytes, lens tissue, colon, and stomach.

autochthonous behavior See under *behavior*.

autogeneic autogenous.

autogenous Self-generated; originated within the body, as an autograft. As applied to bacterial vaccines, the term denotes vaccines made from the patient's own bacteria, as opposed to stock vaccines, which are made from standard cultures.

autograft A graft of tissue transplanted from one portion of the body to another in the same individual.

autoimmune disease (autosensitization) A condition in which antibodies are produced by an individual against his own tissues. The criteria of autoimmune disease are as follows: (1) there should be demonstrable circulating or cell-bound antibodies, (2) the antigen should be identified, (3) the same antigen should produce antibodies in an experimental animal, and (4) similar changes should appear in an actively sensitized animal injected with the same antigen.[93, 129] See also *autoantibody*.

Some evidence implicates autoimmunity in the following diseases. *Man:* chronic thyroiditis (Hashimoto's disease), systemic lupus erythematosus, autoimmune hemolytic anemia, idiopathic thrombocytopenic purpura, rheumatoid arthritis, polyarteritis, scleroderma, dermatomyositis, post-rabies encephalitis, myasthenia gravis, paroxysmal hemoglobinuria, glomerulonephritis, and lupoid hepatitis.

The dog: systemic lupus erythematosus, chronic thyroiditis, thrombocytopenic purpura, and autoimmune hemolytic anemia.

The mouse: NZB mouse disease, runt (homologous) disease, and lymphocytic choriomeningitis.

The mink: Aleutian disease (plasmacytosis).

The horse: equine infectious anemia and viral arteritis.

autoimmune hemolytic anemia See under *anemia*.

autoimmunization The production in an organism of reactivity to its own tissues, with appearance of certain clinical and laboratory manifestations as a result of the altered immunological response. See *autoantibody* and *autoimmune disease*.

autologous Related to self; designating products or components of the same individual organism. See *autogenous*.

autolysis The digestion of dead or degenerated cells by endogenous enzymes, as in postmortem destruction of cells, tissues, and organs. This process is mainly due to the release of hydrolytic enzymes from lysosomes (q.v.).

autophagic vacuole (cytolysome; cytosegresome; autolytic vacuole) An area of focal cytoplasmic degradation or autolysis which becomes surrounded by membrane, resulting in a vacuole containing recognizable cytoplasmic remnants. See *residual body* and *lysosome*.

autopolyploid 1. Having more than two chromosome sets as a result of redoubling of the chromosomes of a haploid individual or cell. 2. An individual or cell having more than two chromosome sets as a result of redoubling of the haploid set.

autoradiography (radioautography) Visualization of radioisotopes within tissues by their effect on photographic emulsions. In experimental biology, the technique is principally applied as microautoradiography by coating a thin section of tissue with a sensitive emulsion and allowing it to be exposed so that the cellular location of isotopes can be visualized. Some of the materials used and the activities studied are listed in the accompanying table.[153] Other isotopes used in autoradiography are thorium, uranium, lead, mercury, gallium, copper, ruthenium, hafnium, fluorine, iron, potassium, cadmium, bromine, sodium, zinc, bismuth, and zirconium.

autosexing In avian genetics, the deliberate breeding of sexual dimorphism associated with sex-chromosome linkage groups for the purpose of identifying the sex of chicks by inspection of down feather pattern. Early, rapid, and accurate determination of sex by external inspection is important in domestic birds and, for these reasons, breeds with sex-linked genes controlling feather color have been developed in the chicken and certain pigeons.[112]

autosome See *chromosome*.

autotransplant autograft.

AUTORADIOGRAPHIC MATERIALS AND THEIR USES

ISOTOPE	ACTIVITY STUDIED
Calcium (^{45}C)	Bone mineralization
Carbon (^{14}C)	Synthesis of any substance that incorporates carbon
Gold (^{198}Au)	Function of Kupffer cells of liver
Iodine (^{131}I)	Thyroid function
Phosphorus (^{32}P)	Bone growth, calculi, viral replication
Plutonium (^{239}Pu)	Periosteum, endosteum
Polonium (^{210}Po)	Dying cells
Radium (^{226}Ra)	Bone metabolism
Strontium (^{90}Sr)	Bone metabolism
Sulphur (^{35}S)	Synthesis of sulfated mucopolysaccharides of connective tissue, mucus-secreting cells, follicular fluid of ovary, cartilage; ethionine and methionine uptake
Tritium (^{3}H)	
thymidine	DNA synthesis
uridine	RNA synthesis

auxochrome A chemical group which, if introduced into a chromogen, will convert the latter into a dye.

aversive See under *stimulus*.

avian 1. Relating to birds. 2. Any member of the chordate class Aves, which comprises the birds. It is subdivided into 27 orders, with 160 families, and some 1800 genera. All names of orders end in "formes" and all family names end in "idae." One or more subpopulations called subspecies have been recognized for some species, resulting in a third word in the full scientific name, e.g., *Turdus migratorius achrusterus*, the southern robin.

avian distemper Newcastle disease.

avian encephalomyelitis See under *encephalomyelitis*.

avian infectious laryngotracheitis See *laryngotracheitis*.

avian leukosis See under *leukosis*.

avian pest Newcastle disease.

avian trichonomiasis See under *trichonomiasis*.

avian vibrionic hepatitis See *vibrionic hepatitis*, under *hepatitis*.

avitaminosis D (cage paralysis, simian bone disease, osteodystrophia fibrosa) A well-defined clinical syndrome of limb distortion, kyphosis, multiple fractures without calcified callus, elevated serum alkaline phosphatase, lack of cortical bone, and osteodystrophia fibrosa. It affects New World nonhuman primates on diets apparently adequate in (plant source) vitamin D_2. Although such diets are sufficient for the maintenance of Old World monkeys and the anthropoid apes, New World monkeys appear unable to metabolize dietary sources of vitamin D_2 to the required D_3, especially in the absence of ultraviolet light or direct sunlight. An adequate level of vitamin D_3 for New World primates has been calculated to be 1.25 I.U. per gm. of diet.[126, 128]

avoidance Strongly aversive behavior on the part of an animal when exposed to a situation in which it had previously received a stimulus such as an electric shock. The response is manifested by running or pulling away from the source of the stimulus.

  gradient of a., a measure of the strength of running or pulling away from an aversive stimulus exhibited by an animal which has been repeatedly presented with that stimulus. The strength of the behavior is inversely proportional to the distance from the aversive stimulus, and this function is referred to as gradient of avoidance.

avoidance-avoidance See under *conflict*.

avoidance conditioning See under *conditioning*.

axenic Not contaminated by or associated with any foreign organisms; used in reference to pure cultures of microorganisms or cells, or to germ-free animals.[86] See *gnotobiote*.

axenite A germ-free animal.[80]

axenobiosis Germfreeness.[86] Cf. *gnotophoresis*.

axolotl A salamander, *Ambystoma mexicanum*, found only in Mexico. It is used in the laboratory for research in embryology and regeneration, and is very susceptible to fungal diseases of the skin.

axoneme 1. The internal portion of the trypanosome flagellum, which originates from the blepharoplast. 2. The axial thread of the chromosome where the combination of genes are located.

axostyle The axial rod of a protozoon which functions as a support.

aye-aye A nocturnal lemur, *Daubentonia madagascariensis* (single genus and species), inhabiting the forest and bamboo thickets of Madagascar. See *primate*.

azaserine An antibiotic produced along with 6-diazo-5-oxo-L-norleucine by species of *Streptomyces*. Both substances have been studied because of their oncolytic activity, but they also have antibacterial and some antifungal potency. Their mode of activity is not completely understood, but they probably inhibit purine synthesis.[36, 49]

azathioprine (Imuran)   A purine analog

used as an immunosuppressant and anti-tumor drug.

azo- A prefix indicating presence of the group—N : N—.

azo blue An acid dye of the dis-azo group. Solubility at 15° C.: water 25 per cent, absolute alcohol 0.02 per cent, and glycerol 7 per cent. It is used with titan yellow and quinalizarin for magnesium in plant cells.[57]

azoprotein An antigen prepared by coupling diazonium salts of aromatic amines such as arsanilic acid and sulfanilic acid with proteins. The resultant compound possesses antigenic activity specific for the diazotized fraction.

azoturia (Monday morning disease) A condition that occurs in heavily muscled horses when they exercise too heavily after a few days of rest. Large amounts of myoglobin are released from the muscles and appear in the urine. Severe nephropathy occurs, which may be due to the toxic effects of the myoglobin, but which may also involve intravascular coagulation in the renal glomeruli. It resembles crush syndrome of man.

azure A methyl thionine dye used for the detection of epidermophytic infections.[153]

   a. A, an asymmetrical dimethyl thionine dye used as a nuclear stain.[37]

   a. B, a trimethyl derivative of thionine, used to stain Negri bodies.[37]

   a. C, a monomethyl thionine used to stain sections of formalin-fixed material.[37]

azurophilic granule A large oval or round cytoplasmic structure found in lymphocytes; sometimes applied to toxic granules in neutrophils.

B

Babesia (formerly *Piroplasma*) A genus of pear-shaped protozoan parasites which occur in the erythrocytes of mammals, usually two organisms within each cell. They were the first organism shown to be transmitted by an arthropod vector, the tick. This epochal discovery was the work of Smith, Kilborne, and Curtice during their studies of Texas cattle fever in the late 19th century.[136] See table.

baboon Any member of the group of primates made up principally of three genera: *Papio*, *Papop*, and *Theropithecus*. See *primate*.

baby pig encephalomyelitis See under *encephalomyelitis*.

bacillary paralysis See under *paralysis*.

bacillophobia A morbid fear of disease-producing microorganisms.

Bacillus anthracis See *anthrax*.

bacitracin An antibiotic produced by certain strains of *Bacillus licheniformis* that interferes to some extent with cell wall and protein synthesis but acts primarily as an inhibitor of cell membrane function. It is highly effective in topical administration against many gram-positive organisms but has little effect on the gram-negative bacteria except *Neisseria*. Because of its renal toxicity, it is not used as a systemic antibiotic.[36, 49]

backcross The mating of an offspring of the first generation of a hybrid mating with one of the parents. See *breeding system*.

bacteria Microorganisms of the class Schizomycetes (fission fungi). For a comparison of the bacteria and other microscopic forms, see *microorganism*.

bacterial competence The transitional physiological state of a bacterial cell that enables it to be transformed during exposure to DNA. Competence is present during the optimal phase of the growth cycle, with the production of a macromolecular activator that changes the cell surface. Cells in the

DISEASES CAUSED BY *Babesia*

AGENT	VECTOR	HOST	DISEASE
B. bigemina	*Margaropus annulatus*	Cow	Texas cattle fever
B. bovis	*Ixodes ricinus*	Cow	Similar to Texas fever
B. argentina	*Margaropus*, possibly *Rhipicephalus*	Calf	Cerebral babesiosis
B. mutasi	Dermacentor, *Hemaphysalis*, *Rhipicephalus*	Sheep, goat	Carciag in Eastern and southeastern Europe
B. ovis	*Rhipicephalus*	Sheep, goat	Mild form of carciag
B. caballi	Dermacentor, *Hyalomma*, *Rhipicephalus*	Horse	Equine piroplasmosis
B. equi	Same as above	Horse	Equine piroplasmosis
B. canis	Dermacentor, *Rhipicephalus*, *Hemaphysalis*	Dog	Similar to piroplasmosis (Texas fever)
B. gibsoni	*Rhipicephalus*, *Hemaphysalis*	Dog	Piroplasmosis in Asia and Africa
B. felis	(?)	Cat	Piroplasmosis
B. rodhaini	(?)	Rodent	Piroplasmosis

stage of competence may be preserved by freezing in 15 per cent glycerol.[32]

bacteriocin   A group of highly specific antibacterial proteins produced by certain strains of bacteria, and active against other strains of the same species. They possess an extremely narrow spectrum of activity. The colicins (q.v.) have been the most extensively studied. One particle (molecule) appears to be sufficient to kill one cell. The mechanism is unknown, but the particles appear to react with receptors in the bacterial cell wall. Effects on the cell may be multiple. Rather than blocking a specific enzyme as do the antibiotics, they may interfere with the regulatory circuits of the cell.[49]

bacteriolysis   Disintegration of microbial cells, such as *Vibrio cholera*, which occurs during incubation with the serum of animals previously inoculated with the same organism. Also seen in vegetative bacteriophage infections.

bacteriophage (phage)   A virus that infects bacterial cells.[32]

   temperate b., a bacterial virus that can produce either an overt infection which destroys the host cell by lysis or a latent infection in which nucleic acid is injected but no intracellular virions are formed. The genome or its replica becomes inserted into the bacterial chromosomes (lysogenic conversion) and is referred to as prophage. A bacterial cell with this type of infection is called lysogenic and can be induced to produce phage particles by treating it with metabolic inhibitors, x-rays, ultraviolet light, etc. Lysis and release of phage progeny can then occur.

   virulent b., a bacterial virus that can produce overt infection only; it is formed when nucleic acid is injected into a sensitive cell, resulting in lysis.

Balantidium   A genus of protozoa of the subclass Ciliata which parasitize the intestine of the monkey, swine, cow, and man.

baleen   See *cetacean*.

ballistophobia   A morbid dread of missiles.

Bamberger-Marie disease   Hypertrophic pulmonary osteoarthropathy. This disease is seen quite frequently in dogs and has been reported in other species of animals, including horses, and is usually associated with a neoplasm of the thoracic cavity in a fashion similar to that seen in man.

bandicoot   See *marsupial*.

Bang's disease   Infectious abortion in cattle caused by *Brucella abortus*. See under *abortion*.

Barbary ape   A species of primates, *Macaca sylvana*, native to Africa and the Rock of Gibraltar; they are tailless monkeys.

barnacle   See *crustacean*.

baro-   A combining form denoting relationship to weight or pressure.

barophilic   Growing best under high atmospheric pressure; said of bacterial cells.

Barr body   Condensed chromatin (heterochromatin) in the interphase nuclei of somatic cells; it is derived from the late replicating sex chromosomes. In most mammals it is seen only in cells of the female, where it appears as a dark-staining mass against the inner surface of the nuclear membrane of epithelial, hepatic, or muscle cells or as a paranucleolar mass in neurons. The number of Barr bodies in a cell is usually one fewer than the number of X chromosomes present. In species in which the X and Y chromosomes are unusually large, as in the golden hamster or chinchilla, two Barr bodies are present in both sexes. Other exceptions occur when unusual sex-determining mechanisms are operative, as in the meadow vole, in which the normal female has only one X chromosome, yet the female has one Barr body while the XY male has two. Differences between male and female interphase nuclei are not observed in most tissues of rodents, birds, reptiles, or amphibians; they have been seen in rat embryos, chickens, crustaceans, and insects. See also *Lyon hypothesis* and *drumstick*.[121]

Bartonella   A genus of the family Bartonellaceae (q.v.). *B. bacilliformis* is the etiologic agent of the anemic (Oroyo fever) and eruptive (verruga peruana) types of bartonellosis in man.

Bartonellaceae   A family of organisms closely related to the rickettsiae, whose members are often pleomorphic (rod-shaped, coccoid, ring-shaped, filamentous, or beaded), gram-negative microorganisms, and which are the agent of disease in man and anomen (see table on page 34).[159]

bartonellosis   An infection caused by any of the group of organisms referred to as the bartonella. *Haemobartonella*, *Grahamella*, or *Eperythrozoon*. See *Bartonella*.

basic dye   An organic dye that binds and stains negatively charged molecules such as acid mucopolysaccharides and nucleic acids.

basophilic   Staining readily with basic dyes.

basophobia   Morbid fear of walking, or fear of being unable to walk.

bathmophobia   Morbid fear of stairways or steep slopes.

batho-, bathy-   Combining form meaning deep, or denoting relationship to depth.

bathochromy (bathochromic effect)   A shift in the peak of the absorption curve of a dye in solution toward longer wavelength.[37]

BCG vaccine (bacillus of Calmette and Guerin)   A living culture of *Myobacterium tuberculosis* var. *bovis* rendered avirulent by prolonged cultivation on glycerinated bile medium. The vaccine has been used to produce immunity against tuberculosis in many species of animals, including monkeys and man. The development of BCG vaccine represents one of the outstanding examples of benefits to the field of human health by cooperative research between workers in human and veterinary medicine. Calmette was a physician, Guerin a veterinarian.[36]

bee paralysis   See *acute* and *chronic paralysis* under *paralysis*.

behavior   The entire complex of observable,

DISEASES CAUSED BY BARTONELLACEAE

SPECIES	HOST	DISEASE
Bartonella bacilliformis	Man	Bartonellosis, Oroyo fever, Carrion's disease
Eperythrozoon coccoides	Mouse, rat, hamster, rabbit	(?)
E. felis	Cat	Feline infectious anemia
E. ovis	Lamb, sheep	Anemia
E. suis	Swine	Anaplasma-like disease of eperythrozoonosis
E. wentoni	Cow (in South Africa)	(?)
Grahamella	Anomen	Grahamellosis of rodents
Hemobartonella bovis	Cow	(?)
H. canis	Dog	Infectious anemia
H. felis	Cat	Infectious anemia
H. muris	Rat	Anemia
H. tazzeri	Guinea pig	(?)
H. spp.	Man	Hemolytic-uremic syndrome

recordable, or measurable activities of an animal as it reacts to its environment.[58, 158]

acquired b., behavior that is dependent upon conditioning and learning, especially when it occurs as a function of the presence of previously ineffective stimuli.

aggressive b., a class of behavior that includes both threat and attack.

agonistic b., a broad group of behavior patterns that include attack, threat, appeasement, and flight.

allochthonous b., behavior that is not activated by its own drive, but as the consequence of the frustration of behavior activated by some drive other than that which most often controls it. See *displacement activity.*

appeasement b., a group of behavior patterns (exclusive of flight or aggression) that terminate attack upon an animal by another animal of the same species.

appetitive b., a term used to characterize an inferred or anticipated consummatory act in animals.

attack b., a class of responses in an animal that may cause injury or possibly death of the attacked animal if the behavior continues. Such patterns include biting, clawing, striking with the wings, etc.

autochthonous b., a behavior pattern activated by internal drives of the animal; the opposite of allochthonous behavior.

emotional b., an arbitrary class of responses that is defined differently for different species; e.g., in the rat, such behavior would cover activities such as freezing, trembling, vocalizing, urination, and defecation. In the pigeon, it would cover cooing and wing-beating.

escape b., activity of an animal to remove itself from the location of a specific stimulus. Stimuli effective in producing escape behavior are usually the same as those identified as negative reinforcing stimuli, or aversive stimuli.

flight b., the effort of an animal to escape from proximity to another animal that is exhibiting threat or attack behavior.

imitative b., behavior that is not species-specific but occurs after one animal is exposed to or placed in the environment of another animal which exhibits that behavior, and when it can be demonstrated that the behavioral patterns of the first animal are the stimuli for the responses of the second. Cf. *mimetic b.*

inborn b., see *species-specific b.* and *unlearned b.*

innate b., see *species-specific b.* and *unlearned b.*

mimetic b., behavior pattern of an animal placed in the environment of another animal, the first animal thereafter behaving in the same fashion as the animal with which it was placed. It differs from imitative behavior in that the response in mimetic behavior is species-specific.

operant b., the total of operant responses in the behavior repertoire of the animal.

purposive b., behavior as considered with respect to its goals.

respondent b., the total of respondents in the behavior repertoire of an animal.

ritualized b., see under *response.*

species-specific b., the group of behavior patterns exhibited by a large majority of the members of a species in similar environment and under similar conditions. See also *unlearned b.*

spontaneous b., behavior that occurs in the apparent absence of any stimuli recognizable as able to set the occasion for the occurrence of the behavior.

threat b., any pattern of behavior which has been shown to produce flight behavior in another animal usually of the same species.

unlearned b. (instinctive, inborn, or innate behavior), species-specific behavior for which no antecedent stimulus can be determined, or which has been demonstrated experimentally to be independent of, and unmodified by, the operation of variables incurred in conditioning and learning, such as the occurrence of reinforcing stimuli.

verbal b., behavior involving the vocalization or writing of words, or response to spoken or written words.

behavior chain A sequence of behavioral stimuli and responses that can be observed repeatedly in an animal with only minor variations.

behaviorism A school of psychology based upon a purely objective observation and analysis of human and animal behavior without reference to the testimony of consciousness.[158]

behaviorist A scientist who investigates the behavior of animals objectively and attempts to relate these observations into classifications or systematic analyses. Cf. *ethologist*.

behavior pattern A set of responses that can be observed as statistically organized in time and manifesting some degree of consistency in the sequence in which they occur.

behavior repertoire The set or profile of behavior characteristic of a species or of a single member of a species.

belonephobia Dread of needles and pins.

Bence-Jones protein A light-chain fraction of gamma globulin found in the urine of patients with multiple myeloma.

benthic Living on the seabed.

benzpyrene A carcinogenic polycyclic hydrocarbon, $C_{20}H_{12}$.

Bergmann's rule The principle that, given wide geographical range, warm-blooded animals of a single species achieve larger size in the colder areas of the range than in the warmer areas; that is, size varies inversely with temperature.

beriberi A form of polyneuritis caused by deficiency of thiamine. It is marked by spasmodic rigidity of the lower limbs, with muscular atrophy, paralysis, anemia, and neuralgic pains. See also *thiaminase, bracken fern poisoning*, and *Chastek's paralysis*.

Berry-Dedrick phenomenon Genetic interaction between viruses. Stimulated by the work on pneumococcal transformation between heat-inactivated and live pneumococcal strains of differing capsular types, G. P. Berry and H. M. Dedrick in 1936 described a reactivation phenomenon between rabbit Shope fibroma and myxomatosis viruses which was the first experimental demonstration of genetic interaction between viruses. They heated extracts of myxoma lesions between 56° and 85° C. for 30 minutes. This treatment completely inactivated the virus; but a mixture of heat-inactivated myxoma virus and live fibroma virus injected into laboratory rabbits produced a substantial proportion of myxoma lesions. This result has been repeatedly confirmed but the results were often irregular. It was necessary to use two successive hosts in order to bring out the transformation phenomenon. The first injection produced a mild disease intermediate between fibroma and myxoma (fibromyxoma). Extracts of these lesions inoculated into a second rabbit produced typical myxoma.[30]

Bertiella An anoplocephalid tapeworm transmitted by mites and characterized by a cyclophyllidean life cycle. *B. studeri* is a common parasite of primates and man.[21] See *cestodiasis*.

beta-glucuronidase See *glucuronidase*.

Bettlach May disease A paralysis of adult honeybees, reported chiefly from Switzerland, caused by poisonous substances in the pollen of *Ranunculus* species (buttercups). Buttercup pollen is collected by the bees only when no other forage is available. The poisoned bees cannot fly, but twirl rapidly or turn somersaults, and die from three to five days after feeding on the pollen.

bi- A combining form meaning two or twice.

bibliomania Abnormally intense desire to collect books.

biebrich scarlet An acid dye of the dis-azo group, widely used in histology.[37, 57]

bilateral symmetry The condition in which an animal's body when divided along a central plane can be divided into two parts, each of which is an approximate mirror image of the other.

bili- A combining form denoting relationship to the bile.

binomial system Scientific method of naming animals and plants with two terms, indicating genus and species. The genus is capitalized and both terms are italicized.

bio- A combining form denoting relationship to life.

bioincrassination The concentration of material by taking greater quantities of the other constituents from the mixture by a biological action.[86]

biological control The use, by man, of living organisms to control (usually meaning to suppress) undesirable animals and plants. Some authors consider biological control to be a part of natural control, and use the term to refer to that action of parasites, predators, or pathogens on a host or prey population which produces a lower general equilibrium position than would prevail in the absence of these agents. Certain nonorganismal biological factors, such as metabolic and genetic diseases, when used in control may be included in the concept of biological control. Biological control involving the use of microorganisms is usually called "microbial control."

biologically pure The state of an organism existing with no direct contact with other living species or their biologically distinctive products. The term may be abbreviated to Bp. Such animals are in the monobiotic state, which is purer than germ-free.[86]

Biological Society of Washington U.S. National Museum, Washington, D.C. 20560.

Biological Stain Commission, Inc. University of Rochester Medical Center, Rochester, N.Y. 14620.

bion An individual living organism. Also used as equivalent to germ-free animal. See also *germ-free*.

bionics The study of specialized animal systems that might possibly be converted to man-made analogs.

biosphere   1. That part of the earth which is occupied by living matter.   2. The sphere of action between an organism and its environment.

biotic insecticide   An organism used to suppress a local insect pest population. To some, the word "insecticide" implies a more-or-less temporary action, comparable to that of a chemical insecticide. Others object to "insecticide" as minimizing the difference between chemical and biological control and as being a source of confusion with purely chemical products. In the case of microorganisms used for this purpose, the term "microbial insecticide" is sometimes preferred.

biotron   A building containing laboratories designed to study both plants and animals under carefully controlled environments.

bipectinate   Bearing comblike projections on each side, especially in birds.

birefringence   See *anistotropic*.

bis-   A prefix signifying two or twice.

Bismarck brown   A basic dis-azo dye. Solubility at 15° C.: water 15 per cent, absolute alcohol 3 per cent, glycerol 20 per cent. It is used as a nuclear stain and for mast cell granules and mucoproteins.[57, 153]

Biston betularia   The peppered moth, used to study industrial melanism in which, through selective pressure from predators, darker individuals are favored to survive in soot-darkened environment. Over many generations darker genotypes reproduce in greater numbers.

bittern   See *ciconiiform birds*.

Bittner mammary tumor virus (milk factor; milk agent; milk influence)   An agent found by Bittner at the Jackson Laboratory in the milk of an inbred mouse line (strain A) with a high incidence of mammary tumor (88 per cent). Bittner showed that the foster-nursing of strain A females by mice of an inbred line (BA) with a low incidence of mammary tumors would reduce the incidence of spontaneous mammary tumors in strain A females. Since these fundamental observations were made, it has been shown by other workers that, although numerous other variables—e.g., sex, age, hormonal effects, and genetic constitution—are important in influencing susceptibility to mammary carcinoma, it is unequivocally the result of a virus infection, and for that reason is of great historical importance. Inability to propagate the virus in vitro has impeded its characterization, but it is known that the virus is inactivated by trypsin, may be stored by lyophilization, is inactivated by heating to 56° C. for 30 minutes, can be concentrated by ultracentrifugation, and may be neutralized by heteroimmune serum. It appears to be an RNA virus. The virus-induced carcinoma can be transplanted as isografts.[27, 53, 114, 127] See *oncogenic viruses*, and see *classification*, under *virus*.

Bittner's milk factor   See *Bittner mammary tumor virus*.

black brood   See *American foulbrood*, under *foulbrood*.

black disease   Infectious necrotic hepatitis of sheep caused by migrating fluke larvae associated with a clostridial infection; it is a fatal disease of sheep, and occasionally of man.

black-egg disease   See *melanosis*.

blackhead   A highly fatal infectious disease of young turkeys, produced by the protozoon *Histomonas maleagridis* and characterized by enterohepatitis and discoloration of the comb. A mild form occurs in chickens, pheasants, quail, and peafowl. The disease is transmitted by the cecal nematode *Heterakis gallinae*, which can pass the organism through the ovum.[16]

blackleg   An infectious disease of sheep, cattle, and goats characterized by emphysematous muscular and subcutaneous swellings and nodules. It is caused by *Clostridium chauvoei*.

blacksnake   See table accompanying *snake*.

blasticidin S   One of a group of antibiotics produced by species of *Streptomyces* which inhibit both gram-negative and gram-positive bacteria and certain fungi. Its effects are exerted through inhibition of protein synthesis.[36, 49]

blasto-   A combining form denoting relationship to a bud or budding, particularly to an early embryonic stage, as to a primitive or formative element, cell, or layer.

blastomycosis   Chronic suppurative granuloma of the respiratory tract and skin caused by organisms of the genus *Blastomyces*.

blending inheritance   Hereditary pattern in which parental characters blend in the offspring in an intermediate level rather than segregating into different phenotypes favoring one parent or the other.

blepharoplast   The small section of chromatin found in the various stages of the life cycle of trypanosomes. The flagellum originates from this structure.[109]

blood group chimerism   The result of exchange during gestation of hematopoietic cells between dizygotic twins because of common placental blood circulation. Each becomes tolerant to the cells of the other and continues to produce both blood types after birth. It is commonly seen in twin calves (see *freemartin*) and in marmosets, but has also been observed in sheep, goats, pigs, and man. Such chimeras can be experimentally produced by treatment with x-irradiation and subsequent injection of living bone marrow.

blood spot   A blood clot of variable size found on the surface of the yolk of a chicken egg, originating from minute hemorrhages of the follicle when the ovum is released from the ovary. They are considered undesirable, and such eggs are detected by candling and removed prior to marketing. Meat spots are also small clots, but are found free within the albumin of chicken eggs and are believed to originate within the uterus when the albumin is secreted around the yolk.

blood values   The average values of the normal constituents of the blood of various animals. See *hemogram*.

blowhole   A modified nasal orifice at the top

of the head, common to cetaceans, being paired orifices in the mysticetes (baleen whales) and single in the odontocetes (toothed whales and porpoises).

blue disease A rickettsial disease of the larvae of the Japanese beetle, *Popillia japonica,* and of other related scarab larvae. The causative agent is *Rickettsiella popilliae.* The name of the rickettsiosis derives from the bluish appearance of the diseased grubs.

blue tongue of sheep (catarrhal fever; sore muzzle) A viral disease of sheep that usually is characterized by fever, stomatitis, lameness, and a mortality rate which may vary from 7 to 50 per cent. Active infection or vaccination with attenuated virus during early pregnancy produces a high incidence of anomalies of the brain and heart in lambs. The disease is caused by an arbovirus, transmitted by flies of the genus *Culicoides.*[142]

B-melanosis See *melanosis.*

Bodansky unit The quantity of phosphatase required to liberate 1 mg. of phosphorus ion in an hour of incubation with a substrate of sodium B-glycerophosphate.

boomslang See table accompanying *snake.*

Bordetella A genus of microorganisms of the family Brucellaceae, order Eubacteriales, made up of minute motile or nonmotile gram-negative coccobacilli. Some are primary pathogens, while others act as opportunists in secondary infections.[36, 142] (See table.)

Borna disease A fatal enzootic encephalitis of horses, cattle, and sheep, caused by a virus.

Borrelia A genus of actively motile microorganisms of the family Treponametaceae, made up of loosely spiraled and irregular cells which generally taper terminally into fine filaments.[16, 142] See table.

Bos A genus of ruminant mammals that includes the domestic cow, *B. taunus,* the Brahman cow, *B. indicus,* and the yak, *B. grunniens.*

botryomycosis A purulent granuloma of horses, camels, and sometimes cattle, caused by *Staphylococcus aureus.*[16]

botulism A type of food poisoning caused by a toxin produced by the growth of *Clostridium botulinum* in improperly canned or preserved foods, especially in spoiled tissues used as animal food. The symptoms are essentially those of paralysis: disturbances in vision and difficulty in locomotion. The tongue becomes paralyzed, and swallowing becomes impossible because of pharyngeal paralysis. Respiratory paralysis finally terminates the disease.

b. toxin, a poisonous protein produced by *Clostridium botulinum.* There are six immunologic types: type A affects man, mink, and birds; type B, man, mink, and sometimes birds; type C, man, mink, sometimes birds, and ruminants; type D, man and ruminants; types E and F, man.[16]

Bp Biologically pure.

brachy- A combining form meaning short.

brachyosis A bacterial disease of certain species of *Malacosoma* (tent caterpillars), caused by *Clostridium brevifaciens* and *Clostridium malacosomae.* These anaerobic bacteria multiply especially in the anterior half of the larval midgut, causing a form of dysentery, sluggishness, shortening of the larval body, and death of the younger larvae. Older larvae may survive the disease.

bracken fern poisoning Poisoning occurring in horses and cattle after prolonged ingestion of bracken fern (*Pteridium aquilinum*). The toxic fraction is thought to be thiaminase, which causes granulocytopenia, thrombocytopenia, and hypoplastic anemia. In the horse, poisoning is manifested by a severe central nervous system disturbance.

bradsot (braxy) An acute disease of lambs and young sheep caused by *Clostridium septicum* and characterized by gastritis of the abomasum and a high mortality rate. Cold weather seems to be a factor in susceptibility to the disease.

brady- A combining form meaning slow.

bradyauxesis See *heterauxesis.*

bradykinin A kinin composed of nine amino acids and contained in the globulin fraction of blood plasma. See table accompanying *allergy.*

bradytelic See *evolutionary rate.*

brand A mark made on the skin with a hot iron especially to identify livestock such as cattle and horses. Also a stigma or mark of disgrace formerly placed on criminals with a hot iron. Cf. *freeze brand.*

braxy Bradsot.

breeding system Any system of mating. The genetic consequences of various breeding systems have been intensively studied and categorized. (See also *congenic* and *coisogenic.*) Some of these systems may be defined as follows:[51]

Backcross mating: the mating of a homozygote and a heterozygote (e.g., +/+ × +/a).

Cross mating: the mating of unlike homozygotes (e.g., +/+ × a/a).

DISEASES CAUSED BY *Bordetella*

SPECIES	HOST	DISEASE
B. bronchiseptica	Dog, cat, rabbit, guinea pig, rat, swine, occasionally man	Bronchopneumonia, other respiratory disease
B. parapertussis	Man	Whooping cough
B. pertussis	Man	Whooping cough

DISEASES CAUSED BY *Borrelia*

SPECIES	VECTOR	HOST	DISEASE
B. anserina	Argus persicus, A. miniatus	Guinea fowl, sparrow, canary	Avian spirochetosis
B. recurrentis	Tick, louse	Mouse, rat, hamster, man	Relapsing fever
B. theileri	Margaropus decoloratus, Phipicephalus evertri	Sheep, horse	Febrile attacks

Diallel cross mating: the set of all possible matings between several genotypes defined as individuals, substrains, or strains, to reveal the nature of a given multiple-factor genetic trait.

Harem (pen) mating: the practice of maintaining a breeding male and a variable number of breeding females in a cage. The females may or may not be removed prior to parturition.

Inbred-derived offspring: progeny produced by the indiscriminate mating of pairs of animals within an inbred strain; not necessarily the mating of brother and sister.

Inbreeding: a system of breeding that employs matings designed to attain maximum homozygosity, e.g., matings of full siblings, or parent and offspring. See *inbred strains* for a more rigorous definition.

Incross mating: the mating of like homozygotes (e.g., +/+ × +/+).

Intercross mating: the mating of heterozygotes (e.g., a/+ × a/+).

Random mating: a system of breeding that implies the employment of methods designed to maximize heterozygosity, e.g., by selection from tables of random sample numbers. Such a system attempts to avoid unwitting bias in the selection of breeding pairs. In large populations, random breeding preserves the gene frequency generation after generation. In populations of small size the expected results of a random system may differ, owing to the random fixation or loss of alleles at each locus at a rate that varies inversely with the number of the population. These changes have been variously called the inbreeding effect, random drift, genetic drift, and the Sewall-Wright effect.

Single-pair mating: the practice of maintaining a breeding pair (and their progeny till weaned) in a single cage for their breeding lifespan.

Strain cross mating: the mating between inbred strains of animals to produce hybrids.[51]

Breyere-Moloney virus   The virus causing lymphoid leukemia in BALB/c and C3H mice, and in Osborne-Mendel rats. It was found in a plasma cell tumor in an adult C3H mouse that had been treated (as a suckling) with methylcholanthrene.[114]

brilliant cresyl-blue   A stain used for reticulated cells and platelets, and which can be treated with sulfurous acid to produce a reagent that can be substituted for Schiff's reagent in the Feulgen reaction.[57, 153]

brisket disease (high altitude disease) A common condition of cattle and occasionally sheep pastured at altitudes above 7600 feet. Similar to "miner's disease" of man (seen in the Andes Mountains), it is characterized by cardiac hypertrophy, chronic passive congestion, and ventral edema.[142] The disease has been produced experimentally in pigs.

British thermal unit (B.T.U.)   The amount of heat necessary to raise the temperature of 1 pound of water from 39° to 40° F.

5-bromo-2′-deoxyuridine (BUDR)   A halogenated pyrimidine that interferes with synthesis of viral DNA, but has no effect on riboviruses; also used as an immunosuppressant.

bromophenol blue   A stain used for differentiating living and dead sperm in fowl semen and as a stain for basic proteins.[57, 153]

5-bromouracil   A pyrimidine analog with mutagenic capability.

bronchitis   Inflammation of the bronchial tubes.

   infectious b. (chick b.; gasping disease), a viral disease of chicks two days to three or four weeks of age, characterized by listlessness, depression, gasping, and rales. The bronchitis virus has been cultivated in chicken embryos, and two antigenic types have been shown.

brood   1. A hatch of young birds. 2. The young of bees before they issue from the brood cells.   3. The pupae of ants.

brooder pneumonia   See *aspergillosis.*

brown fat   A type of adipose tissue found in many rodents that is morphologically, histogenetically, and physiologically distinct. Grossly, this tissue is formed of compact, light-brown bodies that develop from specific embryonic anlagen; no new areas appear postnatally. Lobes of this tissue are found (in the mouse) between the scapulae, in the axillae, in the cervical region along the jugular veins, adjacent to the thymus, along the thoracic aorta, at the hilus of the kidney, and alongside the urethra. The large paired lobes in the interscapular depression have been called *hibernating glands.* Brown fat is physiologically more active than white fat but there is no evidence that it secretes hormones, and it does not function as a gland of hibernation in the mouse. Histologically this tissue is composed of groups of polygonal cells containing lipid droplets in a coarsely granular cytoplasm. The fat droplets are not coalescent, and the nuclei are central.[51]

brown hypertrophy of the cere In psittacine birds, especially budgerigars, hypertrophy of the cere is a common occurrence, with great variation in severity. The cere, which is generally soft and blue (in males) or light brown to pink (females), becomes cornified. The tissue proliferates and the normally flat cere becomes elevated and hornlike. Except for occlusion of the nares, this process of unknown etiology does not affect the bird, and it usually does not require treatment.[112]

Brown-Pearce tumor (epithelioma of Brown-Pearce; Brown-Pearce carcinoma) An anaplastic carcinoma originating in the scrotum of a rabbit inoculated in both sides of the scrotum with testicular tissue from a rabbit infected with *Treponema pallidum*. The procedure was done in the laboratories of W. Brown and L. Pearce at The Rockefeller Institute (now University). The tumor developed in 1921, about five years after local chancre formation at each inoculation site. Brown and Pearce believed the tumor to have originated in eczematous scrotal skin, but this view is not held by all; some believe it could have originated in the testis. The tumor may be serially transplanted by a variety of routes, the intratesticular and intraocular (of Greene) being the most popular because of the nearly 100 per cent successful growths. Considerable difference in biologic behavior is experienced in different laboratories. A. E. Casey found in 1932 that enhancement of tumor growth was occasioned by pretreatment with stored refrigerated (but nonviable) tumor tissue ten days prior to inoculation with viable tumor tissue. Casey termed the agent in stored tumor tissues the XYZ factor. A considerable body of information about tumor immunology has been accumulated with the use of the Brown-Pearce tumor, and it is widely used in experimental oncology.[150]

Brown snake See table accompanying *snake*.

Brucella A genus of microorganisms of the family Brucellaceae, made up of nonmotile, short, rod-shaped to coccoid, gram-negative encapsulated cells.[16] See table.

brucellosis See under *abortion*.

Brugia A genus of nematodes of the superfamily Filaroidea. *B. malayi* infects man, other primates, and cats. *B. pahangi* is found in the lymphatic system of the cat, dog, and wild animals, including the tiger. *B. guyanensis* and *B. beaveri* are the first members of this species to be reported in the Western Hemisphere.[21]

bryozoan Any member of the phylum Bryozoa. These animals are known as moss animals because of their tufted, branched colonies, only a few millimeters high, attached to solid objects in shallow sea water. They are bilaterally symmetrical, nonsegmented, with a complete digestive tract and well developed coelom lined with peritoneum. They have no respiratory or circulatory system. Many of the extinct species had a short geologic life but wide geographic range, and thus are useful in dating strata brought up in drill cores. Representative living species include *Bugula, Membranipora,* and *Pectinatella*.

bumblefoot Subcutaneous abscess of the footpad in domestic and captive wild birds. Injuries to the feet, to which the birds are perhaps predisposed as a result of improper flooring or sanitation, become repeatedly infected with various organisms, most commonly species of *Staphylococcus,* and chronic inflammation results. Satisfactory treatment consists of curettage and application of antiseptics.[11, 112]

Bunostomum A genus of hookworms. *B. phlebotomum* is the hookworm of cattle; *B. trigonocephalum,* of sheep and goats.

buphthalmia See *congenital glaucoma* under *glaucoma*.

bursa of Fabricius A lymphoid organ of the bird that develops as an outpouching of the cloacal epithelium and later becomes surrounded by lymphoid cells. It has a thymuslike role, being responsible for the development of cells that produce humoral antibody. It involutes, becoming atrophic and functionless in adult life—a fact made use of by conservationists in judging the age of pheasants in the field. The age is determined by the depth to which a measured probe can be inserted into the bursa. The rabbit appendix develops in similar fashion and may also function as a source of antibody-producing cells.[48] See also *thymus* and *central lymphoid tissue*.

bush baby A member of the genus *Galago* or *Galagoides*. See table under *primate*.

bushmaster See table accompanying *snake*.

busulfan (Myleran) An alkylating agent used as an oncolytic drug.

Diseases Caused by *Brucella*

Species	Host	Disease
B. abortus	Man, cow	Undulant fever, infectious abortion
B. canis	Dog, man	Epidemic canine abortion, human infections (in laboratory workers)
B. melitensis	Goat, man	Malta or Mediterranean fever
B. ovis	Ram	Ram epididymitis
B. suis	Swine	Infectious abortion

buthioprine   A purine analog used as an immunosuppressant and an oncolytic drug.

butyr-   A combining form denoting relationship to butter.

butyrinase   An enzyme of the blood serum that is capable of catalyzing the hydrolysis of butyrin.

B-virus   See *herpesvirus B*.

C

CA   Croup associated. See table under *simian virus*.

caco-   A combining form meaning bad, or ill.

cacodylate buffer   A solution used with fixatives for electron microscopy.

cage paralysis   See *avitaminosis D*.

calciphylactic   Pertaining to calciphylaxis.

calciphylaxis   An induced, but not necessarily immunologic, type of hypersensitivity in which — during a "critical period" after sensitization by a systemic calcifying factor (e.g., vitamin D compounds, parathyroid hormone) — topical or systemic treatment with certain challengers (e.g., egg white, egg yolk, metallic salts) causes selective calcinosis in various tissues and organs. If an animal is appropriately sensitized with a systemic calcifying factor, two forms of calciphylaxis can be induced: (1) topical calciphylaxis, which is induced by the direct application of the challenger to the responsive tissue and (2) systemic calciphylaxis, in which the challenger is distributed throughout the organism (as after intravenous or intraperitoneal administration) and produces a response in diverse tissues for which it has an affinity.

calf diphtheria   An infection of the mouth, pharynx, and larynx of calves caused by *Spherophorus necrophorus*.

calf pneumonia   See under *pneumonia*.

calf scours   A gastrointestinal disease of young calves caused by enteropathogenic strains of *Escherichia coli* and characterized by severe diarrhea. Colostrum or normal serum confers protection to young calves. Enteropathogenic strains of *E. coli* may also cause abortion in sheep and mares, septicemia and diarrhea in lambs, granulomatous lesions in chickens (Hjarre's disease), and edema disease in swine and young pigs.

calico cat (tortoiseshell cat)   A cat with fur of three colors: black, white, and orange. Most cats affected with this genetic condition are females; affected males are usually sterile. See also *chromosomal aberration*.

California Academy of Sciences   Department of Paleontology, University of California, Berkeley, Calif. 94720.

California encephalitis   See under *encephalitis*.

Callitroga hominivoras (screw worm)   A genus of flies the larvae of which are parasitic and may cause myiasis (q.v.). The lesions are caused by the larvae, which feed upon living tissues and may produce serious effects in open wounds on the skin or by invasion of the nasopharnyx. An interesting and important contribution to the control of parasites occurred in the study of this fly in which the males were made sterile by exposure to irradiation. When treated males mated with females, infertile eggs were produced and, as the female only mates once, the life cycle was broken. Another member of this group is *C. macillarion*, which is not a myiasis-causing agent but lives primarily as a scavenger in soil or may become a secondary wound invader.

callosity   A circumscribed thickening of the skin with hypertrophy of the horny layer, due to friction, pressure, or other irritation.

     ischial c., leathery patches found over the ischial tuberosity (buttocks) of many of the higher Old World primates.

CAM   Chorioallantoic membrane.

Camelus   The genus containing the camels; *C. bactrianus* is the two-humped camel, and *C. dromedarius* the one-humped camel or dromedary.

canary   See *passeriform birds*.

canary diphtheria   Canary pox.

canary pox (canary diphtheria; Kikuth's disease)   A poxvirus disease of canaries, the agent being classified in the avian subgroup of the poxviruses, and given the binomial *Borreliota fringillae*. Experimentally the disease has been transferred to species other than canaries, but it is generally accepted that it is spontaneously infectious only for *Serinus* species and their near relatives. Clinically, canary pox manifests itself as a slowly spreading respiratory disease with a productive conjunctivitis. It is characterized by a high mortality rate and a course of three to ten days. Acute cases may have minimal lesions but, typically, proliferative skin lesions (pocks) form first on the eyelids, and later about the commissures of the beak and skin of the head. Other lesions include those of pneumonia, air sacculitis, pericarditis, and perihepatitis. Diagnosis is established by the finding of typical intracytoplasmic inclusions in sections stained with hematoxylin and eosin and by isolation of the virus in eggs followed by serological identification.

cancer chemotherapy   The treatment of neoplastic diseases with oncolytic substances; see *antimetabolite* for list of oncolytic chemicals.

"cancer eye"   See *epidermoid carcinoma*, under *carcinoma*.

cancer-inducing virus   See *oncogenic virus*, and see *classification* under *virus*.

Candida (formerly *Monilia*)   A genus of

yeastlike fungi characterized by producing mycelia but not ascospores.

Candida albicans A pathogenic species that causes thrush in human infants. It can also be a secondary invader and produce skin and systemic infections in debilitated hosts. It may also be found in the oral mucosa of calves and colts. Thrushlike lesions of birds such as chickens, pigeons, turkeys, pheasants, and grouse are very common and serious.[16]

canine distemper (Carre's disease) A viral disease of young dogs which may be aggravated by superimposed infection with *Bordetella bronchiseptica*. Distemper is a highly contagious disease, manifested by a diphasic fever, coryza, and later bronchitis and bronchopneumonia, severe gastroenteritis, and nervous signs. It also occurs in wolves, foxes, coyotes, dingoes, raccoons, ferrets, and mink. The agent is in the paramyxovirus group and crosses antigenically with rinderpest and measles virus (see *vaccine*). It invades the brain, causing demyelination and inflammation. The condition is important in studies of the viral encephalitides because of the possibility that there may be involved a combination of immunologic mechanisms and direct invasion of the central nervous system by the viral agent. Also the phenomenon of giant cell formation may be of great biological significance.[142] See *giant cell pneumonia* and *heterokaryon*.

canine herpesvirus infection A fatal disease of very young puppies, caused by a member of the herpes group of viruses and in which characteristic intranuclear inclusion bodies can be seen in the liver, kidney, and lung tissues. The virus has been cultivated in dog kidney cells.[16]

canine papillomatosis See *papilloma*.

canine venereal tumor See *venereal tumor*.

Canis familiaris The domestic dog.

canker (of pigeons) See *trichomoniasis*.

cannabis The dried flowering tops of the hemp plant, *Cannabis sativa*, known popularly as marihuana, hashish, and bhang.

Cap-Chur gun Trademark for an air rifle that fires an automatic syringe and is commonly used to inject wild or captive animals in the heavy muscles of the rump or shoulder. It is effective up to about 40 yards. Various drugs may be used to sedate or immobilize animals, including succinylcholine chloride, nicotine, and gallamine (see *anesthesia*).

Capillaria A genus of nematodes parasitic in mammals and birds. C *hepatica* usually infests the liver of rodents. C. *aerophila* is found in the lungs of foxes, C. *annulata* in the esophagus and crop of turkeys, chickens, and other wild birds. C. *plica* appears in the kidneys and urinary bladder of dogs and foxes. C. *bursata* and C. *caudinflata* are important parasites of the small intestine of chickens and other birds. C. *columbae* inhabits the small intestine of pigeons. C. *brevites* and C. *bovis* are parasitic for cattle and

sheep, and C. *linearis* has been found in the intestines of cats.[21]

capon A castrated domestic chicken.

Capra hircus The domestic goat.

caprimulgiform birds Members of the avian order Caprimulgiformes, which includes the nighjars, nighthawks, and goatsuckers; they are long-winged nonpasserine birds that fly at twilight.

capsid The protein coat that surrounds the nucleic acid of a virus.

capsomere A cluster of structure units (q.v.) in the capsid of a virus.

capsule In insect virology, the protein material surrounding the granulosis-virus rod. The "granule" is the inclusion body characteristic of the virus infection known as granulosis, produced in the infected tissue cells.

capuchin monkey A member of the genus *Cebus*. See *primate*.

capybara (carpincho) A large rodent member of the family Caviidae, genus *Hydrochoers*. There are two species: H. *isthmius*, which weighs about 65 lb. and is found in Panama, and H. *drochacris*, which weighs up to 100 lb. and originates to the east of the South American Andes. It is semiaquatic and has partially webbed toes, hooflike nails, sparse hair, and cleft upper lip. It feeds on plants and sometimes grains, melons, and squashes.

carapace The exoskeleton covering the dorsal surface of an animal, as a turtle.

O-carbamyl-D-serine An antibiotic isolated from a strain of *Streptomyces* that interferes with the synthesis of bacterial cell wall. See *D-cycloserine*.[36, 49]

carbol crystal violet A basic triphenyl dye that has three methylated amino groups, contains carbolic acid, and is used to stain fibrin in blood smears.[57, 153]

carbomycin See *macrolide*.

carbon dioxide sensitivity A disease of adult fruit flies (*Drosophila*), caused by sigma virus (q.v.). The presence of sigma virus in a fly is not harmful so long as the insect is not exposed to pure carbon dioxide. However, even a very brief contact with pure carbon dioxide gas is lethal to infected (sensitive) flies. The virus is transmitted to the offspring by the gametes of one or both parents, especially the female.

carboxyl The radical, or group, —COOH, occurring in nearly all organic acids.

carboxylase (pyruvic decarboxylase) An enzyme of the Embden-Meyerhof pathway that catalyzes the conversion of pyruvate to oxalacetate. Acetyl coenzyme A, thiamine pyrophosphate, and Mg^{++} are co-factors.

carboxylesterase An enzyme that catalyzes the hydrolysis of the esters of carboxylic acids.

carboxypeptidase An exopeptidase that acts on the peptide bond of terminal amino acids possessing a free carboxyl group.

carcinoid A yellow circumscribed tumor occurring in the small intestine, appendix, stomach, or colon.

carcinoma   A malignant new growth made up of epithelial cells tending to infiltrate the surrounding tissues and give rise to metastases. See also table accompanying *neoplasm.*

Bashford c. 63 (tumor No. 63; carcinoma 63 of Bashford), an undifferentiated carcinoma that arose spontaneously in the mammary gland of a non-inbred mouse in the laboratory of E. F. Bashford, of the Imperial Cancer Research Fund, London, in 1907. The tumor grows progressively in 100 per cent of non-inbred mouse hosts, killing them in 28 to 42 days. It is transplanted at 10 to 14 day intervals.[150]

epidermoid c., a malignant neoplasm derived from the epidermis and seen in the skin, mouth, esophagus, lung, rumen, urinary tract, and other epithelial surfaces. In anomen, one of the commonest forms is "cancer eye" of Hereford cattle, which occurs as an invasive carcinoma in the nonpigmented portion of the eyelid or conjunctiva. Its incidence is much greater at high altitudes or in regions that have many days of sunlight, as in southwestern United States. It is believed to be related to exposure to solar radiation.

gastric c. 342, originally, a carcinosarcoma of the gastric wall induced in a three-month-old rat by the injection of 20-methylcholanthrene, in the laboratory of H. L. Stewart at the National Cancer Institute in 1949. The tumor lost its sarcomatous elements by the fourth transplant generation and is now considered to be a carcinoma. It grows subcutaneously, without metastases, in 100 per cent of rat hosts, killing the animals in about 90 days.[150]

c. No. 1 (canine carcinoma No. 1), a tumor that arose spontaneously in a five and a half year old Boxer dog presented to M. Allam and his associates at the University of Pennsylvania School of Veterinary Medicine in 1954. It was located in the ventral cervical region and has been classified as a thyroid carcinoma. Transplantation of this tumor requires a state of immunologic incompetency induced by whole body x-irradiation of puppy recipients. Steroid therapy and nitrogen mustard administration are insufficient preparation for this purpose in approximately 50 per cent of cases (about the same as in untreated puppies). This tumor is one of the few transplantable tumors of large animals.[150]

pulmonary c., a malignant epithelial neoplasm of the lung. In anomen, adenocarcinomata of the bronchiolar-alveolar epithelium are more common than squamous cell (bronchogenic) carcinoma, which is commonest in man. Some strains of mice show a high incidence of pulmonary adenoma.[142] See also *pulmonary adenomatosis*, under *adenomatosis.*

V2 c. (VX2 carcinoma), an anaplastic carcinoma developed as a result of malignant transformation in the cells of a Shope papilloma carried by a rabbit of the genus *Orycto-lagus.* Observed originally by Kidd and Rous in a Dutch belted male rabbit that had been infected with Shope papilloma virus some nine to eleven months previously, the carcinomas arising at three of the infection sites were experimentally propagated in other Dutch belted rabbits, and have since been transmitted to domestic rabbits of many breeds.

These same investigators found an antibody response capable of neutralizing Shope papilloma virus in vitro in the serum of every rabbit in which the transplanted tumor grew. They further found that antigenic components of the virus were detectable for at least the first 22 transplant generations (a period of years) of the V2 carcinoma. Tests for antibody were discontinued during the period 1942 to 1946. When the carcinoma was in its forty-sixth transplant generation (1946), it was found that the carcinoma was no longer able to induce antibody against the Shope papilloma virus, although it was morphologically indistinguishable from the earlier generations. It has not been determined whether the virus still persists in the carcinoma in an antigenically incomplete or masked form. The carcinoma is widely used in experimental oncology.[30, 150]

carcinomatosis   Carcinosis; the condition of widespread dissemination of cancer throughout the body.

carcinophobia   1. Morbid dread of becoming affected with cancer.   2. Delusion of being affected with cancer.

carcinosarcoma   A mixed tumor combining the elements of carcinoma and sarcoma.

Flexner-Jobling c. (Flexner-Jobling carcinoma; Flexner-Jobling tumor), a tumor arising spontaneously in the seminal vesicle of a white male stock rat in the laboratory of S. Flexner and J. W. Jobling at The Rockefeller University in 1906. Both Flexner and Jobling were in doubt as to the precise histologic classification of this tumor. As it stabilized after successive transplant generations, it became progressively less differentiated and is now classified as a carcinosarcoma. It grows successfully in most rat strains, beginning to grow in 100 per cent of hosts, but regressing in approximately 25 per cent. It kills the host in three to ten weeks both by invasion and by metastasis.[150]

Walker c. 256 (Walker rat tumor, Walker sarcoma 256), a spontaneous carcinosarcoma that arose in the region of the mammary gland of an albino rat in the laboratory of G. Walker at Johns Hopkins University in 1928. It grows progressively in most rat stocks, becoming palpable one week after subcutaneous transplantation and killing the host within six weeks. Several cellular types of Walker carcinosarcoma are recognized, among them the "carcinomatous variant" composed of sheets of principal cells, and the "sarcomatous variant" composed of interlacing bundles of spindle and stellate cells. Within any given Walker tumor 256, varying proportions of the cell types may be seen, with an increase in the sarcomatous variant as the tumor ages. This process has been termed "healing."[150]

carinate Keel-shaped, or in the case of birds, having a keel-shaped process on the breast bone.

carnassial teeth The shearing last upper premolar and first lower molar teeth of members of Carnivora.

carnivorean lethargy See *torpor.*

carnivorous Flesh-eating.

carotene See *lipochrome.*

carotenism In birds, an abnormality of carotenoid pigmentation that may result from changes in normal distribution of carotenoid pigments, an increase in amount or change in color of the pigment, or from replacement of melanin by carotenoid pigments in an area that is normally melanic. See also *leucism* and *schizochroism.*[112]

carotenoid leucism See *leucism.*

carotenosis Yellowish discoloration, especially of adipose tissues, due to consumption of carotene pigments, which are precursors of vitamin A. The condition is normal in the horse and in certain breeds of cattle. Common sources of carotene pigments are carrots, sweet potatoes, leafy vegetables, milk fat, body fat, and egg yolk.

carp pox See *fishpox.*

Carre's disease See *canine distemper.*

Carrion's disease Bartonellosis, an infectious disease occurring in the valleys of the Andes Mountains in Peru, Chile, Bolivia, and Columbia. It appears in an acute febrile anemic stage (Oroya fever) followed in several weeks by a nodular skin eruption (verruga peruana). It is caused by *Bartonella bacilliformis*, which is transmitted by the sandfly, *Phlebotomus verrucarum.*

cartilaginous fishes (elasmobranchs) Members of the chordate class Chondrichthyes (Elasmobranchii). The sharks, rays, and chimeras are the lowest living vertebrates with complete and separate vertebrae, movable jaws, and paired appendages. All are predaceous and most are marine. The shark is of major biological interest because some of its basic anatomical features appear in early embryos of the higher vertebrates. The skin is tough, covered with minute placoid scales, and contains many mucous glands. Fins are both median and paired, pelvic fins having claspers in males. The mouth is ventral with many enamel-capped teeth. The skeleton is cartilaginous, and the notochord persistent. The heart is two-chambered (atrium and ventricle) with sinus venosus and conus arteriosus. Erythrocytes are oval and nucleated. There are ten pairs of cranial nerves.

The cartilaginous fishes are higher than the cyclostomes in having a scale-covered body, two pairs of lateral fins, movable jaws, three semicircular canals in each ear, and paired reproductive organs and ducts. They are lower than bony fishes in having a cartilaginous skeleton without bone, placoid scales, separate gill clefts, and no air blad-

der. The living elasmobranchs include the order Selachii, composed of the suborder Squali (the sharks) and suborder Batoidea (the rays, skates, and devilfish); and the order Holocephali (the chimeras).

caryo- See *karyo-.*

casease A proteolytic enzyme derived from bacterial cultures, which hydrolyzes albumin and the casein of milk and cheese.

casque An enlargement of the dorsal surface of the upper bill of a bird.

cassowary See *casuariiform birds.*

castrate To remove or destroy the testes or ovaries.

casuariiform birds Members of the avian order Casuariiformes, comprising the cassowary and emu. They are large flightless birds, having small wings and heavy legs with three toes.

cata- A prefix signifying down, lower, under, against, along with, very.

catalysis Change in the velocity of a chemical reaction produced by the presence of a substance (a catalyst) that does not form part of the final product.

catecholamine One of a group of similar compounds having a sympathomimetic action, the aromatic portion of whose molecule is catechol, and the aliphatic portion an amine. Such compounds include dopamine, norepinephrine, and epinephrine.

cathepsin A proteolytic enzyme contained in lysosomes (q.v.).

cat-scratch disease (cat-scratch fever; nonbacterial regional lymphadenitis) An ulceroglandular disease of man, probably caused by an organism of the psittacosis-lymphogranuloma group (*Chlamydia*) although this is disputed. The organism has never been isolated, but the cat appears to be the mechanical carrier of the infectious agent. Rodents may also be a source of infection.[16, 156]

cauliflower disease Soft papillomatous neoplasms of the mouth and head of European eels, *Anguilla vulgaris.* Histologically the lesion is a fibroepithelioma, superficially resembling cauliflower, without inclusions. It has not been experimentally transmitted.[114]

Cavia A genus of rodents including the guinea pig, or cavy.

cavy Guinea pig.

Celebes black ape A member of the species *Cynopithecus niger.* See *primate.*

celestin blue A basic quinone dye. Solubility at 15° C.: water 2 per cent, absolute alcohol 15 per cent, and glycerol 8 per cent. It is used to demonstrate acid mucopolysaccharides, to stain nuclei acids, and as a counterstain in diazo coupling method for N-acetyl-β-glucoaminidase.[57, 153]

cell Any of the minute structures which are the living units of all plants and animals and which make up organized tissues in multicelled organisms. They consist of a circumscribed mass of cytoplasm containing a nucleus and surrounded by a plasma membrane and sometimes additional layers such as cell wall and capsule. In some of the low forms of life, such as bacteria, a morphological nucleus is absent, although nucleoproteins and a functioning genome are present.[38]

cell cycle　See *synthesis,* under *deoxyribonucleic acid.*

cellulase　An enzyme that hydrolyzes cellulose to cellobiose. It is secreted by certain bacteria and fungi which destroy wood.

ceno-　A combining form meaning (1) new or (2) empty or (3) denoting relationship to a common feature or characteristic.

cenophobia　Morbid dread of large open spaces.

cenotophobia　Fear of novelty; neophobia.

centi-　A combining form denoting relationship to 100; usually used in naming units of measurement to indicate one-hundredth (10^{-2}) of the unit designated by the root with which it is combined.

centipede (hundred-legged worm)　An arthropod of the subphylum Mandibulata, class Mryriapoda, subclass Chilopoda. Centipedes are slender, elongate, segmented, and flattened dorsoventrally. The first somite bears a pair of four-jointed poison claws. Each of the remaining 14 to 172 somites, depending on the species, bears a pair of seven-jointed walking legs. Their prey, usually an insect, is killed or immobilized by poison ducted from glands into the poison claws. When man is "bitten," it is usually as a result of defensive or accidental action. The venom may be a direct toxin and/or an allergen. Examples are the giant desert centipede, *Scolopendra heros,* and the southern centipede, *S. viridis.*

central lymphoid tissue　Lymphoid tissue that develops in close association with the digestive tract; it includes the thymus, bursa of Fabricius, the appendix, tonsils, Peyer's patches, and the sacculus rotundus. The immunological role of these tissues varies greatly between species, but in general the thymus is closely related to cellular immunity, while other central lymphoid tissues are more important to humoral antibody production.[48, 93]

centrifugation　The process of separating the lighter portions of a solution, mixture, or suspension from the heavier portions by centrifugal force.

　density gradient c., any of several methods of separating molecules or particles of distinct but similar size, shape and specific gravity. A gradient, frequently of sucrose or cesium chloride, is formed in a tube with the greatest density at the bottom. The material to be separated is layered over the top of the gradient and after centrifugation, samples can be removed at different levels, each of which contains a separate population of material depending on its buoyant density.

　equilibrium density gradient c., a method in which the specimen is spun for several days, and forms a band in the area where the density of the specimen and the solution are equal. This effect is unrelated to size or shape of the particle.

　rate zonal density gradient c., a method

of analysis employed in determining the physical properties of viruses, subcellular particles, and macromolecules. This method utilizes an inert solute or density gradient such as sucrose or cesium chloride. The sample is layered at the top of the gradient and spun down with the ultracentrifuge to separate the components of the sample, based on their sedimentation constants, which are a function of particle size, shape, and density.[32, 64]

centro-　A combining form indicating relationship to a center, or to a central location.

centromere　The region where the arms of a chromosome meet.

cephalo-　A combining form denoting relationship to the head.

cephalodymus　A twin monstrosity with a single or united head.

cephalopod　See *mollusk.*

cephalosporin　A group of antibiotic substances first isolated from a species of *Cephalosporium,* which act by interference with cell wall synthesis in a manner similar to that of penicillin. Derivatives of cephalosporin exhibit considerable activity against both gram-positive and gram-negative microorganisms, perhaps because of their great ability to penetrate to the bacterial cell wall.[34, 49]

cephalothoracopagus　A double monster consisting of two similar components united in the frontal plane, the fusion extending from the crown of the head to the middle abdominal region.

cercarial dermatitis　Swimmer's itch.

cercus　A jointed process arising on the abdomen of some invertebrates.

cere　Fleshy protuberance over the upper part of the bill of some birds. Especially in budgerigars the cere is sexually dimorphic, being pigmented in mature males and dull brownish in the young of both sexes and the mature female. See also *brown hypertrophy of the cere.*

cerebrospinal nematodiasis　See under *nematodiasis.*

Cestoda　A class of Platyhelminthes comprising the tapeworms (q.v.), or cestodes, which have a head or scolex and segments or proglottids. See table.

cestode　Any member of the class Cestoda.

cestodiasis　Infestation by flatworms of class Cestoda (tapeworms) common in most vertebrate animals, including man. Transmission of these worms to man from infected meat of swine and cattle comprises an important public health hazard. See table of common cestode parasites, see *zoonosis* (Addendum II), and *echinococcosis.*

cetacean　Any member of the mammalian order Cetacea. The order is comprised of two suborders, the Mysticeti, or baleen whales, and the Odontoceti, or toothed whales. The baleen consists of rows of horny plates that depend from the roof of the mouth; it is used to strain the food (various small marine flora and fauna collectively called krill) from the sea water. The Mysticeti embrace about

Cestode	Definitive Host	Intermediate Host	Main Characteristics
Pseudophyllidea			
Dibothriocephalus latus (=*Diphyllobothrium latum*)	Man, dog, cat, mink, bear, other fish-eating mammals	Fish	Extremely large; 3-10 meters long; consisting of 3000 or more proglottids; scolex 2.5 mm. long; 1 mm. wide; eggs 70μ by 45μ, operculate
Diplogonoporus grandis	Normally a parasite of whales, occasionally in man	– – –	1.4-5.9 meters long; two sets of reproductive organs per proglottid; eggs 63-68μ by 50μ, operculate
Spirometra erinaceieuropaei	Dog, cat, man	– – –	85-100 cm. long; multiple testes larger than those of *D. latus*; vitellaria numerous; eggs 57-60μ by 33-37μ, operculate
S. mansonoides	Dog, cat (usually bobcat)	Cyclops, mouse	Rarely over 1 meter long; scolex 200-500μ wide; bothria shallow; cirrus and vagina open independently on ventral surface; eggs 65μ by 37μ, operculate
Ligula intestinalis	Fish-eating birds, occasionally man	Fish	Specimens found in humans small, less than 80 cm. long
Cyclophyllidea (Anoplocephalidae)			
Bertiella studeri	Monkey, ape, man	– – –	275-300 mm. long; 10 mm. wide; scolex subglobose, set off from strobila; eggs irregular in outline, 45-46μ by 50μ, nonoperculate
Anoplocephala magna	Horse	Oribatid mite	350-800 mm. long; 20-50 mm. wide; 400-500 testes per mature proglottid; eggs 50-60μ in diameter, nonoperculate
A. perfoliata	Horse	Oribatid mite	10-80 mm. long, 10-20 mm. wide, scolex 2-3 mm. in diameter with lappet behind each sucker
Paranoplocephala mamillana	Horse	Oribatid mite	6-50 mm. long; 4-6 mm. wide; suckers slitlike; eggs 50-88μ in diameter, nonoperculate
Moniezia expansa	Sheep, goat, cow	Mite	Up to 4-5 meters long, 1 cm. wide; two sets of reproductive organs per proglottid; proglottid much wider than long; 100-400 testes per segment; eggs 50-60μ in diameter, nonoperculate
M. benedeni	Sheep, goat, cattle	Mite	Up to 4 meters long, larger scolex than *M. expansa*
Thysanosoma actinioides	Sheep, cattle	Oribatid mite	150-300 mm. long; large and prominent suckers; proglottids broader than long with fringe along posterior margin; two sets of reproductive organs per proglottid; eggs expelled in capsules; each egg 19.25μ to 26.95μ in diameter, nonoperculate
Aporina delafondi	Pigeon	– – –	70-160 mm. long, no rostellum, genital pore irregularly alternate, 100 testes per proglottid
Taeniidae			
Taenia solium	Man	Pig	Up to 2-7 meters long; scolex quadrate with diameter of 1 mm.; rostellum armed with double row of hooks; eggs 31-43μ in diameter, nonoperculate
(*Cysticercus cellulosae*)	Various animals, including man	Rat, mouse, rabbit	Ovoid, whitish, 6-18 mm. long
Taenia taeniaformis	Cat, dog, man	– – –	15-60 cm. long, 5-6 cm. wide, armed rostellum, double row of usually 34 hooks
(*Cysticercus crassicollis*)	Rat	– – –	– – –

(Table continues)

*Adapted from T. C. Cheng: The Biology of Animal Parasites. W. B. Saunders Co., Philadelphia, 1964.

CESTODE	DEFINITIVE HOST	INTERMEDIATE HOST	MAIN CHARACTERISTICS
Taeniidae – Cont'd			
Taenia hydatigena	Dog	Ruminants	Up to 5 meters long, 4-7 cm. wide, scolex armed with double row of 26-44 hooks, 600-700 testes per segment, gravid uterus with 5-10 lateral branches
T. ovis	Dog, fox, wolf	Sheep	Approximately 1 meter long, scolex armed with two rows of 24-36 hooks, 300 testes per proglottid, gravid uterus with 20-25 lateral branches
T. tenuicollis	Dog, cat, fox, mink	Sheep	Up to 70 mm. long, large suckers, 237-303μ in diameter, two rows totaling 48 hooks, eggs 17-20μ in diameter
T. pisiformis	Dog, cat, rabbit, fox, wolf	Rabbit, squirrel	500 mm. long; 5 mm. wide; scolex with double row of 34-48 hooks; genital pores alternate irregularly; gravid uterus with 8-14 branches; eggs 36-40μ long, 31-36μ wide, nonoperculated
Taeniarhynchus saginatus	Man	Cow	10-12 meters long, no rostellum, unarmed, 1000-2000 proglottids, eggs similar to those of *T. solium*
Multiceps multiceps	Dog, fox, coyote, man	Sheep, goat	Up to 1 meter long, 5 mm. wide, scolex armed with double row of 22-32 hooks, approximately 200 testes per proglottid, gravid uterus with 9-26 lateral branches, eggs 31-36μ in diameter
M. serialis	Dog, occasionally man	Rabbit	70 cm. long, 3-5 cm. wide, rostellum with double row of 26-32 hooks, gravid uterus with 20-25 lateral branches
Echinococcus granulosus	Man, dog, fox	Man, cow, swine, sheep, etc.	Hydatid cysts with thick two-layered wall, filled with fluid (adult morphology given in text)
Hymenolepididae			
Hymenolepis nana	Rat, mouse, man	– – –	25-40 mm. long, 1 mm. wide, short rostellum with 20-30 hooks in one ring, three testes, eggs 30-47 mm. in diameter
H. diminuta	Rat, mouse, man, dog	Arthropods	200-600 mm. long, 1-4 mm. wide, rostellum unarmed, eggs 60-80μ by 72-86μ
H. carioca	Chicken, turkey	Beetles	300-800 mm. long, 500-700μ wide, rostellum unarmed
H. cantaniana	Chicken, turkey, quail	– – –	2-12 mm. long, rostellum shorter than that of *H. carioca*, otherwise the two species are similar
Fimbriaria fasciolaris	Chicken, duck, pigeon	– – –	14-85 mm. long, with pseudoscolex
Dilepididae			
Dipylidium caninum	Dog, cat, fox, occasionally man	Flea, louse	15-70 cm. long, 3 mm. wide, conical rostellum, armed with 30-150 hooks, 200 testes per proglottid, eggs in capsules, each egg 35-60μ in diameter
Choanotaenia infundibulum	Chicken, turkey, pheasant	Beetles	Up to 20 cm. long, 1-2 mm. wide, posterior proglottids much wider than anterior ones, rostellum with single row of 16-20 hooks
Amoebotaenia sphenoides	Chicken, turkey	Earthworm	2-4 mm. long, entire worm roughly triangular in shape, rostellum with single row of 12-14 hooks, uterus lobed
Metroliasthes lucida	Turkey	Grasshopper	Up to 20 mm. long, 1.5 mm. wide, scolex unarmed, uterus as two simple round sacs

COMMON CESTODE PARASITES (*Continued*)

CESTODE	DEFINITIVE Host	INTERMEDIATE Host	MAIN CHARACTERISTICS
Davaineidae *Raillietina cesticillus*	Chicken, pheasant	Beetles	100-130 mm. long, 1.5-3 mm. wide, scolex broad and flat and about 100μ in diameter, rostellum armed with double row of 400-500 hooks
R. tetragona	Chicken, turkey	Ants	Up to 250 mm. long, 1-4 mm. wide, rostellum with double row of 90-130 hooks, suckers armed with 8-12 rows of hooklets, 6-12 eggs in single capsule
R. echinobothrida	Chicken, turkey	Ants	Up to 250 mm. long, 1-4 mm. wide, rostellum with double row of 200-250 hooks, suckers with 8-15 rows of hooklets
R. salmoni	Rabbit	– – –	85 mm. long, 3 mm. wide, retractile rostellum with double row of hooks
R. retractilis	Rabbit	– – –	35-105 mm. long, 3 mm. wide, short neck, rostellum with two rows of hooks, genital pore unilateral
Davainea proglottina	Chicken	Snail	Up to 4 mm. long, usually only 2-5 proglottids, rostellum with 66-100 small hooks, one egg per capsule
D. meleagridis	Turkey	– – –	Up to 5 mm. long, composed of 17-22 proglottids, rostellum with double row of 100-150 hooks, suckers armed with 4-6 rows of hooklets
Mesocestoididae *Mesocestoides latus*	Cat, skunk, raccoon	– – –	12-30 cm. long, 2 mm. wide, scolex unarmed, vitellaria bilobed in posterior region of proglottid
M. lineatus	Dog	– – –	30 cm. to 2 meters long, genital atrium midventral

a dozen species, none prominent in research. The odontocetes, rather than subsisting on krill, consume chiefly fish and squid. The Odontoceti is composed of about 70 species, including the toothed whales, porpoises, and dolphins. The term dolphin is used in the European literature in equivalence to the English and American term porpoise. Of the approximately 40 species of porpoises, the Atlantic bottlenose, *Tursiops truncatus*, is the most prominent research cetacean.[45c]

Chagas' disease Trypanosomiasis of man, mainly children, caused by *Trypanosoma cruzi* and widely distributed in South America, Central America, and Mexico. Cats, dogs, opossums, monkeys, armadillos, bats, foxes, squirrels, and wood rats are considered to be reservoir hosts.[159]

chalcomycin An antibiotic produced by species of *Streptomyces* that is active against certain gram-positive bacteria but relatively inactive against gram-negative organisms and fungi. It inhibits protein synthesis.[36, 49]

chalk brood A disease of larval honeybees, caused by the fungus *Ascosphaera apis*. Infected larvae usually die within the first two days after their cells have been sealed. The cadavers dry up to a hard, shrunken, chalk-like lump. Under suitable conditions, fungal fruiting bodies and spores form at the surface of the larval remains.

charadriiform birds Members of the avian order Charadriiformes, a group of shorebirds that includes the snipes, plovers, gulls, terns, the sandpiper, the phalarope, and the auk.[154]

Chastek's paralysis Thiamine deficiency of foxes caused by enzymatic destruction of the vitamin by thiaminase in raw fish.

Chediak-Higashi syndrome (Steinbrinck syndrome) An inherited defect of cytoplasmic granule formation involving the lysosomes and perhaps other cellular organelles, first seen as giant granules in peripheral blood leukocytes. Affected individuals have poor ability to defend themselves against bacterial infections. Because melanin granules are abnormally dispersed, resulting in dilution of color, the term partial albinism has been used, but the disorder is not a truly defective synthesis of melanin. It affects man, mink, cow, and mouse.[44, 70] See also *Aleutian mink*.

cheek teeth Premolar and molar teeth.

chelate To combine with a metal in weakly

dissociated complexes in which the metal is part of a ring. By extension, applied to a chemical compound in which a metallic ion is sequestered and firmly bound into a ring within the chelating molecule.

chemotaxis   The movement of an organism or cell in response to a chemical concentration gradient.

    negative c., movement of an organism or cell from a region of high concentration to a region of low concentration of a specific chemical compound or element.

    positive c., movement of an organism or cell from a region of low concentration to a region of high concentration of a specific chemical compound or element.

Cheyne-Stokes psychosis   See under *psychosis.*

Cheyne-Stokes respiration   Breathing characterized by rhythmic waxing and waning of the depth of respiration, with regularly recurring periods of apnea.

chemotherapy   The treatment of disease by chemical agents.

    cancer c., see *antimetabolite.*

chicken   See *galliform birds.*

chickenpox (varicella)   An acute communicable disease, principally of young children, caused by a poxvirus, and marked by slight fever and an eruption of macular vesicles, which appear in crops and are superficial and rarely umbilicated. The disease runs a very mild course, occasionally leaving some scarring.

Chilomastix   A genus of protozoan intestinal parasites of the family Chilomastigidae. *C. mesnili* parasitizes the large intestine of man. *C. bettencourti* is found in rats and mice (see *protozoan parasites,* under *rat.*), *C. cuniculi* in rabbits, *C. intestinalis* in guinea pigs, *C. caprae* in the goat, and *C. gallinarum* in poultry.[109]

chimera   1. An individual exhibiting chimerism. 2. A cartilaginous fish (q.v.).

    mericlinal c., an organ composed of two genetically distinct tissues one of which partly surrounds the other.

chimerism   The state of being composed of cells of different chromosome number or genotype derived from more than one zygote. This may occur in utero when blood or germ cells are acquired from a twin via placental vascular anastomoses, a common occurrence in freemartins and marmosets. Fusion of early embryos or double fertilization of an egg and polar body may explain other chimeras. Recipients of nonisogeneic tissue transplants become chimeras if the grafted tissue is accepted. Cf. *mosaicism* and see *blood group chimerism.*

chimpanzee   One of the great apes. *Pan troglodytes* is the greater chimpanzee, and *P. paniscus* the lesser chimpanzee. See *ape primate.*

CHINA virus   An acronym suggested for *ch*ronic *i*nfectious *n*europathic *a*gents.[14] See *slow virus.*

chinchilla   A genus of small rodents of the family Chinchillidae. The chinchilla (*C. lani-*

ger or *brevicaudata*) inhabits the mountains of Peru, Bolivia, Chile, and Argentina. It has a slender body, with flattened large head, a broad snout, large eyes, rounded ears, and beautiful pale gray fur with dusky overtones. The Peruvian or royal chinchilla was hunted extensively for its valuable fur and is now nearly extinct. The Chilean chinchilla is raised in captivity. The Bolivian type is still fairly numerous. They are vegetarians and eat seeds, fruits, grains, herbs, and moss.

chinook salmon disease   A host-specific viral disease of hatchery-reared young chinook salmon, *Oncorhyncus tshawytscha.* Affected fish are lethargic, show exophthalmia, and darkened pigmentation. There is loss of motor stability, and hemorrhages develop dorsally behind the head, at the fin bases, and at the opercles, isthmus, and eyes. Mortality may exceed 60 per cent. The lesions consist of necrosis of kidney, liver, and pancreas, with anemia. Both nuclear and cytoplasmic inclusions have been observed. Because of the temperature dependency of the host, the mortality rate shows seasonal periodicity.[114]

chiropody   Former name for podiatry.

chiropractic   A system of therapeutics based upon the claim that disease is caused by abnormal function of the nervous system. It attempts to restore normal function by manipulation and treatment of the structures of the human body, especially those of the spinal column.

chitinase   An enzyme that hydrolyzes chitin to N-acetyl glucosamine.

Chlamydia   A group of obligate intracellular organisms (formerly known as the psittacosis-lymphogranuloma group or *Bedsonia*), which can produce minute, spherical basophilic bodies in reticuloendothelial cells. Considered evolutionary forms originating from gram-negative bacteria, they possess a cell wall containing muramic acid, and they reproduce by binary fission.[36] For a comparison of *Chlamydia* and other microscopic forms, see *microorganism. Chlamydia* causes psittacosis and ornithosis in birds and man; meningopneumonitis; mouse pneumonitis; feline pneumonitis; bovine enteritis and encephalitis (Buss disease), enzootic abortion, pneumonitis, and arthritis in sheep; and lymphogranuloma venereum, trachoma (inclusion conjunctivitis), and pneumonitis in man.

chlamydospore   Fungal spore formed from swollen, thick-walled hyphal elements.

chloramphenicol   An antibiotic produced by a species of *Streptomyces.* It was the first broad-spectrum antibiotic introduced into medical use and also the first antibiotic to be completely synthesized in the laboratory. It inhibits the growth of most bacteria and of rickettsiae and organisms of the *Chlamydia* group. Its activity is directed against protein synthesis by inhibition of peptide chain extension, rather than of the initial process of the biosynthesis of protein molecules. Its use in treatment of disease has been limited because of its ability to produce blood dyscrasia. One of these, an acute type, is dose-dependent and reversible but the other, which occurs in very low incidence, is an aplastic anemia that has a fatal outcome. The greater sensitivity of bacterial systems, as compared to mammalian cells, to inhibition by chloramphenicol is probably due to the conformation of a specific ribosomal site.[36, 49]

chlorantine fast green An acid tris-azo dye. Solubility at 15° C.: water 5.25 per cent, absolute alcohol 0.5 per cent, and glycerol 7 per cent. It may be used to destain tissues already stained with acid fuchsin and light green SF, and to stain fungal cell walls.[153]

chlorazol azurine An acid dis-azo dye. Solubility at 15° C.: water 1.5 per cent, absolute alcohol 0.1 per cent, and glycerol 4.25 per cent. It is used for herbarium specimens.[153]

chlorazol black An acid tris-azo dye. Solubility at 15° C.: water 6 per cent, absolute alcohol 0.1 per cent, and glycerol 2 per cent. It is used to stain connective tissue and the nuclei and chromosomes of plants.[37, 153]

chlorazol fast pink An acid dis-azo dye. Solubility at 15° C.: water 1.3 per cent, absolute alcohol nil, and glycerol 8 per cent. It is used to stain fungal cell walls, unmineralized bone, and tooth matrix.[153]

chlorazol paper brown An acid dis-azo dye. Solubility at 15° C.: water 4.5 per cent, absolute alcohol 1.5 per cent, and glycerol 8.5 per cent. It is used to stain plant tissue.[153]

chloro- A combining form meaning green.

chloroleukemia 123 (Shay's leukemia) A transplantable leukemia. An experiment involving the gastric instillation of 20-methyl-cholanthrene in Wistar stock rats by Shay and his colleagues at Temple University, Philadelphia, in 1951 resulted in the induction of granulocytic leukemia in three rats. It was found to be transplantable to seven-day-old suckling rats using whole blood or a brei of liver or spleen cells. In the three original leukemic animals, there were no solid tumors, but all subsequent transplant hosts developed both myelogenous leukemia and greenish solid tumors which infiltrated various tissues. The tumor may be carried in various laboratory strains of *Rattus norvegicus*, in which there is an 80 per cent success rate in injected sucklings, with a latent period of about seven weeks. Under ultraviolet light, the chloromas exhibit a red fluorescence owing to protoporphyrin, as do those of man.[150]

chloroma A malignant green tumor arising from myeloid tissue, associated with myelogenous leukemia and occurring anywhere in the body. Besides containing green pigment, which has no clear metabolic role and is principally myeloperoxidase (verdoperoxidase), chloroma tissue demonstrates a bright red fluorescence under ultraviolet light.

chlorophyll unit A group of about 2000 chlorophyll molecules that participate in the reduction of one molecule of carbon dioxide in photosynthesis.

chloroplast Any of the chlorophyll-bearing bodies of plant and animal cells.

choice point A position in a maze at which an experimental animal must make one choice exclusive of all others.

cholangiohepatoma A tumor consisting of abnormally mixed masses of liver cord cells and bile ducts.

cholanthrene A pentacyclic hydrocarbon, $C_{20}H_{14}$, of great carcinogenicity.

chole-, chol-, cholo- Combining form denoting relationship to the bile.

cholecystokinase An enzyme in the blood that catalyzes the decomposition of cholecystokinin.

choleophosphatase An enzyme in the pancreas and in intestinal secretions that liberates choline from lecithin.

cholera See *hog cholera.*

cholerase An enzyme developed by the spirillum of cholera and capable of destroying it.

cholesterol A fatlike, pearly substance, a monatomical alcohol, $C_{27}H_{45}OH$, crystallizing in the form of acicular crystals, and found in all animal fats and oils, in bile, blood, brain tissue, milk, yolk of egg, the medullated sheaths of nerve fibers, the liver, kidneys, and adrenal glands. It constitutes a large part of the most frequently occurring type of gallstones, and occurs in atheromatous lesions of the arteries. High blood cholesterol levels are thought to be of pathogenetic importance in atherosclerosis (q.v.).

choline dehydrogenase (choline oxidase) A pyridine nucleotide enzyme that catalyzes the dehydrogenation of choline, utilizing NAD as a co-enzyme.

chondrioid Mesosome.

chondro-, chondr- Combining form denoting a relationship to cartilage.

chondroadenoma An adenoma containing cartilaginous elements.

chondroangioma An angioma containing cartilaginous elements.

chondroblastoma A tumor the cells of which tend to differentiate into cartilage cells. The term includes chondroma and chondrosarcoma.

chondrocarcinoma A carcinoma containing cartilaginous elements in its stroma.

chondrodystrophy Achondroplasia.

chondroma A hyperplastic growth of cartilage tissue.

chondromyxoma Myxoma containing cartilaginous and mucous elements.

chondrosarcoma Sarcoma with cartilaginous elements; a cartilaginous tumor characterized by rapidity of growth.

Chordata A phylum of animals comprising five subphyla, all having the following features in common (at least in embryonic life; many features are altered or absent in adult forms): bilateral symmetry, three germ layers, a segmented body, complete digestive tract, and well developed coelom. Three char-

Major Divisions of the Phylum Chordata

Subphylum	Class	Common Name
Hemichordata	1. Enteropneusta	Tongue worms
	2. Pterobranchia	– – –
	3. Graptozoa	Graptolites
Tunicata	1. Larvacea	– – –
	2. Ascidiacea	Ascidians
	3. Thaliacea	Chain tunicates
Cephalochordata	1. Leptocardii	Lancelets
Agnatha	1. Ostracodermi	Ancient armored fishes
	2. Cyclostomata	Cyclostomes, e.g., lampreys
Gnathostoma	Pisces (Superclass)	
	1. Placodermi	Ancient fishes
	2. Chondrichthyes	Sharks and rays
	3. Osteichthyes	Bony fishes
	Tetrapoda (Superclass)	
	1. Amphibia	Amphibians
	2. Reptilia	Reptiles
	3. Aves	Birds
	4. Mammalia	Mammals

acteristics distinguish them from all other animals: a single dorsal tubular nerve cord, a notochord, and pharyngeal pouches or gill slits. The subphyla and their classes are listed in the accompanying table.

chordate Any member of the phylum Chordata.

chordo- A combining form denoting relationship to a cord.

chordoblastoma A tumor the cells of which tend to differentiate into cells like those of the notochord.

chordoma A malignant tumor arising from the embryonic remains of the notochord.

chorio- A combining form denoting relationship to the chorion.

chorioadenoma Adenomatous tumor of the chorion; destructive placental mole; called also *c. destruens, invasive mole*, and *malignant mole*.

choriocarcinoma Carcinoma developing from the chorionic epithelium.

chorioepithelioma Chorionic carcinoma; a tumor formed by malignant proliferation of the epithelium of the chorionic villi and including chorioadenoma, choriosarcoma, choriocarcinoma, and syncytioma.

choreomania Dancing mania.

Christmas disease See *hemophilia*.

chromaffinoma Any tumor containing chromaffin cells.

chromargentaffin Staining with chromium salts and impregnable with silver; said of certain cells of the mucous membrane of the intestinal tract.

chromatin A portion of nucleus that can be readily stained, forms a network of nuclear fibrils, and is composed of DNA combined with a protein. It is the carrier of inheritance genes.

chromatography Any of several methods of separating mixtures of chemical materials by taking advantage of the fact that they migrate through certain substances at slightly different rates. Some of the methods are paper c., column c., thin layer c., and gas c.

    column c., an ion-exchange method used for the fractionation of proteins and based on the electrostatic binding of proteins to a cellulose resin suspended in buffer and packed into a column. Diethylaminoethyl (DEAE) cellulose is commonly used as the anion exchanger and carboxymethyl (CM) as the cation exchanger. Elution of the absorbed proteins is accomplished by either changing the pH of the buffer or increasing its molarity. This technique is useful for the preparation of pure IgG and to separate immunoglobulin fragments.[32]

    exclusion c., see *gel filtrations*.

chromatoidal body A cytoplasmic inclusion that stains like chromatin and is found in certain amebae.

chromatophobia Morbid aversion to certain colors.

chromic acid-Schiff reaction A staining technic employed to demonstrate polysaccharides in tissue sections which have a high content of 1,2-glycol groups, mainly glycogen. Colloid material of the pituitary and thyroid glands can also be stained.[153] Cf. *periodic acid-Schiff reaction*.

chromo-, chrom-, chromato- Combining form denoting relationship to color.

chromogen Any substance which may give origin to a coloring matter.

chromomycin One of a group of antibiotic substances—which also includes olivomycin and mithramycin—that possess anticancer and antibacterial properties. All three act by inhibition of the synthesis of RNA in bacterial and animal cells.[36, 49]

chromosomal aberration Any abnormality in structure or number of chromosomes. They occur in many species. Some are associated with specific disease syndromes, such as neoplasms; some are lethal and detected only in embryos or fetuses; others are associated with mental retardation; still others are related to chemical or physical damage to somatic cells.[6, 65, 67, 84, 142] Some of the terminology used to describe such aberrations is as follows:

    heteroploidy: possession of a complement

of chromosome number other than the normal or euploid number

aneuploidy: duplication or loss of only certain chromosomes, as in *monosomy,* the loss of one entire autosome

trisomy: gain of one entire autosome, as in Down's syndrome (mongolism) in man

polyploidy: duplication of complete extra sets of chromosomes, as in *tetraploidy,* the presence of four sets of autosomes and four sex chromosomes

deletion: loss of a portion of a chromosome from a cell

inversion: rearrangement of genetic material within a chromosome without loss or gain

translocation: rearrangement of genetic material between nonhomologous chromosomes

chimerism: see *chimerism*

mosaicism: see *mosaicism,* and see below.

sex c. a., aberrations involving only the sex chromosomes; among the most commonly diagnosed aberrations, probably because they are the most easily recognized, are:

Turner's syndrome: absence of one X chromosome in the female (XO); seen in many species, and results in infertility except in the mouse. In the meadow vole it is the normal female state.

Klinefelter's syndrome: presence of extra X chromosomes in the male (XXY, XXXY, XXXXY, etc.). Male tortoiseshell (calico) cat is the counterpart of the condition in man. Results in infertility.

XYY syndrome: presence of an extra Y chromosome in the male. Seen in man and mouse; results in infertility in the mouse.

XXX syndrome: presence of an extra X chromosome in the female. Those affected may be fertile, but to a reduced degree.

Mosaicism is commonly seen in animals having chromosomal aberrations, especially when the sex chromosomes are involved. Such manifestations of chromosomal aberrations as infertility, depend upon the type of aberration, the presence of mosaic cells along with normal cells, and the distribution of abnormal cells within the tissues, as well as which chromosome is abnormal. See *mosaicism.*

chromosome Any of the small dark staining bodies located in cell nuclei, composed of DNA and basic proteins and which result from condensation of the nuclear chromatin of cells at the time of mitosis or meiosis. They contain the genes or hereditary factors. The number of chromosomes is usually constant for each species.[6, 31, 65, 75, 121] (See table on page 52.)

Autosomes are those chromosomes present as paired elements in all normal animals of a species, excluding the sex chromosomes.

Sex chromosomes are those chromosomes present in different forms in males and females of a species. They carry information for development of the reproductive system

(male or female), in addition to many other factors. The heterogametic sex has two morphologically unlike sex chromosomes, while the homogametic sex has two morphologically identical sex chromosomes. When the male of a species is heterogametic, the male sex chromosomes are designated as X and Y chromosomes, the female sex chromosomes as X and X; this is the situation in almost all mammals. When the female is heterogametic, the female sex chromosomes are designated as Z and W chromosomes, the male sex chromosomes as Z and Z; this is the case in birds and some reptiles. In a few species of marsupials and artiodactyls in which the male is heterogametic but has one more chromosome than the female, the sex chromosomes of the male are designated as X, Y_1, and Y_2. In such cases, the X and Y chromosomes probably represent sex chromosomes combined with autosomes by translocation.

lampbrush c., a type of chromosome found in the oocytes of many vertebrates and invertebrates during the diplotene stage of the first meiotic division and in spermatocyte nuclei of *Drosophila.* They are thickened in appearance because of distended loops of DNA extending from their surface. They probably indicate active sites of DNA-dependent RNA production.[31, 75, 121]

late-replicating X c., in mammalian cells, only one X chromosome is believed to be functional during interphase and cannot be visually identified. Additional X chromosomes, if present, form condensed masses known as Barr bodies and are nonfunctional. Such chromosomes complete replication later than the functional X and the autosomes. See *Barr body, Lyon hypothesis,* and *drumstick.*

Philadelphia c., an abnormal chromosome found in human patients suffering from chronic granulocytic leukemia.

sex c., See *chromosome.*

chromosome bridge A dicentric chromosome that bridges between the diverging chromosomes in anaphase because its two centromeres are moving toward opposite poles.

chromosome diminution (chromosome elimination) The deletion of certain chromosomes from somatic cells but with retention in germ cells, as in *Parascaris equorum.*

chromotrope Any of a group of acid dyes capable of altering the color of a metachromatic dye.

chronic Persisting over a long period of time, as opposed to acute.

chronic bee paralysis See *chronic paralysis,* under *paralysis.*

chronic respiratory disease See under *respiratory disease.*

chrono- A combining form denoting relationship to time.

chronobiology The scientific study of the effect of time on living systems.

chronophobia A morbid fear of time: a common psychoneurosis in prison inmates.

chrysoidin Y A basic mono-azo dye. Solubil-

CHROMSOME COMPLEMENT OF SOME COMMON SPECIES*

SPECIES		DIPLOID NUMBER OF CHROMOSOMES (2N)	SEX CHROMOSOMES	
Common Name	Scientific Name		Female	Male
Ass	Equus asinus	62	XX	XY
Mule	E. mulus	63	XX	XY
Horse	E. caballus	64	XX	XY
Prezewalsky horse	E. caballus prezewalskii	66	XX	XY
Mrs. Hartmann's mountain zebra	E. zebra hartmannar	32	XX	XY
Man	Homo sapiens	46	XX	XY
Rhesus monkey	Macaca mulatta	42	XX	XY
Chimpanzee	Pan troglodytes	48	XX	XY
Gorilla	Gorilla gorilla	48	XX	XY
Mouse	Mus musculus	40	XX	XY
Chinese hamster	Cricetulus griseus	22	XX	XY
Dog	Canis familiaris	78	XX	XY
Cat	Felis catus	38	XX	XY
Rabbit	Oryctolagus cuniculus	44	XX	XY
Guinea pig	Cavia cobaya	64	XX	XY
Goat	Capra hircus	60	XX	XY
Sheep	Ovis aries	54	XX	XY
Cattle	Bos taurus	60	XX	XY
Camel	Camelus bactrianus	74	XX	XY
Zebu	Bos indicus	60	XX	XY
Pig	Sus scrofa	38	XX	XY
Fox	Vulpes fulva	38	XX	XY
Mink	Mustela vision	30	XX	XY
Opossum	Didelphis virginiana	22	XX	XY
Parakeet	Melopsittacus undulatus	58	WZ	ZZ
Turkey	Meleagris gallopava	80	WZ	ZZ
Duck	Anas platyrhyncha domestica	80	WZ	ZZ
Chicken	Gallus gallus	78	WZ	ZZ
Honeybee	Apis Mellifera	32†	WZ	ZZ
Gopher snake	Drymarchon corais couperi	36	WZ	ZZ
Leopard frog	Rana pipiens	26	(?)	(?)
North American alligator	Alligator mississippiensis	32	(?)	(?)
Chameleon lizard	Anolis carolinensis	36	(?)	(?)

*Adapted from H. A. Smith and T. C. Jones: Veterinary Pathology. 3rd ed. Lea & Febiger, Philadelphia, 1966.

†16 in drones.

ity at 15° C.: water 5.5 per cent, absolute alcohol 4.75 per cent, glycerol 12.5 per cent. Combined with Albert's iodine solution, it is used to stain volutin in *Corynebacterium diphtheriae,* and to stain mitochondria and the Golgi apparatus.[37, 153]

ciconiiform birds Members of the avian order Ciconiiformes, a group of long-legged, long-necked wading birds, which includes the herons, bitterns, storks, ibises, and flamingos.

circulin An antibiotic; see *polymyxin.*

Cittotaenia An anoplocephalid tapeworm characterized by a cyclophyllidean life cycle; it parasitizes rabbits and hares.[21]

cladogram A diagram that describes the branching of an evolutionary tree.

claustrophobia Morbid dread of being shut up in a confined space.

clear heads (disease of) See *gattine.*

cleistothecia Basket-like structure of fungi in which are formed asci and ascospores.

climacophobia Morbid fear of stairs or of climbing.

cline Variation in characteristics of populations of a single species in different locations along its range, indicating gradual phenotypic change.

cloaca (avian) In birds, the cloaca is a terminal chamber of both entodermal and ectodermal derivation into which the digestive tract and urogenital ducts empty. The rectum enters midventrally into an area called the coprodeum. The latter is separated by a fold from a dorsal area (the urodeum) into which the ureters and oviduct, or in the case of the male the deferent ducts, enter. Both the urodeum and coprodeum are in open communication with a common chamber (the proctodeum), which terminates in the sphinctered vent to the outside. On the middorsal wall of the proctodeum near the vent, there is a cul-de-sac entrance to the cloacal bursa of Fabricius (q.v.).

clonal selection The theory that antibody formation occurs initially by contact of antigen with antibody-like sites found on the surface of lymphoid cells. Secondary response occurs when an excess number of cells, which are formed after primary stimulation, successfully capture the antigen. Tolerance is explained through the disappearance of a particular clone after contact with an antigen that occurred during early life. The ability to form antibody with macrophage-extracted RNA has introduced new

Diseases Caused by *Clostridium*

Species	Host	Disease
C. botulinum	(See *botulism*)	
C. chauvoei	Cow, sheep	Blackleg
C. hemolyticum	Cow	Bacterial icterohemoglobinuria, "red water"
C. novyi	Sheep	Black disease, occasionally malignant edema in other species
C. perfringens	Lamb, sheep	Dysentery "struck," pulpy kidney disease
C. septicum	Sheep	Braxy, malignant edema in other species
C. tetani	Horse, cow, swine, sheep, man, and other species	Tetanus infection

possibilities to this theory of immune response. See also *synthesis of antibody,* under *antibody.*

clone   A group of identical cells descended from a single ancestor.

Clostridium   A genus of schizomycetes, family Bacillaceae, order Eubacteriales, made up of obligate anaerobic or microaerophilic, gram-positive, spore-forming, rod-shaped bacteria, with spores of greater diameter than the vegetative cells. The spores may be central, terminal, or subterminal.[16] (See table.)

Cloudman melanoma S91   See under *melanoma.*

Cnemidocoptes   See *scaly leg.*

coagulase   An enzyme that accelerates the formation of blood clots, but is not involved in in-vivo coagulation of human blood.

cobra   See table accompanying *snake.*

cobra factor   A protein in cobra venom which, when added to serum, causes selective inactivation of the C′3 fraction of complement.[93]

cocarboxylase (thiamine pyrophosphate)   A diphosphoric acid ester of thiamine (vitamin B_1) that functions as a required coenzyme of carboxylase.

cocarcinogen   An agent that increases the effect of a carcinogen by direct concurrent local effect on the tissue.

Coccidia   An order of protozoa of the subphylum Sporozoa, commonly parasitic in the epithelial cells of the intestinal tract, but also found in the liver and other organs (see table).[142]

Coccidioides immitis   A species of pathogenic fungus of the order Endomycetales, which in tissue or exudates appears as a spherical, thick-walled, endospore-filled organism and, in culture at room temperature, as a fluffy, white, cottony fungus. It is the causative agent of coccidioidomycosis.[36]

coccidioidin   An extract of filtrate of broth culture of *Coccidioides immitis;* used for skin sensitivity tests in the diagnosis of coccidioidomycosis.[16]

coccidioidomycosis   An infectious disease of the respiratory tract. The first or primary stage is an acute respiratory infection known as Valley fever, San Joaquin fever, or desert fever. The secondary or chronic stage is a progressive, disseminated, usually fatal condition referred to as coccidioidal granuloma. The causative agent is *Coccidioides immitis.*[36]

coccidiosis   A disease caused by intracellular protozoan parasites of the order Coccidia,

Examples of Tissue Localization of Coccidia[142]

Host	Organism	Tissue
Man	Isospora hominis	Intestine
Chicken	Eimeria tenella	Ceca
	E. necatrix	Small intestine, ceca
	E. brunetti	Small intestine, ceca
	E. acervulina	Small intestine, ceca
Dog, cat	Isospora bigemina, I. felis	Intestine
	Eimeria canis, E. felina	Intestine
Cattle	E. zurnii	Intestine
Sheep, goat	E. parva	Intestine
Swine	E. scrofae	Intestine
	Isospora suis	Intestine
Geese	Eimeria truncata	Renal tubules
Equidae	Klossiella equi	Renal tubules
Rabbit	Eimeria steidae	Intrahepatic bile ducts
	E. magna	Duodenum, ileum
	E. perforans	Duodenum
	E. media	Duodenum
	E. irresidua	Duodenum, ileum

which affects the epithelial cells of the intestine, liver, and occasionally other organs.[11, 142]

rabbit c., an important parasitic gastrointestinal disease in the colony husbandry of domestic rabbits. As the standards of hygiene have been elevated, and with the practice of rearing young rabbits on wire-bottomed hutches, this disease has diminished from its former importance as a leading cause of death. The misinterpretation of hepatic coccidiosis lesions in the rabbit has been a frequent source of confusion in their use as experimental animals. The life cycle of the parasite begins as oocysts are passed in the feces. They require two to three days for sporulation before they are infective, and then five to eighteeen days before completing both the sexual and asexual phases of multiplication, depending on the species. Affected animals are treated with sulfaquinoxaline in the drinking water at the 0.04 per cent level for two seven-day courses one week apart.

coccobacilliform body   See *Mycoplasma.*

cock   Postpubertal male of various avian species, especially gallinaceous birds.

codominant   Denoting genes whose alleles are expressed individually in the heterozygote. The classic example is the A and B blood group locus in man, where both A and B properties are immunologically demonstrable on heterozygous, AB erythrocytes. Incomplete dominance is a blending of the heterozygote such that the character is intermediate between the two homozygotes, and should be distinguished from codominance.[51]

codon   The nucleotide triplet that specifies the amino acid to be placed in correct position in polypeptide formation.

coel-   A combining form denoting relationship to a cavity.

coelenterate   Any member of the phylum Coelenterata, considered the lowest animal forms with definite tissues. The symmetry is radial, and two forms are distinguished: (a) polyps, in which the body is tubular, one end being closed and forming a foot by which it attaches to a solid object, and the other end containing a central mouth, and (b) medusae, which are free-swimming with an umbrella shape, margined with tentacles, having a central mouth on the ventrum. All forms are equipped with stinging cells (nematocysts). Three classes are recognized: Hydrozoa includes *Hydra, Obelia,* and *Physalia* (Portuguese man-of-war); Scyphozoa, the jellyfishes (e.g., *Aurelia*); and Anthozoa, the sea anemones and corals.

coelioanastomosis   A surgical method for the preparation of parabiosis by the establishment of a common peritoneal cavity between the parabionts.[45]

coenzyme   A nonprotein factor required to be bound lightly to the protein portion (apoenzyme) before it becomes a complete enzyme (holoenzyme).[90, 118]

coffee senna   A poisonous plant, *Cassia occidentalis,* which causes myodegeneration in skeletal and cardiac muscle characterized by loss of mitochondrial matrix and fragmentation of cristae.

cognition   That operation of the mind by which we become aware of objects of thought or perception, including understanding and reasoning.

coisogenic   The term applied to strains of inbred animals genetically identical except for a difference at a single genetic locus. Since true coisogenicity describes an ideal state difficult to define with certainty, another term (congenic) is used to describe the practical approximation of the coisogenic state.[51]

colchicine   An alkaloid obtained from *Colchicum autumnal,* occurring as pale yellow amorphous scales or powder; used in the treatment of gout, and to treat cell cultures to arrest mitosis in metaphase by interference with formation of the spindle, so that chromosome spreads can be prepared.

colicin   Bacteriocin (q.v.) produced by certain strains of Enterobacteriaceae.[49]

coliform birds   Members of the avian order Coliiformes, composed of a single family, the Coliifae, which includes the mousebird or coly.

colistin   An antibiotic; see *polymyxin.*

collagen   The main supportive protein of skin, bone, cartilage, and connective tissue.

collagenase   An enzyme that catalyzes the destruction of collagen.

College of American Pathologists   Suite 1100, 230 N. Michigan Ave., Chicago, Ill. 60601.

Colorado Scientific Society   P.O. Box 15164, Denver, Colo. 80215.

color blindness   Defective color vision due to reduced or absent visual pigments. Complete loss of color vision is known as achromatopsia and is inherited as an autosomal recessive trait. Incomplete color blindness is known as dyschromatopsia and is inherited as a sex-linked recessive trait. Color blindness is also distinguished according to the color (or colors) involved.

colostrum   A thin milky fluid secreted by the mammary gland about the time of parturition, which is rich in antibodies and capable of conferring passive immunity to the newborn.

colubrid   See table accompanying *snake.*

Colubridae   See table accompanying *snake.*

columbiform birds   Members of the avian order Columbiformes. The order is composed of three families, including the extinct Raphidae (including the dodo) and the Columbidae (pigeons and doves), a family of great agricultural and research importance. In general, even under domestication, columbiform birds are monogamous and tend to mate for life, the males partaking in nest building and caring for the squabs (young). The helpless young are fed for the first few days with pigeon milk (see under *milk*) in all members of Columbidae. Although the family contains many important species, including turtle doves and ringdoves, the rock dove (*Columbia livia*) is the most important: from it the domesticated varieties have been derived. The breeds include the Roman, tumbler, Jacobin, fantail, pouter, and carrier pigeons. One breed, the white carneau, is of particular importance in research because of its predilection to spontaneous atherosclerosis.[23]

column chromatography See under *chromatography.*

comedocarcinoma A carcinoma of the breast composed of ductlike acini filled with hardened secretion.

cometophobia Morbid fear of comets.

commensalism A symbiotic relationship between a host and its parasite in which the host provides the habitat and food. The host is physiologically independent of the parasite and suffers no damage. Some examples are the bacteria and protozoa found in the alimentary canal of man and marine animals such as anemones and crabs.[159] See *symbiosts.*

complement A lytic substance in normal serum that combines with antigen-antibody complex, producing lysis when the antigen is an intact cell. Symbol C'. It is differentiated into four components: C'_1, a euglobulin containing carbohydrate that is the midpiece of complement, precipitated by passing CO_2 through serum diluted 1:10 or by dialysis of serum against distilled water. C'_2, a mucoglobulin that is the end-piece of complement, remaining in solution after C'_1 is precipitated. C'_3, a heat-stable component of complement that is inactivated by treatment with yeast, zymin, or cobra venom. C'_4, a heat-stable component of complement that is inactivated by treatment with ammonia or hydrazine, or by shaking with chloroform or ether. It is the carbohydrate portion of C'_2, containing labile carbonyl groups.[129]

complement deficiency Inherited deficiency of various fractions of complement. Many forms have been described in guinea pig, rabbit, and mouse.[93]

complementary color That portion of the spectrum absorbed by an object, as opposed to the portion reflected, the latter being the color by which it is identified (e.g., in a red object, the red is reflected and its complementary color, blue-green, is absorbed).[153] See *wavelength* (table).

complementary gene See under *gene.*

complementation Enhancement of viral infection resulting from a mixed infection, especially when one of the viruses is defective and another (helper virus) assists by supplying or restoring the activity of a viral gene.[39] Cf. *interference.*

complement unit The least quantity of complement that will hemolyze a definite amount of red blood corpuscles in the presence of an amboceptor unit.

concanavalin A globulin of jackbean that can agglutinate erythrocytes of animals. Agglutination is due to the reaction with terminal nonreducing sugar residues present on red cell mucopolysaccharides.

condensing enzyme See under *enzyme.*

conditioned See *conditioned response,* under *response; conditioned* and *reinforcing stimulus,* under *stimulus;* and *conditioned suppression.*

conditioned suppression The experimental procedure in which a neutral stimulus is presented during the performance of a given pattern of behavior, followed by a strongly aversive stimulus, and which is repeated until there is a decrease in response strength during the presentation of the initially neutral stimulus.

conditioning In behavioral science, a general term for the development of a conditioned response to a stimulus. The technique was derived from the classical experiments of Pavlov and his observations of increasing salivation when a dog was presented with food as a reinforcing stimulus.[158]

approximation c., a special type of operant conditioning in which the ultimate conditioning objectives are approached by steps (e.g., if a dog is desired to jump against or over a wall, the first step may be to reinforce a head turn toward the wall, then a body turn, and so forth, until reinforcement results in the desired response.)

avoidance c., an experimental procedure in which the occurrence of the response prevents the administration of any negative reinforcing stimulus, which would otherwise occur shortly after the onset of the conditioned stimulus.

counter-c., the experimental procedure of producing and conditioning a second and antagonistic response to the original conditioned or discriminated stimulus.

escape c., in operant conditioning, a situation in which an animal must make a specific response in order to terminate a noxious stimulus. The most usual measurement taken is latency of response (reaction time) from the beginning of the presentation of the noxious stimulus.

instrumental c., a term applied to operant conditioning when the conditioned response is instrumental in producing a reinforcing stimulus for the animal. For instance, the animal is not free to give the response except when the experimenter chooses, as by opening a door so that the animal can run out.

operant c., the experimental procedure of giving an animal a reinforcing stimulus immediately following the occurrence of a given preexisting response. Conditioning is present only if the response then increases in magnitude, or relative frequency, or decreases in latency (reaction time) as a consequence of this operation.

pseudo-c., the phenomenon seen in an animal that responds to the conditioned stimulus in the same way that it responds to the unconditioned stimulus before the two have been paired; pseudoconditioning is possibly related to stimulus generalization.

sensory c., an experimental procedure of repeatedly and consecutively presenting an animal with two stimuli to both of which it is indifferent, and then conditioning the animal to respond to the second of the two. *Sensory preconditioning* is said to occur if the animal is then observed to respond to the first in the absence of the second.

strength of c., 1. the magnitude of response to a given conditioned stimulus. 2. resistance to the extinction of a conditioned response. See *experimental extinction* under *extinction*.

Conference of Research Workers in Animal Diseases College of Veterinary Medicine, University of Minnesota, St. Paul, Minn.

conflict In behavioral science, a term applied when the stimuli for two incompatible responses are presented simultaneously under conditions in which either presented alone would yield the response.

approach-approach c., the situation in which two stimuli, toward either of which the subject animal would move when presented alone, are presented simultaneously but in different locations so that approach to one takes the animal away from the other.

approach-avoidance c., the situation in which two stimuli, toward one of which the subject animal would move when presented alone and from the other of which it would actively run, are presented together at the same, or approximately the same, location.

avoidance-avoidance c., the situation in which two stimuli, from either of which the subject animal would move if presented alone, are presented simultaneously but in different locations so that escape from one places the animal in the presence of the other.

congenic Denoting inbred strains of animals produced by the continued crossing of a gene from one stock onto the inbred (and therefore isogenic) background of another. It is presumed that the foreign gene is accompanied by and is part of a foreign chromosome segment. A strain derived in this fashion approximates but never achieves true coisogenicity and is referred to as a *congenic strain*. The inbred strain to which repeated crosses have been made is the *inbred partner*. A congenic strain and its inbred partner are referred to as a *congenic pair*. If the foreign gene in the congenic partner is a histocompatibility gene, so that members of the congenic pair mutually resist transplants of each other's tissues (e.g., tumors), the congenic strain is a *congenic resistant* (*CR*) *strain* and the pair a *congenic resistant* (*CR*) *pair*.[51]

congenital Denoting a condition that exists at or before birth but is not necessarily genetically transmitted, although it may be.

congenital viral infection Any viral infection passed from the female parent to the offspring either by transplacental transmission or by infection during passage through the birth canal.[39, 106] The accompanying table shows the incidence of some of these infections.

Congo red A metachromatic anionic dye.

THE OCCURRENCE AND EFFECTS OF CONGENITAL INFECTIONS WITH VIRUSES*

VIRUS GROUP	EXAMPLE	EFFECT ON FETUS
Poxvirus	Smallpox (man)	Fetal death (abortion)
Herpesvirus	Cytomegalovirus (man)	Severe neonatal disease
		Cerebral damage and prolonged viruria in survivors
	Equine rhinopneumonitis	Abortion in mares and in guinea pigs
	Herpes-like virus (dogs)	Acute hemorrhagic disease
Parvovirus	H1 (hamsters)	Fetal death with developmental defects
	RV (rats)	Fetal death and resorption; hepatitis and cerebellar hypoplasia in newborn
Leukovirus	Avian leukosis (chickens)	Inapparent; prolonged viremia, immunological tolerance, eventually leukosis (rarely)
	Murine leukemia (mice)	Inapparent; prolonged viremia, eventual leukemia (sometimes)
Unclassified	Lymphocytic choriomeningitis (mice)	Inapparent; prolonged viremia, immunological tolerance
	Hog cholera vaccine (pigs)	Edema and limb malformation
	Blue tongue vaccine (sheep)	Lambs stillborn or with symptoms of CNS disease
	Rubella (man)	Usually non-lethal, congenital defects, prolonged viremia, no immunological tolerance
	Scrapie (sheep)	Slowly progressive infection with signs of CNS disease in adult sheep
	Aleutian disease (mink)	Hypergammaglobulinemia, plasmacytosis

*Adapted from F. Fenner: The Biology of Animal Viruses. Academic Press, New York, 1968.

Solubility at 15° C.: water 5 per cent, absolute alcohol 0.75 per cent, glycerol 4 per cent. It is used to demonstrate amyloid in tissue sections, and is the only anionic dye that shows hypochromic shifts in tissue sections and solutions of certain basic compounds. Amyloid deposits stained with Congo red exhibit pink fluorescence when examined with a fluorescent microscope at a wavelength of 365 mμ.[57, 153]

conidia (pl. of *conidium*)   Lateral or terminal fungal spores that are shed from the hyphae.

Connecticut Society of Pathologists   310 Cedar Street, New Haven, Conn. 06510.

consecutive sexuality   The condition in which individuals are males at one stage of life and females at another.

consummatory act   A behavior pattern that most often terminates a given sequence of behaviors, such as eating, copulation, etc.

consummatory stimulus   See under *stimulus*.

contact inhibition   A poorly understood mechanism that causes cells in culture to stop growing when they come in contact with one another. Loss of contact inhibition usually indicates transformation to a state of malignancy.

contagious disease   A disease that is communicable by contact with an individual suffering from it or with some secretion of such an individual or with an object touched by him.

contagious ecthyma of sheep   A poxlike disease of sheep and goats characterized by the appearance of papules and vesicles on the skin of the lips and occasionally around the nostrils and eyes. Secondary infection by *Cochliomyia americana* (the screwworm fly) and *Spherophorus necrophorus* may occur.

contagious equine abortion   See under *abortion*.

contagious pneumonia of calves   See under *pneumonia*.

contagious stomatitis   See under *stomatitis*.

control   A standard against which experimental observations may be evaluated, as a procedure identical in all respects to the experimental procedure except for absence of the one factor that is being studied.

conventional animal   A polycontaminated animal as found in its usual environment, as the rats in a stock colony maintained with little regard to the species of microorganisms associated with it. The term may be abbreviated to Cv.[86] Cf. *gnotobiote*, *axenic*, and *bion*.

convergence (convergent evolution)   The appearance of similar structures or adaptation in organisms which are unrelated but which are adapted to the same mode of life.

copperhead   See table accompanying *snake*.

coprodeum   See *cloaca (avian)*.

coraciiform birds   Members of the avian order Coraciiformes, which includes the kingfishes, bea-eaters, rollers, hoopoes, and hornbills; they are characterized by a strong sharp bill and syndactylous third and fourth toes.

coral snake   See table accompanying *snake*.

cordycepin   An antibiotic produced by a fungus, *Cordyceps*, which inhibits *Bacillus subtilis*. Its mode of activity is not well understood, but it appears to interfere with nucleic acid synthesis by participating as a component in polynucleotide structure, a fact which may have considerable biological significance. Its primary activity, however, may be in the inhibition of purine metabolism.[36, 49]

cormorant   See *pelecaniform birds*.

corpora allata   A pair of small glandular bodies that are in close association with the cerebral ganglia of larval insects and that secrete the "juvenile hormone," which allows molts to occur by inhibiting growth and metamorphosis. The action of this hormone is counteracted by the molting and pupation hormones, which are produced by the cerebral ganglia.[111]

Corynebacterium   A genus of microorganisms of the family Corynebacteriaceae, order Eubacteriales, made up of straight to slightly curved, gram-positive rods, which are generally aerobic but may be microaerophilic or even anaerobic. The cells may be clublike in form and tend to arrange themselves in parallel or "palisade" formations. See table.[142]

cottony   Indicating a surface of a colony of fungi covered with loose, cottony, or tufted aerial hyphae.

Diseases Caused by *Corynebacterium*

AGENT	HOST	DISEASE
C. equi	Foal, swine	Purulent pneumonia in foals; tuberculous lesions in swine
C. kutscheri	Mouse	Pneumonia, generalized infections
C. pseudotuberculosis	Sheep, horse, cow	Caseous lymphadenitis, ulcerative lymphangitis, suppurative lymphangitis
C. pyogenes	Cow	Mastitis, metritis
	Swine	Pneumonia
	Sheep, goat	Joint infectious and purulent pneumonia
	– – –	Miscellaneous pyogenic infections in many species
C. renale	Cattle, horse, sheep	Pyelonephritis

Council of Biology Editors, Inc.   24 W. Hunting Towers, Alexandria, Va. 22314.

Council on Medical Television, Inc.   Box 3163, Duke University Medical Center, Durham, N.C. 27706.

counterconditioning   See under *conditioning*.

Cowdria ruminantium   A rickettsial organism that produces a disease of cattle, sheep, and goats known as heartwater. It is transmitted by the tick *Amblyomma hebraeum*.

cowpox (vaccinia, poxvirus officianalis)   A viral disease which affects mainly cattle, but also occasionally man (in whom the disease is called vaccinia), particularly farmers producing skin lesions on the hands known as "milker's modules." Observations of this disease led William Jenner to deduce that immunity to smallpox resulted from exposure to cowpox virus.[16] See also *poxvirus*.

Coxiella burnetii   See *Rickettsia*.

cozymase   NAD.

CPE   Cytopathogenic effect.

Crabtree effect   The inhibition of oxygen consumption when glucose is added to tissues that have a high rate of aerobic glycolysis. A characteristic effect exhibited by tumor cells.[90] It is the converse of the Pasteur effect.

cranio-   A combining form denoting relationship to the cranium or skull.

craniopagus   A double monster united at the heads.

craniopharyngioma (craniopharyngeal duct tumor; Rathke's pouch tumor; suprasellar cyst; pituitary adamantinoma or ameloblastoma)   A tumor arising from cell rests derived from the hypophyseal stalk or Rathke's pouch, frequently associated with increased intracranial pressure, and showing calcium deposits in the capsule or in the tumor proper.

craniorachischisis   Congenital fissure of the skull and spinal column.

crayfish   See *crustacean*.

crayfish plague   Krebspest.

creatinase   An enzyme that catalyzes the degradation of creatine into urea and ammonia.

crepuscular   Pertaining to twilight; active at dusk and shortly before dawn.

cresomania   Hallucinations consisting in the imagination of the possession of great wealth.

cresyl fast violet   A basic dye. Solubility at 15° C.: water 9.5 per cent, absolute alcohol 6 per cent, and glycerol 11.5 per cent. It is used to stain root tip smears and for nerve cells in celloidin sections.[37, 153]

Creutzfeldt-Jakob disease (spongiform encephalopathy)   A degenerative lesion of the cerebral cortex of man, which may be of viral etiology. See *slow virus*.

crista   A projection or ridge. In cytology, the folded inner membrane of mitochondria.

Cristispira   A large, flexible, undulating spiral organism of the family Spirochaetaceae, order Spirochaetales, found in the intestinal tract of oysters and other mollusks.

Crithidia   A genus of protozoan organisms of the family Trypanosomatidae found as parasites in the intestines of certain insects. Because of their fastidious culture requirements, they are potentially valuable as a bioassay tool.[159]

Crocker tumor 180 (mouse sarcoma 180; Crocker sarcoma 180; sarcoma 180)   A tumor that arose spontaneously as a carcinoma in the axilla of a white laboratory mouse. It was found at necropsy in 1914 in the laboratory of W. H. Woglom at the Crocker Laboratory in New York City. The tumor was carried by serial transplantation, but by 1919 the histologic pattern became altered to resemble that of a sarcoma. It is not strain-specific, growing rapidly in 90 per cent or more of injected mouse hosts, regressing in the rest. Tumor-bearing hosts die 18 to 28 days after inoculation. The tumor is both locally invasive and metastatic. Crocker sarcoma 180 is transplantable intraperitoneally to newborn rats, which usually die within a week with widespread metastases.[150]

Crohn's disease   Regional ileitis; see under *ileitis*.

crossing over   Exchange of genes between homologous chromosomes.

Crotalidae   See table accompanying *snake*.

croup-associated virus (CA virus)   See *simian virus*.

crustacean   Any member of phylum Arthropoda, subphylum Mandibulata, class Crustacea. The class is characterized by a head consisting of five fused somites with two pairs of antennae, one pair of jaws, and two pairs of maxillae. The body usually has a dorsal carapace and ends in a telson containing the anus. The exoskeleton is calcareous; the appendages often biramous. Respiration is accomplished by gills or through body surface, excretion by antennal (green) glands; there are no malpighian tubules. Sex openings are paired and anterior, the eggs usually being carried by the female. Development usually involves larval stages. Most species are aquatic (marine and fresh water), but some are terrestrial. At least 25,000 species are known. (See table.)

cryo-   A combining form denoting relationship to cold.

cryobiology   The science dealing with the effect of low temperatures on biological systems.

Cryogenic Society of America   7712 24th Street, Westminster, Calif. 92683.

cryoicthyozoose virus   See *contagious stomatitis*, under *stomatitis*.

cryophilic   Psychrophilic.

cryostat   An instrument designed to maintain carefully controlled low temperatures for cutting frozen tissue sections.

cryptic coloration   Body coloring having a camouflaged pattern.

crypto-   A combining form meaning hidden or concealed, or denoting relationship to a crypt.

cryptocephalus   A fetal monster with an inconspicuous head.

Cryptococcus neoformans (*Torula menin-*

A CLASSIFICATION OF CRUSTACEA

SUBCLASS	ORDER	EXAMPLES
1. Branchipoda	Anostraca	Brine and fairy shrimp, (e.g., *Artemia salina*)
	Conchostraca	– – –
	Cladocera	Water fleas (e.g., *Daphnia pulex*)
	Nostraca	– – –
2. Cephalocarida	– – –	– – –
3. Ostracoda	Cladocopa	– – –
	Myodocopa	– – –
	Platycopa	– – –
	Podocopa	– – –
4. Copepoda	Branchiura	– – –
	Eucopepoda	Mostly small parasitic forms (e.g., *Salmincola*)
	Mystacocarida	– – –
5. Cirripedia	Thoracica	Barnacles
	Acrothoracica	Barnacles
	Apoda	Barnacles
	Rhizocephala	Rhizocephalans (parasitic on crabs)
	Ascothoracica	Ascothracicans (parasitic on corals)
6. Malacostraca	Nebaliacea	– – –
	Anaspidacea	– – –
	Mysidacea	Opossum shrimps (e.g., *Mysis*)
	Cumacea	– – –
	Tanaidacea	– – –
	Isopoda	Sowbugs, pill bugs, wood lice
	Amphipoda	Beach fleas, whale "lice"
	Stomatopoda	Mantis shrimps
	Euphausiacea	– – –
	Decapoda	Lobsters (e.g. *Homarus*), crayfish (e.g., *Astacus* and *Cambarus*), prawns, crabs, shrimps

igitidis) A yeastlike, nonmycelial budding fungus which forms a characteristic polysaccharide capsule. It frequently penetrates the central nervous system, producing a subacute or chronic infection of the meninges, and occasionally involves the skin, lungs, or other organs.

Cryptosporidium A genus of protozoan parasites. *C. muris* and *C. parvum* infest the mouse. See *protozoan parasites,* under *rat.*

cryptozoite A stage of the malaria parasite (*Plasmodium*) which originates from the sporozoite and develops in liver cells. It is also known as the exoerythrocytic stage or the tissue stage, for it is in the liver that the cryptozoite undergoes asexual multiplication and produces cryptozoic merozoites, which enter other liver cells and form a second generation known as metacryptozoites, that finally produce the metacryptozoic merozoites, which invade erythrocytes. This cycle takes eight days.[109, 159]

crystalliferous Producing or bearing crystals; especially as applied to a number of *Bacillus* species which, in addition to the endospore, produce a crystal or crystal-like inclusion in the sporulating cell. One of the best known crystalliferous bacteria capable of infecting insects is *Bacillus thuringiensis.*

crystal violet Gentian violet.

ctenophore Any member of the phylum Ctenophora, free-swimming marine animals with transparent gelatinous bodies. Their symmetry is biradial. They have an oral-aboral axis, three germ layers, a digestive system, and a primitive sense organ (statocyst). Those with comblike plates are called combjellies; those with lengthwise ridges are known as sea walnuts.

ctetology That branch of biology which treats of acquired characters.

cuckoo See *cuculiform birds.*

cuculiform birds Members of the avian order Cuculiformes. One family, the Cuculidae, contains a parasitic subfamily, the Cuculinae, in which the eggs are incubated, hatched, and reared by the parasitized host species. The order contains the cuckoos, roadrunners, anis, and turacos.

Culicoides A genus of biting flies of the family Heleidae, which act as intermediate hosts for filarial worms and are capable of transmitting viral diseases such as blue tongue of sheep, African horse sickness, and fowlpox.

culture 1. The propagation of microorganisms or of living tissue cells in special media conducive to their growth. 2. A growth of microorganisms or other living cells. 3. To induce such growth.

culture dialysis See under *dialysis.*

Curvularia geniculata A fungus reported to be the etiologic agent of maduromycosis of the feet of the dog.

Cushing's syndrome A syndrome resulting from excessive secretion of cortisone and hydrocortisone, caused by adrenocortical hyperfunction due to hyperplasia, adenoma, or carcinoma; pituitary hyperfunction due to basophilic adenoma; or ectopic production of corticotropin. It is characterized by obesity, hypertension, and striae over the abdomen, thighs, and arms. In females, there may be signs of masculinization, including hirsutism, deep voice, and amenorrhea.[142]

Cv Conventional animal.

C60 virus See *Manaker leukemia virus.*

cyanism An abnormal amount of blue pigmentation in birds resulting from melanocarotenoid schizochroism.[112]

Cycas circinalis One of several species of cycads, palmlike plants that contain toxic glycosides with hepatotoxic and carcinogenic capability. Others in the group are of the genera *Bowenia* and *Macrozamia.* Ingestion causes progressive ataxia and paralysis in cattle. Mild, ill-defined degenerative changes can be found in the spinal cord. The syndrome has been studied because of its possible relationship to human amyotrophic lateral sclerosis.

cyclic neutropenia A repeated pattern of precipitous drop in the number of circulating neutrophilic leukocytes. The process probably involves an arrest in maturation and release of cells from bone marrow. The mechanism is not understood. Seen in man and as a recessive inherited trait in gray collies.

cyclo- A combining form denoting round or recurring. Often used with particular reference to the eye, or to the ciliary body of the eye.

cycloheximide One of a group of antibiotics isolated from various species of *Streptomyces* and derived from the glutarimide molecule. They are noted for their antifungal properties but are toxic to a broad spectrum of microorganisms. They interfere with protein synthesis by prevention of the transfer of amino acids from the aminoacyl-s-RNA to polypeptide chain.[36, 49]

cyclophosphamide (Cytoxan) An aklylating agent used as an immunosuppressant and oncolytic drug.

cyclopia A developmental anomaly characterized by a single orbital fossa. In honeybees, a deformity of hereditary origin, consisting of a fusion of both compound eyes at the vertex of the head. Also seen in lambs born to ewes which have eaten *Veratrum californicum* (false hellebore).

D-**Cycloserine** An antibiotic isolated from a species of *Streptomyces* which interferes with cell wall snythesis by inhibition of the incorporation of D-alanine into the nucleotide precursor of mucopeptide. It has a broad spectrum of activity, although it is in general more effective against gram-positive than against gram-negative organisms. It is closely related to and may be produced simultaneously with O-carbamyl-D-serine.[36, 49]

cyclostome A chordate of the class Cyclostomata. All forms are aquatic and jawless, and are believed to be the lowest group of living vertebrates. Typically the body is long, slender, and round, but compressed posteriorly. The mouth is located ventroanteriorly and is suctorial. The skull is cartilaginous, the notochord persists, and the vertebrae are represented by small neural arches (arcualia) over the notochord. The heart is two-chambered, with an atrium and ventricle; the blood contains leukocytes and circular nucleated erythrocytes. The skin is smooth, without scales, and the mouth has horny teeth.

Two orders are recognized: (1) Petromyzontia, which contains the lampreys, e.g., *Entosphenus* and *Ichthyomyzon.* Most species are parasitic on fish and some, e.g., *Petromyzon*, the sea lampreys, have become major hazards to fish life in the St. Lawrence River and N.Y. Finger Lakes; and (2) Myxinoidia, which contains the hagfishes, e.g., *Eptatretus* and the slime eels, *Myxine.*

cygnet See *anseriform birds.*

cynanthropy Delusion in which the patient considers himself a dog or behaves like a dog.

cyno- A combining form denoting relationship to a dog, or meaning doglike.

cynomologous monkey *Macaca irus;* see *primate.*

cynophobia Morbid fear of dogs.

cypridophobia 1. A morbid fear of becoming infected with venereal disease. 2. Morbid fear of sexual intercourse.

cyst A sac filled with fluid. In parasitology, a nonmotile infective stage of a protozoon or intermediate larval form of helminth.

cystadenoma Adenoma associated with cystoma.

cystencephalus A fetal monster with a membranous sac in place of a brain.

cysticercosis The special name given to the presence of the larvae of certain tapeworms in the tissues of man or anomen. The seriousness of the effect upon the host depends upon the organs involved and the number of parasitic cysts formed. Some types involve vital organs such as the liver, heart, or brain. Among the commonest forms of this disease are *Cysticercus bovis* (larvae of *Taenia saginata,* the beef bladderworm), *C. cellulosae* (the larvae of pork bladderworm, the agent of pork measles, which is the intermediate stage of *Taenia solium*). The adult of this worm occurs in the small intestine of man (cestodiasis).

Cysticercus The genus name given to larval forms of tapeworms.

    C. bovis, see *cysticercosis.*

    C. cellulosae, see *cysticercosis.*

    C. (Taenia) fasciolarus, see *helminth parasites,* under *rat.*

    C. ovis, the intermediate stage of the tapeworm *Taenia ovis,* the adult of which occurs in dogs, foxes, wolves, coyotes, and other carnivores.

    C. (Taenia) serialis, see *helminth parasites,* under *rat.*

    C. tenuicollis, the intermediate stage of a tapeworm, *Taenia tenuicollis,* the adult of which occurs in dogs and other carnivores.

cystic fibrosis A congenital hereditary disease of man for which no animal counterpart has yet been discovered; it is characterized by abnormal chloride secretion in saliva, chronic respiratory disease, and fibrosis of the pancreas.

cysto- A combining form denoting a relationship to a sac, cyst, or bladder, most frequently used in reference to the urinary bladder.

cystoadenoma   A tumor containing cystic and adenomatous elements.

-cyte   A word termination denoting a cell, the type of which is designated by the root to which it is affixed, as *elliptocyte, erythrocyte, leukocyte,* etc.

cyto-   A combining form denoting relationship to a cell.

cytobiology   The biology of cells.

cytochemistry   The scientific study of the chemical organization and activity of the cell.

cytogenetics   The branch of genetics devoted to the study of the cellular features of heredity, for example, chromosomes and genes.

cytology   The scientific study of cells, their origin, structure, and functions.[38]

cytomegalovirus infection   Any disease caused by morphologically similar viruses of the herpesvirus group that infect guinea pigs, rats, mice and other rodents, subhuman primates, and man. The viruses are biologically related in the sense of pathogenesis and organ (salivary gland and kidney) predilection, but are antigenically distinct and apparently host-specific. In anomen, the infection is usually subclinical. In man, two forms of infection are recognized. The first parallels the type seen in animals; i.e., the disease is clinically silent and epidemiologically widespread. Typical cytomegalic inclusion bodies are seen in the kidney tubules and the salivary gland duct epithelium. Viruria may be detected by virus isolation in tissue culture or by exfoliative cytology of urine sediments for as long as two years after serologic evidence of infection appears. Giemsa stain is the method of choice for demonstrating inclusions. The second form, disseminated cytomegalic disease, is seen in infants six months of age or younger. Clini-

cal symptoms include hepatosplenomegaly, jaundice, chorioretinitis, and calcifications of the central nervous system with mental retardation. Infected stillborn fetuses demonstrate that infection may occur in utero. Some of the features of the latter disease may be induced in guinea pigs by intracerebral inoculation of guinea pig cytomegalovirus. Guinea pig infections provide a useful model for human cytomegalovirus infections.[64, 106, 114]

cytopathic   Pertaining to or characterized by pathological changes in cells.

cytopathogenic   Capable of producing pathological changes in cells.

cytopathogenic effect (cytolytic effect; CPE)   The effect of cell destruction by viruses, seen as visible plaques or islands of degeneration in monolayer cultures of susceptible cells.

cytopathology (cellular pathology)   The study of cells in disease.[38, 74]

cytoplasmic polyhedrosis   A viral disease of insects, mainly the larvae of certain *Lepidoptera,* characterized by the formation of polyhedral inclusion bodies (polyhedra) in the cytoplasm of the midgut epithelial cells. See also *polyhedrosis.*

cytopyge   The anal opening of ciliates, located at the posterior end of the body, which serves as the excretory pore for the contractile vacuoles.[109]

cytosine arabinoside (ARA C)   A synthetic nucleoside that inhibits replication of all deoxyriboviruses by interference with the reduction of cytidylic acid to 2-deoxycytidylic acid. Related compounds, arabinosylthymine and arabinosyluracil, occur naturally in the sponge. Also used as an antineoplastic and because of its impairment of cell division, to produce abnormalities of development in the central nervous system of experimental animals.

cytostome   The oral cavity of ciliates.

Cytoxan   Trademark for cyclophosphamide.

D

dacnomania   A morbid impulse to kill.

-dactyly   A word termination denoting relationship to a digit, usually to a finger but sometimes to a toe.

Dasypus novemcinctus   See *armadillo.*

daunomycin   An antibiotic produced by species of *Streptomyces,* which inhibits experimental tumors and is effective against gram-positive bacteria and fungi but relatively ineffective against gram-negative organisms. It interferes with DNA metabolism and possesses antimitotic activity.[36, 49]

Dawson's encephalitis   See under *encephalitis.*

de-   Latin prefix signifying down or from; it is sometimes negative or privative, and is frequently intensive.

de aar disease   A pasteurellosis among veldt rodents of South Africa.

death adder   See table accompanying *snake.*

deaminase   Any of a group of enzymes that cause deamination, or the removal of the amino groups from organic compounds.

deer fly fever   Tularemia.

deer hemorrhagic fever   A viral disease of the Virginia white-tailed deer characterized by multiple hemorrhages and edema in various tissues. An arthropod vector may be involved in the transmission of the disease.[16]

defaunate   To remove from an organism its parasitic, commensalistic, or mutualistic fauna, for which the organism ordinarily serves as a host; e.g., removing flagellates from the alimentary tract of termites, ciliates from the rumen of herbivores, or hookworms from the intestine.

defective virus A virus unable to produce virions without the presence of a helper virus.[39] See *complementation.*

definitive host The host in which a parasite achieves adulthood or sexual maturity.

dehydrogenase Any of a group of enzymes that mobilize the hydrogen of a substrate so that it can pass to a hydrogen acceptor. Dehydrogenases are variously designated according to their specific activity, or the substrate acted upon.[90, 118]

  acetaldehyde d., the enzyme that oxidizes acetaldehyde to acetic acid and H_2O_2.

  aerobic d., one that transfers hydrogen directly to oxygen.

  alcohol d., a pyridine nucleotide enzyme of the Embden-Meyerhof pathway, which catalyzes the conversion of ethanol to acetaldehyde using NAD and Zn^{++} as co-factors.[17]

  D-amino-acid d., a flavin nucleotide enzyme that catalyzes the dehydrogenation of D-amino acids into keto acids with FAD as a coenzyme.

  fatty acid d., dehydrogenase that catalyzes the removal of hydrogen from higher fatty acids.

  formic d., an NAD-requiring enzyme that degrades formic acid into carbon dioxide.

  glucose d., one that catalyzes the oxidation of glucose to gluconic acid.

  glutamic acid d., one that catalyzes the change of glutamic acid into α-ketoglutaric acid.

  glyceraldehyde-3-phosphate d., a pyridine nucleotide enzyme of the Embden-Meyerhof pathway that catalyzes the conversion of D-glyceraldehyde-3-phosphate into 1,3-diphosphoglycerate, using NAD^+ and phosphate as co-factors.[17]

  α-glycerophosphate d., a pyridine nucleotide enzyme of the Embden-Meyerhof glycolytic pathway that converts α-glycerophosphate to dihydroxyacetone using NAD as a coenzyme.[17]

  hexose d., an enzyme that catalyzes the oxidation of hexose to hexonic acid.

  β-hydroxybutyric d., a pyridine nucleotide enzyme active in the glycogenesis of carbohydrates; it converts β-hydroxybutarate to acetoacetate, using NAD as a coenzyme.[17]

  α-ketoglutaric d., an enzyme of the Krebs cycle that catalyzes the conversion of α-ketoglutarate to succinyl coenzyme A, using NAD, thiamine pyrophosphate and lipoic acid as co-factors.

  lactic d., a pyridine nucleotide enzyme of the Embden-Meyerhof glycolytic pathway that converts lactate into pyruvate using NAD as a coenzyme.[17]

  malic d.-NAD, an enzyme of the Krebs cycle that converts L-malate to oxaloacetate, using NAD as a co-factor.

  malic d.-NADP, an enzyme of the glycolytic Krebs cycle that catalyzes the conversion of L-malate to pyruvate, using NADP as a cofactor.

  6-phosphogluconic d., an enzyme of the hexose-monophosphate shunt that catalyzes 6-phospho-D-gluconate into D-ribulose-5-phosphate, using NADP as a co-factor.

  pyruvic d., a pyridine nucleotide enzyme of the Embden-Meyerhof pathway that converts pyruvate to acetyl coenzyme A, using NAD, thiamine pyrophosphate, and lipoic acid as co-factors.

  succinic d. (succinoxidase), an enzyme that catalyzes the dehydrogenation of succinic acid to fumaric acid, using NAD.

  xanthine d. (xanthine oxidase), an enzyme that catalyzes the oxidation of xanthine to uric acid.

deletion Loss of a segment of a chromosome. If the deletion is of an end segment, it is called terminal, otherwise intercalary. Deletion segments may transfer to other arms of the same pair or to other chromosomes.

delusion A false belief that cannot be corrected by reason. It is logically founded and cannot be corrected by argument or persuasion or even by the evidence of the patient's own senses.

deme A local interbreeding group of organisms.

demography The study of mankind collectively, especially of their geographical distribution and physical environment.

demonology The earlier approach to problems of mental disorder, in which evil spirits were believed to possess the patient and exorcisms constituted the treatment.

demonomania Monomania in which the patient considers himself possessed of devils.

demonophobia Morbid fear of demons.

densonucleosis A fatal disease of larvae of the wax moth, *Galleria mellonella,* and certain other insects, caused by a virus which replicates in most tissues of the insect, with the exception of the midgut and nervous system. The nuclei of the infected cells become progressively larger, lose their characteristic structure and, in histological preparations, appear as compact, densely stained masses. The virus particles are isometric, with an average diameter of 20 millimicrons.[148]

dental formula See *estimation of age,* under *age.*

dental malocclusion See *malocclusion.*

dentinoblastoma A tumor of odontogenic origin composed of connective tissue cells of round or spindle shape, among which are islands of irregularly shaped masses of dentin.

dentinoma A tumor of odontogenic origin, consisting mainly of dentin.

deoxy- A prefix used in naming chemical compounds, to designate a compound containing one less atom of oxygen than the reference substance.

deoxyribonuclease (DNAase) An enzyme that catalyzes the depolymerization of deoxyribonucleic acid. Sometimes called *dornase.*

deoxyribonucleic acid (DNA) An organic acid originally isolated from fish sperm and present in all living cells that possess a nucleus. It is composed of a ribose phosphate backbone formed into a double helix by pairs of bases which are bound to each other in specific complementary fashion to maintain the spatial relationships of the two strands of the helix. It functions as the hereditary molecule in all replicating organisms, with the exception of certain viruses which sit on the boundary between life and nonlife and must parasitize other cells in order to replicate.[32, 90]

synthesis of d. a., the process of replication of DNA. During interphase between mitoses, cell populations consist of two main groups. Those with the normal amount of DNA and those with twice that amount. This reflects the cyclic nature of manufacture of DNA in preparation for mitotic division. The phases have been divided into four periods. G_1 (first gap), the post-telophase stage during which DNA is stable; S (synthesis), during which DNA doubles in amount; G_2 (second gap), the preprophase stage during which DNA is again stable; M (mitosis), during which DNA quantitatively halves and is distributed between daughter cells.[31, 61]

deoxyribovirus   A group of viruses containing DNA as their genetic material. See under *oncogenic viruses,* and see *replication of viruses,* under *virus.*

depluming itch   See *scaly leg.*

depolymerization   The conversion of a compound into one of smaller molecular weight and different physical properties without changing the percentage relationships of the elements composing it.

der-   A combining form denoting relationship to the neck.

deradelphus   A fetal monster made up of twins fused at or near the navel, and having only one head.

derencephalus   A fetal monster with rudimentary skull bones and bifid cervical vertebrae, the brain resting in the bifurcation.

derepression   The process by which selected genes are activated. Since most genes are inactive, or repressed, at any given time, it has been postulated that nonstructural genes control the derepression (activation) and inactivation of the genes that are responsible for the structure of polypeptides. See *gene.*

dermato-   A combining form denoting relationship to the skin.

dermatofibrosarcoma   A fibrosarcoma of the skin.

dermatophobia   A morbid dread of having some cutaneous lesion.

dermatomycosis (ringworm; superficial mycosis; favus tinea)   Infection of the hairs, epidermis, and more rarely the dermis by dermatophytes, and the accompanying inflammatory reaction associated with these parasitic fungi. Recently discovered matings between certain imperfect fungi (including *Microsporum, Trichophyton,* and *Keratinomyces*) have elevated them to the perfect status within the Ascomycetes. A certain degree of host specificity exists among the dermatophytic fungi; certain species are more commonly found in man (anthropophilic), some are more commonly found in animals (zoophilic), and others are facultative, being equally at home in the soil (geophilic) or as parasites. In all species, certain individuals exhibit a predilection for dermatomycosis while others do not, even when in an infective environment. In the table the more common animal isolates are arranged by species and frequency, with an indication of the more relevant synonymy. The animal isolates are important in the study of zoonoses.[115, 142]

dermatophyte   An organism of a group of closely related fungi that cause specific infections of man and animals by invading superficial keratinized areas such as the skin, the hair, and the nails. In their parasitic habitat, they show only mycelial fragments and arthrospores located either inside or outside of the hair, whereas in culture they exhibit filamentous colonies with a variety of asexual spores characteristic of the group. The genera in this group are *Trichophyton,*

DERMATOPHYTES AND THEIR HOSTS

DERMATOPHYTE	HOST (FREQUENCY)*	SYNONYMY
Keratinomyces ajelloi	Dog(1), cow(1), horse(1)	– – –
Microsporum audouinii	Dog(1)	– – –
M. canis	Dog(4), cat(4), swine(1), horse(2), rodent(2), simian primate(3)	*M. caninum. M. felineum*
M. distortum	Dog(1), horse(1), simian primate(2)	– – –
M. gypseum	Cat(2), dog(3), swine(1), horse(3) rodent(3), simian primate(1)	*Achorion gypseum*
M. nanum	Swine(2)	– – –
M. vanbreuseghemii	Dog(1), rodent(1)	– – –
Trichophyton equinum	Dog(1), horse(4)	*Microsporum equinum*
T. gallinae	Bird(4)	*Achorion gallinae*
T. mentagrophytes	Cat(2), dog(2), cow(2), sheep(2), swine(2), horse(2), rodent(4), simian primate(3)	*T. asteroides, T. radians, T. quinckeanum, Achorion quinckeanum*
T. rubrum	Dog(1)	*T. multicolor, T. rodhaini*
T. verrucosum	Dog(1), cow(4), sheep(2), horse(2)	*T. album, T. discoides, T. faviforme*

*Frequency: (1) reported, (2) occasional, (3) frequent, (4) usual.

Epidermophyton, and *Microsporum*. See *dermatomycosis*.

Dermestes A genus of carnivorous beetles; see *dermestid beetle*.

dermestid beetle Any member of Dermestidae, a family of carnivorous beetles in the insect order Coleoptera. They are destructive but very useful in the preparation of museum specimens. Skeletal preparations are made by dropping the specimen into a dermestid colony maintained in a glass-enclosed case. The softer parts are eaten, leaving the bony tissues. Larder beetles, genus *Dermestes*, are often used for this purpose.

desert fever See *coccidioidomycosis*.

desmo- A combining form denoting relationship to a band, bond, or ligament.

desmo-enzyme An enzyme that is bound to the protoplasm of the secreting cell and is therefore not easily extractable.[90, 118]

desmolase An enzyme that catalyzes the addition or removal of some chemical group to or from a substitute without hydrolysis, oxidation, or reduction, the group being taken up from or liberated in the free state.[90, 118]

desmosome Platelike densities of the plasma membranes of two adjacent cells, probably a point of adherence. Sometimes called *macula adherens*.[38]

dextrinase An enzyme that catalyzes the conversion of starch into isomaltose.

dextro- A combining form denoting relationship to the right.

dextrocardia Location of the heart in the right hemithorax, with the apex pointing to the right, sometimes associated with transposition (situs inversus) of the abdominal viscera.

dextrogastria Displacement of the stomach to the right.

dextrophobia Morbid dread of objects on the right side of the body.

dia- A prefix meaning through, apart, across, or between.

diabetes mellitus A complex metabolic disorder characterized by impaired ability to oxidize carbohydrates, persistent hyperglycemia, glycosuria, ketosis, impairment in the synthesis of glycogen, protein, and fat, and decreased amounts of extractable insulin in the pancreas. The disease exists in man as a genetically determined entity probably transmitted by a recessive gene. Several other species develop this disease and comprise important experimental models. These include the dog, certain strains of mice, and the Chinese hamster (*Cricetus griseus*). A recent valuable addition to the list of experimental animals is *Psammomys obesus* (the sand rat, or obese sand rat) which develops severe diabetes, especially when maintained on a high caloric diet.[15, 105]

diabetophobia An abnormal fear of diabetes.

diabolepsy A state in which the subject believes he is possessed by a devil or that he is endowed with supernatural powers.

diakinesis See *meiosis*.

diallel cross See *breeding system*.

dialysis The separation of molecules of varying sizes by the difference in their rate of diffusion across a semipermeable membrane. The procedure is valuable for estimating the size of viruses.

   culture d., a technique for culturing of cells or microorganisms either in vivo or in vitro enclosed in membranes or diffusion chambers so that soluble products can be removed and separated from the organisms. Valuable for the study of metabolic products of organisms in culture.

   equilibrium d., a method employed to measure an association constant between a solution that contains antibody molecules and a haptenic group such as 2,4-dinitrophenyl. It utilizes permeable membranes that allow small molecules to dialyze between the two compartments. This general principle is also applied in other experimental systems.

dialyzable Capable of dialysis or of passing through a membrane.

diamond skin disease of swine See *erysipelas*.

dianil blue An acid dis-azo dye. Solubility at 15° C.: water 5 per cent, absolute alcohol 0.01 per cent, and glycerol 11 per cent. It has been used to study corpora lutea and mammary glands.[37, 153]

diapause A period of growth suspension in an insect.

diapedesis The migration of cellular elements from blood vessels through an intact wall, by traversing the intercellular spaces between endothelial cells or, in the case of lymphocytes, by passing through the cytoplasm of the endothelial cells.

diarrhea See *infantile diarrhea of mice*.

diastase A white, amorphous, soluble enzyme produced during the germination of seeds, and contained in malt. It converts starch into maltose and then into dextrose.

diastematocrania Congenital longitudinal fissure of the cranium.

diastematomyelia Congenital longitudinal fissure of the spinal cord, separating the lateral halves.

diastematopyelia Congenital median fissure of the pelvis.

diazo- Prefix indicating possession of the group —N_2—.

6-diazo-5-oxo-L-norleucine See *azaserine*.

diazo reaction The coupling of a diazo compound such as sulfanalic acid with a protein. This results in an antigen which has specificity for the diazo compound and loses its specificity for the protein to which it is coupled. This type of compound has been extremely valuable in producing antigens against specific chemical structures.

   Ehrlich's d. r., a reaction of a pure pink or red color resulting from the action of diazobenzenesulfonic acid and ammonia upon certain aromatic substances found in the urine. It is useful for diagnostic procedures in certain diseases.[160]

Dibothriocephalus latus (formerly *Diphyllo-*

bothrium latum) A platyhelminth member of Family Dibothriocephalidae; it is commonly known as the broad fish tapeworm.[21] See table accompanying *cestode*.

dicephaly A developmental anomaly characterized by the presence of two heads.

dicheiria A developmental anomaly characterized by duplication of a hand.

dichromatism A change of hue of a dye in solution that varies with the concentration of the dye or the thickness of the solution.[57]

dicoumarol An anticoagulant compound, 3,3'-methylenebis[4-hydroxycoumarin] that develops in sweet clover hay. Ingestion causes a disorder first described as sweet clover poisoning in cattle by veterinarians; the chemical factor was later found to interfere with prothrombin formation. Dicoumarol has been widely used as a rodent poison, and also as a therapeutic drug in cases in which reduced coagulability of the blood is desirable.[142]

didactylism The condition of having only two digits on one hand or foot.

Didelphis virginiana See *opossum*.

differential count A count made by observation, on the stained blood smear, of the proportion of the different types of leukocytes and other cells, expressed in percentages. See also *hemogram*.

differentiation 1. The distinguishing of one thing or disease from another. 2. The act or process of acquiring completely individual characters, such as occurs in the progressive diversification of cells and tissues of the embryo. 3. In behavioral science, the process by which a particular response is differentiated; if a reinforcing stimulus is withheld except when a very specific response is given by the subject, the frequency of occurrence of that response will increase, and that of alternative responses, even though they may differ only slightly, will decrease. This is known as a response differentiation, and its outcome is called a differentiated response.

digitigrade Walking on the toes; said of animals, e.g., dogs and cats, that have adopted this form of locomotion.

di Guglielmo's disease A condition originally described as acute erythremic myelosis or erythroid hyperplasia, but later grouped with the myeloproliferative disorders. Erythroblastic leukemia caused by a virus occurs in birds.[70]

dihydrotachysterol (DHT; AT 10) A synthetic sterol that mimics the action of parathyroid hormone. It is used experimentally as a calciphylactic sensitizer and therapeutically to raise blood calcium in cases of tetany.

dikephobia Morbid fear of justice.

dimelia A developmental anomaly characterized by duplication of a limb.

dimethylsulfoxide (DMSO) A chemical byproduct of paper manufacture that has peculiar properties, including ready absorption through the skin; used as a preservative for living cells stored at low temperatures.

dimorphism See *sexual dimorphism*.

dinactin See *nonactin*.

dinornithiform birds Members of the extinct avian Order Dinornithiformes, which includes the moas.

Dioctophyma renale A nematode of the family Dioctophymidae, characterized by a life cycle which involves two intermediate hosts. This parasite is found in the kidney and peritoneal cavity of the dog, mink, fox, and wolf. Pigs, cattle, horses, and man can also be infected. *D. renale* is one of the largest nematodes known: the females may measure up to 103 cm. in length and have a diameter of 12 mm.[21] See also *kidney worm*.

Dipetalonema A genus of filarioid nematodes of the superfamily Filariodea. *D. perstans* infects man; primates are the natural reservoirs of infection. *D. streptocerca* is also parasitic for man. *D. reconditum* is found in dogs.[21]

dipeptidase A peptidase that hydrolyzes only peptide linkages, the amino acids of which bear both free amino and carboxyl groups.

diphycercal Denoting a tail fin that is equally developed on both the dorsal and ventral sides of the vertebral column. See also *heterocercal* and *homocercal*.

diplo- A combining form meaning double, twin, twofold, or twice.

diplotene See *meiosis*.

dipodia A developmental anomaly characterized by duplication of a foot.

diprosopus A fetal monster with a single trunk and normal limbs, but with varying degrees of duplication of the face.

dipsia Thirst. Often used as a word termination, denoting a condition relative to thirst, or the physiological state of the body leading to the ingestion of fluids.

dipygus A fetal monster with double pelvis.

Dirofilaria A genus of nematodes of the superfamily Filarioidea. *D. immitis* is the heartworm of the dog, cat, wolf, and fox (see *dirofilariasis*). *D. magalhaesi* and *D. louisianensis* may affect man.

dirofilariasis Infestation by *Dirofilaria immitis* (the heartworm), a species of nematodes that infect the dog, cat, wolf, fox, and muskrat. The females are viviparous, releasing highly motile microfilariae which appear in the peripheral circulation and can be detected in blood smears. Several genera of mosquitoes, including *Aedes*, *Culex*, and *Anopheles*, have been reported as vectors. The adult parasites, slender threadlike worms, are found in the heart, particularly the right ventricle, and the pulmonary artery. They may also be found in subcutaneous tissue, in the anterior chamber of the eye, and in pulmonary tissues. Infection is common in the southern and eastern parts of the United States, where it constitutes an important background disease for experimenters who use dogs as laboratory animals, this being particularly important in cardiovascular research.[21]

dis- A prefix denoting a reversal or separation, or a duplication.

disaccharidase An enzyme that hydrolyzes disaccharides.

discriminated Denoting a response brought under the control of stimulation by differential reinforcement (see *differentiation*). When applied to a stimulus the term refers to one differentially responded to by an animal.

discrimination A differential response, or the difference in response strength, to two or more stimuli.

discrimination training The experimental reinforcement of a response in the presence of a discriminating stimulus and failure to reinforce it in the presence of other stimuli, leading to a quantitative increase in the response given in the presence of the discriminating stimulus. See *discriminative stimulus*, under *stimulus*.

discriminative See under *stimulus*.

disease A definite morbid process having a characteristic train of symptoms; it may affect the whole body or any of its parts, and its etiology, pathology, and prognosis may be known or unknown.

disease model See *animal model*.

disinhibition In behavioral science, a term applied to the observation, in the course of extinction of a classical conditioned response, that an extraneous stimulus not previously present in the situation can, together with the conditioned stimulus, increase the magnitude of the conditioned response to a level greater than predicted from its magnitude in previous trials.

disintegration See *watery disintegration*.

disjunction The moving apart of chromosomes during anaphase. Failure of disjunction, or nondisjunction (q.v.), occurs as a chromosomal aberration.

disomus A double-bodied fetal monster.

Dispharynx nasuta Proventricular worm of the chicken, turkey, guinea fowl, pigeon, pheasant, ruffed grouse, and other gallinaceous birds.

displacement activity The occurrence of a response belonging to a ritualized sequence of behavior, but out of context in the situation confronting the animal. Such a response is quite often brought on by conflicts, e.g., grooming behavior in the herring gull during disputes of territorial claims.

distemper See *canine distemper*.

distomiasis Infestation with trematode parasites, principally of two families, Fasciolidae and Dicrocoeliidae; also known as fascioliasis, liver fluke disease, fascioloidiasis, and dicrocoeliasis. Some of the important members of this trematode group are *Fasciola hepatica*, which in its adult form is found in the liver, bile duct, and gallbladder of the cow, sheep, horse, goat, dog, rabbit, guinea pig, squirrel, deer, beaver, pig, and man; *Fascioloides magna*, the large liver fluke that occurs in cattle, deer, sheep, moose, the horse, and other animals; *Dicrocoelium dendriticum*, the lancet fluke of the Old World, which is capable of infecting the cow, sheep, goat, horse, camel, deer, elk, pig, rabbit, and man. The life cycle of this group is extremely complex, usually involving a free-living larva and one stage which inhabits a snail.[21]

dizygotic Denoting twins derived from separate ova. They may have separate or fused placental circulation. See *blood group chimerism*.

DNA Deoxyribonucleic acid.

dogfish Any of the cartilaginous fishes of the genera *Squalus* and *Mustelus*, of the chordate class Chondrichthyes, which include the sharks, rays, and chimeras. The dogfish is of considerable biological interest because it has been much studied as an example of chordate characteristics in comparative anatomy. It is also of interest because it maintains the osmolarity of its fluids against sea water by retention of urea (uremia).

Döhle body A lamellar aggregate of rough endoplasmic reticulum that appears in blood neutrophils during severe bacterial infection.

dolphin See *cetacean*.

dominance Expression of a gene in the heterozygous state, resulting in the typical phenotype.

   incomplete d. (partial d.; semidominance), partial expression of a gene in the heterozygous state, resulting in an intermediate phenotype. Cf. *codominance*.

dominant Denoting a gene that is fully expressed when present on only one of a pair of homologous chromosomes.

DON Trademark for 6-diazo-5-oxo-L-norleucine. See *azaserine*.

dopa-oxidase An enzyme that oxidizes dihydroxyphenylalanine to melanin in the skin, producing pigmentation.

doraphobia A morbid dread of the skin or fur of animals.

dormancy Reduced physiological level not well characterized. Cf. *hibernation*.

dornase A shortened term for deoxyribonuclease; sometimes used as a word termination, as in streptodornase.

dose-response curve A curve which when plotted shows the relationship between the dose of a drug or number of organisms and the biological response.

dove See *columbiform birds*.

Down's syndrome Mongolism; see *chromosomal aberrations*.

downy Denoting the surface of a colony of fungi covered with short, sparse to dense, aerial hyphae.

DPN Diphosphopyridine nucleotide, the former name for nicotinamide adenine dinucleotide.

dracunculiasis A disease caused by a species of nematodes (*Dracunculus medinensis*) 20 to 30 inches long; also known as Guinea worms or dragon worms. This parasite usually occurs in tropic or subtropical countries but is occasionally seen in North America, and may infect the dog, horse, cow, wolf, cat, monkey, baboon, and man. The worm matures in the subcutaneous tissue, from which the female deposits her living larvae through a small orifice at the tip of a small nodule formed in the skin by the parasite. The larvae then escape into the water to gain access to the intermediate host, a small copepod of the genus *Cyclops*. The larvae become infective and reach the definitive host when the copepod hosts are swallowed in contaminated drinking water. The larvae are then released from the intermediate hosts into the intestine and migrate to the subcutaneous tissues to reach adulthood.[21]

Dracunculus medinensis (Guinea worm; dragon worm) A nematode of the superfamily Dracunculoidea. See *dracunculiasis*.

drake See *anseriform birds*.

drive A hypothetical state of an animal, which is identified by gross changes in the relative frequency of broad classes of behavior; e.g., an animal is said to exhibit a hunger drive if it actively searches for food. The strength of the drive is related to the strength and frequency of the searching responses.

dromo- A combining form denoting relation to conduction, or to running.

dromophobia Morbid fear of running.

drone broodiness Morbid drone-laying.

drone-laying See *morbid drone-laying*.

dropsy (of fish) An infectious disease of uncertain etiology in domestic carp. Although clinical and epizootiologic evidence suggest a specific bacterial pathogen, the disease may occasionally be transmitted by cell-free filtrates. Antibiotics, however, often effect clinical cure. In Europe, where the disease has been extensively investigated, the majority opinion favors a bacterial cause.[114]

Drosophila See *fruit fly*.

drumstick A teardrop-shaped nuclear lobule present in segmented leukocytes of most female mammals, but absent in males. It is probably analogous to the Barr body of interphase cells and represents late-replicating X chromosome material (see under *chromosome*). A difference between the nuclei of male and female leukocytes is not seen in rats, mice, guinea pigs, chinchillas, or marsupials.

duck See *anseriform birds*.

Dutch shell disease A disease similar to or the same as maladie du pied (q.v.).

dwarfism The state of being an abnormally undersized individual. See *achondroplasia*.

dye A material used for staining or coloring. The dyes used in medicine may be divided into the following classes: (1) acridine, (2) azo, (3) fluorescein, (4) phenolphthalein, (5) triphenylmethane or rosaniline, (6) pyronidine. See individual dyes for description.[57]

anionic d., one in which the auxochromes are negatively charged sulfonic groups. Some ionic dyes are amphoteric and become ionic when the pH is above their isoelectric point.

cationic d., one in which the auxochrome is a positively charged amino group. The electrical charge of this dye is usually mobile and becomes a part of the resonance system which affects the color of the dye.

dys- A combining form signifying difficult, painful, bad, disordered, etc.; the opposite of *eu-*.

dysgerminoma A solid ovarian or testicular tumor derived from germinal epithelium that has not been differentiated to cells of either male or female type.

dysgonic Denoting a slow-growing fungal variant, especially *Microsporum canis* and *M. audouinii*.

dysmelia Malformation of a limb or limbs as a result of a disturbance in embryonic development. The term includes defects of excessive development as well as reduction deformities. See *phocomelia*.

dysplasia (of a joint) (splayleg, in the rabbit; hip dysplasia, in the dog and man) Congenital and presumptively hereditary congenital dysplasia of the hip and/or shoulder joint. The lesions include flattening of the head of the femur (and/or humerus); incorrect angulation of the femoral neck with a corresponding shallowness of the acetabulum (or glenoid fossa of the scapula); subluxation and dislocation, with production of a false joint; and chronic lesions of traumatic osteoarthritis as late sequelae. The condition is regarded as a variant of achondroplasia (chondrodystrophia fetalis), restricted to the hip and shoulder. In its severe lethal form, it has occurred in rabbits, calves, dogs (particularly the German Shepherd) and man.[69]

E

earthworm See *annelid*.

Eaton agent *Mycoplasma pneumoniae*.

E.B. virus Epstein-Barr virus.

ecchymosis An extravasation of blood in the order of 1 cm. in diameter on an epithelial, mucous, or other surface; a small hemorrhage. Cf. *petechia*.

ecdysis The molting of the outer layers of the body covering.

echino- A combining form denoting relationship to spines, or spiny.

echinococcosis A form of cestodiasis caused by cysts of the intermediate stage of *Echinococcus granulosus*, a tapeworm of dogs, foxes, wolves, and other carnivores. This parasite is of importance because of the effects of the larvae upon the intermediate hosts, which include sheep, goats, cattle, horses, deer, moose, and man. In man, echinococcosis (or hydatid disease) is serious because the cysts may reach any part of the body, especially the lung and liver, and also occasionally the brain. They are able to produce multiple cysts by replication within the body and may cause serious tissue damage by pressure on vital organs.[21, 136]

echinoderm   Any member of the phylum Echinodermata, characterized usually by five-parted radial symmetry, typified by the starfish, around an oral-aboral axis. The body wall is calcareous, usually forming a rigid or flexible exoskeleton with external spines. The digestive tract is complete, the coelom includes a water vascular system, and locomotion is accomplished with external tube feet. All forms are marine, usually free-living. A few forms are used as human food. Five living classes are recognized within the phylum: Crinoidea, the sea lilies and feather stars; Asteroidea, the starfishes; Ophiuroidea, the brittlestars and basketstars; Echinoidea, the sea urchins and sand dollars; and Holothuroidea, the sea cucumbers.

Echinolaelaps echidnius   See *arthropod parasites*, under *rat*.

echinulate   Spiny-surfaced fungus, as *Microsporum canis* macrospores.

echolocation   The system by which certain mammals, as bats and porpoises, determine the distance and direction of objects by emitting sounds of a certain frequency that produce an echo.

echovirus (enteric cytopathogenic human orphan virus)   See *picornavirus*.

eclipse phase   The period between infection of a cell and the earliest time when infectious virus can be demonstrated.

ECMO virus (enteric cytopathogenic monkey orphan virus)   See *simian virus*.

ecological niche   The position of an organism in its ecosystem.

ecology   The study of the relationships between an organism, its territorial cohabitants, and the environment.

ecomania   An attitude of mind that is dominating toward members of the family but humble toward those in authority.

ecopartner any species of organisms (whether human, anoman, or vegetable) among the group of species sharing an ecosystem (R. W. Leader).

ecophenotype   A nongenetic modification in response to environment.

ecosystem   The basic fundamental unit in ecology, comprising the living organisms and the nonliving elements interacting in a certain defined area.

ecthyma of sheep   See *contagious ecthyma of sheep*.

ecto-   A prefix denoting situated on, without, or on the outside.

ectocardia   Congenital displacement of the heart, either inside or outside the thorax.

ectoenzyme   An enzyme that is secreted from a cell into the surrounding medium; an extracellular enzyme. Cf. *endoenzyme*.

-ectomize   A word termination denoting deprivation by excision, as in thyroidectomize, adrenalectomize, etc. By extension, used in terms to designate destruction or deprivation by other methods as well.

ectomorphy   A type of body build in which tissues derived from the ectoderm predominate. There is relative preponderance of linearity and fragility, with large surface area and thin muscles and subcutaneous tissue.

ectoparasite   A parasite that lives on the outside of the body of the host.

ectopia   Displacement or malposition, especially if congenital.

ectothrix   A dermatophyte that parasitizes the hair, with vegetative hyphae both inside the hair shaft and on the hair surface, and with arthrospores almost entirely on the surface of the hair. Cf. *endothrix*.

ectrodactyly   Congenital absence of all or of only part of a digit.

ectromelia   1. (Mousepox, maladie du Marchal) A poxvirus infection of laboratory mice (*Mus musculis*), rare in the United States, more common in Europe. The virus is closely related antigenically to vaccinia, smallpox, rabbitpox, and monkey pox viruses. Marchal originally described the disease as occurring in acute and chronic phases, but it is now recognized that the full spectrum of virus-host relationships are seen in spontaneous infections, including latent or inapparent infection. Acute and peracute forms are characterized by general malaise and high mortality following a short incubation period (five to seven days). The gross lesions include massive necrosis of the liver and duodenal hemorrhage. The chronic phase resembles a typical pox disease, with skin eruptions, swelling of the extremities, and gangrenous amputation (ectromelia) of the extremities. Inclusion (Marchal) bodies may be easily demonstrated in the skin, gut, and pancreas, rarely in the liver. Diagnosis may be established by a specific immunofluorescent, or hemagglutination-inhibition, test employing immune (survivor) serum, demonstration of inclusion bodies in typical lesions, and virus isolation in susceptible mice, chick embryo CAM, or tissue cultures. A nonhemagglutinating (IHD-T) variant of vaccinia virus is widely used as a vaccine for mice, which are immunized by tail scarification. The experimental disease in mice has been extensively investigated as a model for poxvirus infections.[27] 2. Gross hypoplasia or aplasia of one or more long bones of one or more limbs. The term includes *amelia, hemimelia*, and *phocomelia*.

edeine   A basic polypeptide antibiotic produced by *Bacillus brevis*, which inhibits gram-positive and gram-negative bacteria, some fungi and yeasts, and mammalian neoplastic cells in tissue culture, by interference with DNA synthesis.[36, 49]

edentia   Absence of the teeth.

EDIM virus　See *infantile diarrhea of mice*.

Egtved virus　The agent of a severe disease of salmonid fishes (variously known as viral hemorrhagic septicemia, infectious kidney swelling, and liver degeneration), with a mortality rate up to 75 per cent. The course is strongly influenced by nutritional factors and temperature. The acute disease is characterized by slow spiral swimming and sluggishness, and by dark pigmentation, exophthalmia, and anemia. The liver is pale, and the kidneys are swollen and exhibit hemorrhages. The disease closely mimics chinook salmon disease. The virus is cultivable in fish cell cultures.[114]

Ehrlichia　A genus of rickettsiae. See table accompanying *Rickettsia*.

Ehrlich tumor　An undifferentiated tumor that originated as a spontaneous carcinoma of the mammary gland in a stock mouse in the laboratory of Paul Ehrlich, Frankfurt, Germany, approximately in 1906. Ehrlich selected a large number of solid tumor variants from the original in efforts to develop early malignancy. The "Frankfurt" tumor is probably the solid variant that was brought to the United States. In 1932, H. Loewenthal and G. Jahn developed an ascites variant by selective transplantation of ascitic fluids of mice inoculated intraperitoneally with cells from solid Ehrlich tumors. Based on this model, ascites variants of many rat, mouse, and chicken strains have been developed. As a result the term "ascites tumor" has come to be associated with a process whereby, following the inoculation of tumor cells into a body cavity, the tumor cells multiply, and there is an effusion of fluid containing a suspension of neoplastic cells. The ascites tumor technic has become a useful experimental tool because, since precise numbers of tumor cells can be implanted, the growth and/or regression of the tumor can be quantified. It is used extensively in this context in cancer chemotherapy programs.[150]

Eimeria　A genus of parasitic protozoa. For various species, see table accompanying *Coccidia*, and see *protozoan parasites*, under *rat*.

elapid　See table accompanying *snake*.

Elapidae　See table accompanying *snake*.

elasmobranch　See *cartilaginous fishes*.

elastinase　An enzyme that dissolves elastic tissue.

electrobiology　The study of electric phenomena in the living body, whether developed by vital or other processes.

electron-dense　Denoting an area of tissue, cells, organisms, or other substance that impedes the passage of electrons, resulting in a relatively unexposed portion of film in an electron micrograph. Density is related to the ability of the area to combine with fixatives and stains such as osmium, gluteraldehyde, lead, etc.

Electron Microscopy Society of America　Sperry Rand Research Center, North Road, Sudbury, Mass. 01776.

electrophoresis　A technic for the separation of charged particles in an electrical field. It requires carefully defined conditions of pH and ionic strength in a supporting medium such as starch, paper, agar, or polyacrylamide gels.[32]

electrothanasia　Death by electricity; electrocution.

embolism　The sudden blocking of an artery or vein by a clot or obstruction that has been carried to the location by the blood current.

　aortic e., impaction of an embolus in the iliac branches of the aorta, seen in middle-aged cats. It is sudden in onset and characterized by partial or complete paralysis of the hind limbs. The emboli are thought to originate in the left atrium of the heart.[142]

embolus　A solid material such as a clot or other plug which is forced into a vessel of smaller lumen and obstructs the circulation. Emboli can be composed of air, neoplastic cells, fat, clotted blood, bacteria, or other materials. Cf. *thrombus*.

embryoma (embryonal carcinosarcoma)　A tumor made up of two or more kinds of tissues which may be well differentiated histologically and sometimes functionally, but are entirely devoid of organization. Teeth and hair are particularly common.

emotion　See *emotional behavior*, under *behavior*.

encephalitis　An inflammation of the brain, which frequently also involves the meninges, in which case it is referred to as meningoencephalitis.

　California e., a nonfatal viral infection of man, rabbits, squirrels, and domestic animals, caused by an arbovirus. The infection is propagated by the mosquitoes *Culex tarsalis* and *Aedes dorsalis*. In addition to the original strain, four new strains of virus have been isolated that could be classified in the California group of viruses.[16]

　Dawson's e. (subacute sclerosing panencephalitis [SSPE]), a progressive disease of the central nervous system of children. The presence of inclusion bodies made up of structures which appear to be nucleocapsids of a myxovirus indicates that it may be caused by a latent viral infection.

　fox e., an acute infectious disease of foxes caused by the virus of infectious canine hepatitis. Affected foxes, usually the young, suffer convulsions and subsequent lethargy, with a possibility of recurrence of convulsions.

　Japanese B e., a viral disease of man and anomen which is prevalent in Japan, Korea, China, and Indochina and may be identical with a disease called Australian X-disease, or Murray Valley encephalitis. The disease is caused by a mosquito-borne arbovirus, and surveys have shown a mild infection of horses, cattle, and swine in endemic areas. Some fatal cases in horses in Malaya and of cattle and swine in Japan have been described.[16]

　Murray Valley e. (Australian-X disease), see *Japanese B e.*

　Russian spring-summer e. (Central European tick-borne fever), a viral infection of man and anomen characterized by an initial influenza-like phase followed by a second stage of meningoencephalitis. Virus may be present in the mammary glands of infected goats, cows, and sheep. The agent is an arborvirus, and the vector and reservoir of infection is the tick *Ixodes ricinus*.[16]

St. Louis e., a viral infection of man that occurs in the central and western parts of the United States. Chickens are easily infected with this RNA arbovirus. The *Culex* mosquito and the red chicken mite (*Dermanyssus gallinae*) could transmit the infection to chickens.[16]

encephalitozoonosis See *nosematosis*.

encephalo- A combining form denoting relationship to the brain.

encephalomalacia Softening of the brain characterized by loss of myelin and the presence of phagocytic cells containing lipid material.

avian e., a disease of young chickens caused by lack of vitamin E and characterized by ataxia and general incoordination. Several areas of the brain, particularly the cerebellum, exhibit severe encephalomalacia, small hemorrhages, and edematous swelling of meninges.[11]

encephalomyelitis Inflammation involving both the brain and the spinal cord.

avian e. (epidemic tremor), a severe disease of young chickens caused by a picornavirus and characterized by degeneration of neurons in the pons, medulla, and anterior horns of the spinal cord. It must be differentiated from avian encephalomalacia.[11]

baby pig e., inflammation of the brain and spinal cord in piglets caused by a virus which produces hemagglutination of chicken erythrocytes and forms multinucleated giant cells in tissue culture. It is characterized by depression, loss of condition, hyperesthesia, incoordination, and occasionally vomiting. Immunologically this disease is different from Teschen's disease, but it is indistinguishable in its histological reaction. See also *porcine e.*

equine e., encephalomyelitis that is widespread in horses throughout the United States, and caused by a virus that is frequently the cause of encephalomyelitis in man. The three principal strains, the viruses of Western, Eastern, and Venezuelan equine encephalomyelitis, are antigenically distinct from each other. All three strains are transmitted by mosquitoes. Wild birds are the principal reservoirs of the infection between outbreaks in the equine and human population. The life cycle in nature is not well understood. Infections of man and horse are probably incidental occurrences unimportant in perpetuation of the virus. The belief that horses may transmit the infection to man is erroneous, the disease always resulting from bites by infected insects.

murine e., Theiler's mouse e.

ovine e., a viral disease of sheep in Scotland and England, also known as louping ill,

which is a descriptive term for the peculiar "louping" gait of affected animals. It occasionally affects man as a nonfatal, mild infection of laboratory workers, and has been experimentally transmitted to mice, pigs, and monkeys. In mice, it is uniformly a fatal disease marked by diffuse encephalomyelitis.

sporadic bovine e. (Buss disease), a disease of cattle, especially young calves, characterized by depression, fever, weakness, emaciation, and prostration. The etiologic agent is a member of the psittacosis-lymphogranuloma (*Chlamydia*) group.

porcine e. (Teschen disease; porcine poliomyelitis), a viral disease of swine that occurs in many countries of central and western Europe, but is not clearly recognized in the Western Hemisphere. Teschen disease is similar to poliomyelitis in man, in that the virus may be isolated from the digestive tract and causes lesions in the ventral columns of the spinal cord. The lesions of the porcine disease are much more severe and extensive in the cerebral cortex and cerebellum than those of human poliomyelitis, and there is no immunological relationship between the two viruses. See also *baby pig e.*

Theiler's mouse e. (Theiler's disease; mouse poliomyelitis; murine encephalomyelitis), a spontaneous encephalomyelitis of mice characterized by progressive flaccid paralysis, particularly of the hind legs. Although in colonies, only a few mice may exhibit symptoms, there may be large numbers without apparent illness which may carry the virus in the intestinal tract. The disease can be exacerbated by nonspecific stresses and also can be detected by intracranial inoculation of filtrate into normal susceptible mice. Because of the possible confusion in interpretation of experiments, mouse colonies should be frequently checked for the presence of this virus.

Enteric infection of newborn mice is common; the neonate acquires the virus early in life and is protected by maternal antibody in milk from the lethal effects of (but not infection by) the virus. This leads to a low-grade persistent intestinal infection accompanied by limited serologic response in adult life. The first isolation, done by Theiler, came from a spontaneously infected mouse with flaccid paralysis of the hind limbs. Theiler's original (TO) isolate when inoculated intracranially elicits acute necrosis of ganglion cells of the anterior horn of the spinal cord and cerebrum, followed by neuronophagia and perivascular cuffing. Clinical signs include ruffled fur, circling, and paralysis. In later experiments, viruses called FA and GDVII were found which could cause clinical "Theiler's disease" and which proved to be antigenically related to the original isolate.

Even in colonies with widespread endemic infection, the incidence of spontaneous mouse poliomyelitis is very low (estimated at 1 to 10 per 10,000), and the occasional infection of the central nervous system, as in human poliomyelitis, represents only a biological accident of little significance in the natural ecology of the agent. Diagnosis is established by the characteristic lesions, isolation of virus from feces, and serologic (hemagglutination-inhibition) evidence of infection.[27, 63]

encephalomyocarditis virus See *reovirus-3.*

encephalopathy Any degenerative disease of the brain.

   mink e., a progressive degenerative disease of the central nervous system affecting mink; it may be a form of scrapie.[14, 44]

encystation A stage in the life cycle of a parasite that involves the change of the trophozoite into a cyst.

endemic 1. Present in a community at all times, but occurring in only small numbers of cases. 2. A disease of low morbidity that is constantly present in a human community. Cf. *enzootic* and *epidemic.*

endo-, end- A prefix denoting an inward situation, within.

endocardial fibroelastosis See under *fibroelastosis.*

endocarditis Inflammation of the endocardium, or lining of the heart. The most common form of this disease is valvular endocarditis, in which the inflammatory lesions are located on the heart valve, sometimes referred to as vegetative endocarditis or cauliflower lesions. The lesions are most frequently caused by the localization of bacteria or occasionally by nematode parasites, as seen in strongyle infections of the horse. The agents of endocarditis in anomen are most commonly *Streptococcus, Shigella, Staphylococcus, Corynebacterium, Erysipelothrix,* and occasionally *Neisseria.* No animal counterpart of rheumatic endocarditis as seen in children has yet been discovered in anomen. See also *valvular fibrosis.*

endocrinology The study of the ductless or endocrine glands and their secretions, which regulate the rate of various physiological processes of the body. These processes are concerned with all phases of health and disease, and there is most likely an endocrine component in all pathologic conditions. The anterior pituitary gland is the hormone-regulating center of most other endocrine glands in the body. And since the anterior pituitary gland receives neurohumoral messages from the hypothalamus, it is also connected with other parts of the central nervous system. Neurohumoral mechanisms are of great importance in the control of endocrine homeostasis. The vast uncharted sea of psychosis, neuroendocrine disorders, and the general adaptation syndrome (q.v.), and how these relate to pathologic manifestations in the body provide some of the most important areas for exploration and elucidation of the interplay between man, anomen, and their environment.[144]

endocytosis Engulfment by a cell of solid or fluid material. Cf. *phagocytosis, pinocytosis,* and *ropheocytosis.*

endoenzyme An intracellular enzyme; an enzyme that is retained in a cell and does not normally diffuse out of the cell into the surrounding medium. Cf. *ectoenzyme.*

Endolimax nana See *protozoan parasites,* under *rat.*

endomitosis Reproduction of nuclear elements not followed by chromosome movements and cytoplasmic division.

endomorphy A type of body build in which tissues derived from the endoderm predominate. There is relative preponderance of soft roundness throughout the body, with large digestive viscera and accumulations of fat, the body usually presenting a large trunk and thighs and tapering extremities.

endo-oxidase Oxidase occurring within a cell, such as a bacterium.

endoparasite A parasite that lives within the body of its host.

endopeptidase A proteolytic enzyme that is capable of hydrolyzing peptide linkages in the interior of the peptide chain.

endoplasmic reticulum (ergastoplasm) A membranous labyrinth within the cytoplasm. It is continuous with the outer nuclear envelope and the plasma membrane. In areas where ribosomes are adjacent to its surface, it is known as rough endoplasmic reticulum. The cavity of the rough form is believed to be the exit for certain cell secretory products, as gamma globulin from plasma cells.[38]

endopolyploid Having reduplicated chromatin within an intact nucleus, with or without an increase in the number of chromosomes (applied only to cells and tissues).

endothrix A fungus causing dermatomycosis in which the growth of mycelium and the formation of spores takes place entirely within the hair shaft. Cf. *ectothrix.*

endotoxin A heat-stable toxin present within the bacterial cell, which is not released into the surrounding environment unless the organism bursts. Endotoxins are found particularly in enteric bacteria, in which they occur as lipid-polysaccharide-polypeptide complexes in the cell wall.

-ene A suffix used in chemistry to indicate an unsaturated hydrocarbon containing one double bond.

engram A lasting mark or trace. A definite and permanent trace left by a stimulus in the protoplasm of a cell or tissue. In behavioral science, a hypothetical locus in the nervous system or a persistent activity presumably anatomically or physiologically identifiable, having developed as a result of some psychic experience. A latent memory picture.

enolase An enzyme of muscle in the Embden-Meyerhof pathway, which converts 2-phospho-D-glycerate to phospho-enol-pyruvate using Mg^{++} as a co-factor.

Entamoeba muris See *protozoan parasites,* under *rat.*

enteritis Inflammation of the intestine, particularly the small intestine.

   mucoid e. of rabbits (bloat; scours), one of the most important spontaneous diseases of dometic rabbits (*Oryctolagus cuniculus*), and one of the least understood. It is a disease of weanling rabbits (the six to twelve week age group), although it may affect older and younger rabbits with less frequency. It is characterized by acute onset with anorexia and weight loss. The posture is hunched, the eyes dull, and the animal is inactive. Thirst is a constant finding as is diarrhea, which extensively soils the hind legs and perineum. The animals appear to be in pain, and tooth-grinding is a common sign. Death occurs in 75 per cent of cases approximately 12 hours after these signs are noticed. Large quantities of albuminoid, gelatinous mucus are observed in the droppings. Necropsy reveals little, other than dehydration and gas-filled intestines. All other organs are grossly normal, but microscopically the source of mucus is seen to be the tremendously hyperplastic globlet cells of the colon and cecum. The diagnosis is based on case history and necropsy findings.

Many approaches have been made to ascertain the etiology of the disease, but those designed to isolate or pass an infectious agent have failed, as have experiments attempting to induce the disease by premature introduction to adult food. Those favoring the latter factor as the cause have named the disease neonatal hypoamalasemia.

One problem complicating progress in the control of mucoid enteritis is the frequent occurrence in rabbits of the same age group of a similar but morphologically distinct entity variously named acute hemorrhagic enterocolitis, hemorrhagic typhlitis, and young rabbit enteritis. It is not understood whether this condition is a morphologic variant (since it behaves epizootiologically in a manner identical to that of mucoid enteritis), or whether it has a separate cause. Nor has it been experimentally reproduced. No treatment or method of prevention or control is known.

regional e., regional ileitis; see under *ileitis.*

viral e. of mink, an acute fatal mucoid enteritis of mink caused by a virus closely related to the feline panleukopenia virus.

entero- A combining form denoting relationship to the intestines.

Enterobius vermicularis A nematode (pinworm) of the superfamily Oxyuroidea that infects only man. The life cycle is direct and takes place within the host's intestine. The infected eggs hatch after they reach the duodenum, and the larvae become mature when they reach the large intestine. This life cycle takes about two months.[21]

enterolithiasis The presence of calculi (enteroliths) in the intestinal tract of an animal. Rectal enteroliths occur as single or agglomerated, spherical or polymorphous concretions in adult queen honeybees.

enterovirus See *picornavirus.*

Entner-Doudoroff pathway The metabolic breakdown of fructose, mannose, and glucose through 6-phosphogluconic acid and 2-keto-3-deoxy-6-phosphogluconic acid to form pyruvic acid and 3-phosphoglyceraldehyde.

entomo- A combining form denoting relationship to an insect, or to insects.

entomogenous 1. Denoting organisms growing in or on the bodies of insects; the term connotes a parasitic or other intimate symbiotic relationship. 2. Derived from insects, their bites, etc.

entomology That branch of zoology which deals with the study of insects.

entomophagous Insectivorous; the consumption of insects or their parts.

entomophilic Pertaining to the associations between insects and plant microorganisms, insects and protozoa, and insects and nematodes.

entomophobia Morbid dread of insects (mites, ticks, etc.).

entomophyte A plant living within or on the body of an insect.

entomophytic Pertaining to almost any relationship between plant microorganisms (bacteria and fungi) and insects.

entophyte A parasitic plant organism living within the body of its host.

envenomization The poisonous effects caused by bites, stings, or effluvia of venomous animals. See names of individual animals.

enzootic 1. Present in an animal community at all times, but occurring in only small numbers of cases. 2. A disease of low morbidity, but constantly present in an animal community. Cf. *endemic* and *epizootic.*

enzootic abortion of ewes See under *abortion.*

enzootic intestinal adenocarcinoma Terminal ileitis of hamsters; see under *ileitis.*

enzootic pneumonia of calves See *calf pneumonia,* under *pneumonia.*

enzyme A protein capable of accelerating or producing by catalytic action some change in a substrate. Enzymes display an unusual degree of specificity with regard to substrate on which they act and the type of action they catalyze.[90, 118] Cf. *apoenzyme, coenzyme,* and *prosthetic group.*

classification of e's, in the past, the naming of enzymes has been done in a very haphazard fashion based on substrate and type of action. The classification recommended by the Commission on Enzymes of the International Union of Biochemistry in 1961 is given in the accompanying table.[90, 118]

condensing e., an enzyme of the Krebs cycle and responsible for the conversion of oxaloacetate to citrate.

inducible e. (adaptable or adaptive e.), an enzyme whose production requires or is markedly stimulated by a specific compound. See *inducer.*

repressible e., an enzyme the production of which can be repressed by certain metabolites.

enzyme defect See *inborn error of metabolism,* under *metabolism.*

enzyme induction The ability of a cell to

MAJOR CLASSES OF ENZYMES

Oxidoreductases	catalyze oxidation reduction reactions
Transferases	catalyze group transfer reactions
Hydrolases	catalyze hydrolytic reactions
Lyases	catalyze reactions involving the removal of a group leaving a double bond, or the addition of a group to a double bond.
Isomerases	catalyze reactions involving isomerization
Ligases or synthetases	catalyze reactions involving the joining together of two molecules coupled with the breakdown of a pyrophosphate bond of ATP or similar triphosphate

produce the specific enzyme required to metabolize a given substrate, such as the induction of β-galactosidase by cells of *Escherichia coli* when grown in the presence of lactose. This mechanism was formerly known as adaptive enzyme formation.

enzyme repression   A decrease in net enzyme activity which may result from the exposure of cells to the product of the enzyme. It is commonly observed in the response of autotrophic bacteria to the presence of an amino acid in their media: the activity of the particular enzymes concerned with the synthesis of the amino acid, e.g., histidine, are selectively decreased. This decrease may result from the inhibition of the enzyme activity by metabolites of subsequent steps in the biosynthetic pathway (allosteric inhibition) or by inhibition of the transcription or translation of the genomic information coding for the enzyme.

eosin   A rose-colored acid xanthene dye derived from coal tar. Solubility at 15° C.: water 44 per cent, absolute alcohol 2 per cent, and glycerol 20 per cent. Used for staining glycogen and galactans, as a counterstain for acetylation-deacetylation technics, and in Verhoeff's elastica stain to demonstrate elastic or collagen fibers. Combined with methylene blue, it is used to stain Negri bodies.[57, 153]

    e. Y, a water-soluble stain, widely used as a plasma stain.[57, 153]

eosinophil   A type of motile phagocytic polymorphonuclear leukocyte with cytoplasmic granules that have strong affinity for acid aniline dyes and contain various hydrolytic enzymes, thus being classified as lysosomes.

eosophobia   Morbid fear or dread of daybreak.

ependymoma A(22)   A tumor developed by selective transplantation of an original mixed cell glioma that was induced by intracranial injection of 20-methylcholanthrene in an inbred mouse of A/St strain. The original tumor was produced in the laboratory of H. M. Zimmerman at the Montefiore Hospital in New York City in 1948, some 354 days after injection. The tumor grows progressively in 100 per cent of A/St strain mice, killing the host approximately 21 days after transplantation, without metastasis.[150]

Eperythrozoon coccoides   See *eperythrozoonosis.*

eperythrozoonosis (murine)   A disease caused by a reticuloendothelial rickettsial parasite of the laboratory mouse, *Eperythrozoon coccoides.* Infections in intact mice are usually inapparent, but splenectomy results in the appearance of large numbers of organisms in the blood. *E. coccoides* is about 200μ in size, appears in the form of delicate rings on stained blood films, is sensitive to organic arsenicals and tetracycline, and has been passed into other susceptible mice and embryonated eggs, but not other media. Spontaneous infections are believed to be horizontally transferred by blood-sucking lice (*Polyplax serrata*).

In experimental infections, a prepatent phase ensues, following which large numbers (exceeding 10^8 eperythrozoa per ml.) may be found in the blood, but then the numbers decline over a period of months, with a variable number of recrudescences, until the infection is eliminated. Complement-fixing, but not neutralizing, antibodies have been found in recovered mice. The affinity of the parasite for the reticuloendothelial system is believed to underlie its prominence in potentiating a number of viral infections, including mouse hepatitis, lymphocytic choriomeningitis, and lactic dehydrogenase-elevating virus disorders, and in increasing the susceptibility of mice to bacterial endotoxin.[20, 159]

ephemeral fever (three-day sickness; bovine epizootic fever)   A viral disease of cattle characterized by high temperature, stiffness, and lameness. The disease appears to be transmitted by biting insects of the genus *Culicoides.*

epicarcinogen   An agent that increases the effect of a carcinogen.

epidemic   1. Attacking many people in any region at the same time; widely diffused and rapidly spreading. 2. A disease of high morbidity that is only occasionally present in a human community. 3. A season of the extensive prevalence of any particular disease. Cf. *epizootic* and *endemic.*

epidemic (epizootic) diarrhea of infant mice   *Infantile diarrhea of mice.*

epidemic tremor   Avian encephalomyelitis; see under *encephalomyelitis.*

epidemiology   The field of science dealing with the relationships of the various factors that determine the frequencies and distributions of an infectious process, a disease, or a physiological state in a human community.

epidermoid   1. Resembling the epidermis. 2. A cerebral or meningeal tumor formed by inclusion of epidermal cells from the skin or mucous membrane.

epidermoma   A cutaneous outgrowth, such as a wart.

Epidermophyton   A member of Fungi Imperfecti that develops a cottony colony with a greenish-yellow aerial mycelium and occasionally attacks the skin and nails of man and causes tinea pedis (athlete's foot).

epigenetics   The science concerned with the causal analysis of development, particularly with studies of the mechanisms by which genes express their phenotypic effects.

epiphyte   1. A plant organism growing upon another plant. 2. A plant organism parasitic upon the exterior of an animal body.

epiphytic   1. Pertaining to or caused by epiphytes. 2. A widely diffused outbreak of an infectious disease in plants.

episome   A genetic element of an accessory nature in addition to the genome. There are two distinct states, the autonomous independently replicating cytoplasmic state and the integrated state characterized by a linkage relationship with the chromosomes. See *temperate bacteriophage*, under *bacteriophage*.

epistatic gene   See under *gene*.

epistemology   The science of the methods and validity of knowledge.

epistemophilia   Marked or abnormal interest in learning.

epithelioma   An epithelial cancer; a malignant tumor consisting mainly of epithelial cells and primarily derived from the skin or mucous surface. See *carcinoma*.

epizootic   1. Attacking many animals (an-omen) in any region at the same time; widely diffused and rapidly spreading. 2. A disease of high morbidity that is only occasionally present in an animal community. Cf. *enzootic* and *epidemic*.

epizootiology   The study of epizootics; the field of science dealing with the relationships of the various factors that determine the frequencies and distributions of infectious diseases among anomen.

epon   A plastic embedding material used in electron microscopy.

eponym   A name or phrase formed from or including the name of a person, as Bang's disease and bursa of Fabricius.

epornithology   The scientific study of diseases of high morbidity that are only occasionally present in a bird community.

epornitic   1. Attacking many birds in any region at the same time. 2. A disease of high morbidity that is only occasionally present in a bird population.

Epstein-Barr virus (E.B. virus; EBV)   A herpesvirus first isolated from Burkitt's lymphoma and studied as a possible cause of infectious mononucleosis and neoplastic disease of lymphoid tissue.

equilibrium dialysis   See under *dialysis*.

equine arteritis   See under *arteritis*.

equine encephalomyelitis   See under *encephalomyelitis*.

equine infectious anemia   See under *anemia*.

equine rhinopneumonitis   See under *rhinopneumonitis*.

equine virus abortion   See *abortion*, and see *rhinopneumonitis*.

Equus   The genus that contains the horse, *E. caballus*, and the ass, *E. asinus*.

eremophobia   Morbid fear of being alone.

erepsin   Any of a group of enzymes in the small intestine that catalyze the hydrolysis of partially digested proteins to produce amino acids. See *peptidase*.

ergasiophobia   1. Morbid aversion to work.

ergastoplasm   Endoplasmic reticulum.

ergo-, ergaso-   A combining form denoting relationship to work.

ergomaniac   A person morbidly desirous of being continually at work.

erotographomania   Morbid interest in writing love letters.

erotomania   Morbid exaggeration of sexual behavior or reaction.

erotophobia   Morbid dislike for sexual love.

error   In behavioral science, any response or set of responses, the occurrence of which delays reinforcement, as entry into a blind alley during maze running.

   anticipatory e., an error in the occurrence of a behavior chain that occupies a position in the chain earlier than that in which it would lead to reinforcement. See *behavior chain*.

   inborn e., see under *metabolism*.

   perseverative e., an error in the acquisition of a behavior chain in which the error occurs at a position in the chain following that in which it would lead to reinforcement. See *behavior chain*.

erysipelas (swine)   Infection associated with *Erysipelothrix insidiosa (rhusiopathiae)* in swine and other anomen, and termed erysipeloid in man. The infection is typically septicemic in acute phases in certain species, e.g., turkeys, domestic swine (diamond skin disease), and research cetaceans, and is usually associated with wound infection in man. *E. insidiosa*, the only medically important member of the genus, is a gram-positive bacillus. Prophylaxis may be accomplished with bacterins or modified live erysipelas vaccines used at six month intervals.[11, 16]

erythrism   The abnormal replacement in birds of all or almost all eumelanin (and possibly phaeomelanin) by erythromelanin, giving rise to a chestnut-red plumage.[112] See also *leucism, melanism,* and *schizochroism*.

erythro-   A combining form meaning red, or denoting a relationship to red.

erythroblastoma   A tumor-like mass composed of nucleated red blood corpuscles.

erythroblastosis   1. The presence of erythroblasts in the circulating blood; erythroblastemia. 2. A disease of fowl marked by an increase in the number of immature red blood cells in the circulating blood; erythroleukosis.

e. fetalis, a hemolytic anemia (q.v.) of the fetus or newborn infant, caused by the transplacental transmission of maternally formed antibody, usually secondary to an incompatibility between the blood group of the mother and that of her offspring. It is characterized by increased numbers of nucleated red cells in the peripheral blood, hyperbilirubinemia, and extramedullary hematopoiesis.

erythrocyte fragility A measure of the resistance of erythrocytes to hemolysis, which may increase or decrease in disease. It is of special interest in idiopathic hemolytic anemia. The approximate normal values for some species are given in the accompanying table.

erythromycin The most important member of the macrolide group of antibiotics. It is a product of a species of *Streptomyces* and has a medium spectrum, being active against many gram-positive bacteria but against only a few gram negative bacteria. The mechanisms of the activity of erythromycin are not well understood but are probably based on interference with protein synthesis at the ribosomal level.[36, 49]

erythrophobia 1. A neurotic manifestation marked by blushing on the slightest provocation. 2. Morbid fear of blushing. 3. Morbid aversion to red.

erythrosin B An acid xanthene dye. Solubility at 15° C.: water 10 per cent, absolute alcohol 5 per cent, and glycerol 12 per cent. It exhibits a bathochromic effect in the presence of a chromotrope. In combination with cyanin, it is used to stain cellulose and lignified tissues.[57, 153]

es Nietsche's term for the metaphysical incomprehensible something at the very bottom of human nature, being lower than the conscious ego and even lower than the Freudian subconscious.

escape See under *behavior* and *conditioning.*

Escherichia coli (*Bacterium coli*) A small gram-negative bacillus normally found in the intestinal tract of man and anomen. Strains containing somatic K antigen appear more toxic and resistant to phagocytosis or action of antibody.[36] Pathogenic strains of *E. coli* cause scours in calves, septicemia and diarrhea in lambs, abortion in mares and ewes, Hjarre's disease (coli-granuloma) in chickens, and edema disease in swine.

-esis Word termination denoting state or condition.

estivation (summer sleep) A dormant physiological state similar to hibernation, so called because animals that manifest it appear to be retreating from seasonal heat and lack of water. The distinction is that estivating animals enter that state to survive hot, dry weather, whereas their counterparts hibernate to pass the winter.

estrogenic activity unit The estrus-producing activity represented in 0.1 microgram of the International Standard estrone.

estrous cycle Cycle of sexual activity. See table of Mammalian Reproduction Data, accompanying *mammal.*

estrus The stage of the estrous cycle at which the female will accept the male and is capable of conception. See table accompanying *mammal.*

ethnography A description of the races of men.

ethnology The science that deals with the races of men, their descent, relationships, etc.

ethologist A scientist skilled in the study of comparative animal behavior, frequently with background training in zoology.

ethology The scientific study of animal behavior, particularly of behavior in the natural state, the evolution of behavior, and its biologic significance.

etiology The study or theory of the causation of any disease; the sum of knowledge regarding causes.

eu- A combining form meaning well, easily, or good; the opposite of *dys-.*

euchromatin The gene-bearing fraction of chromatin, composed of deoxyribonucleic acid and basic protein. Cf. *heterochromatin.*

eugenics Alteration of the human genotype by selective breeding of those found to have desirable genes (positive eugenics) and discouraging reproduction of those possessing undesirable genes (negative eugenics). The greatest problems in achieving this "ideal" situation are, of course, in deciding what is desirable and who shall separate the desirable from the undesirable. Cf. *euphenics.*

Euglena A genus of flagellate protozoa frequently used in genetic studies.

euphenics Control of expression of unfavorable genes by treatment or manipulation; "genetic engineering." Cf. *eugenics.*

euploid 1. Having a balanced set or sets of

Normal Values of Erythrocyte Fragility*

Species	Per cent of Saline Solution	
	Minimum Resistance	Maximum Resistance
Canine	0.50	0.32
Equine	0.56	0.39
Bovine	0.66	0.44
Feline	0.72	0.46
Ovine	0.76	0.40
Caprine	0.74	0.60

*Adapted from O. W. Schalm: Veterinary Hematology. 2nd ed. Lea & Febiger, Philadelphia, 1965.

chromosomes, in any number. 2. An individual or cell having a balanced set or sets of chromosomes, in any number.

European viper See table accompanying *snake*.

euthanasia A term taken from the Greek *eu* (well) and *thanatos* (death), but in practice used to mean painless death. Different connotations, however, are used for certain circumstances. The infliction of painless and presumably desired death for the alleviation of suffering comes closest to the original intent of the word. The words euthanasia and sacrifice are both used for the deliberate killing of experimental animals at the termination of an experiment or for the purpose of postmortem examination. Neither expresses precisely the scientific purpose involved. "Mercy killing" is a lay expression for euthanasia.[45]

euthenics Improvement of the well-being and efficiency of mankind by control of environmental factors.

evolution 1. An unrolling. 2. A process of development in which an organ or organism becomes more and more complex by the differentiation of its parts; a continuous and progressive change according to certain laws and by means of resident forces.

    e. of immune response, see *phylogeny of immunoglobulins*, under *immunoglobulin*.

evolutionary rate The comparative rapidity of evolution of a species. Rapid evolution is referred to as tachytelic, slow rate is bradytelic, and expected or average rate is horotelic.

ex- A prefix meaning away from, without, or outside, and sometimes used to denote completely, as in exacerbation.

excitation An act of irritation or stimulation, as of a nerve or a muscle. In behavioral science, a hypothetical state of an animal said to account for the occurrence of a response, and presumed to vary directly with the magnitude of response.

excystation A stage in the life cycle of a parasite in which a motile metacystic trophozoite is released.

exencephalia A developmental anomaly characterized by an imperfect cranium, the brain lying outside of the skull.

exhaustion In behavioral science, a hypothetical process thought to account for the process of adaptation or habituation of a species-specific response. It presumes that a response drains off or consumes a certain quantity of energy, thus raising the threshold and reducing the frequency and magnitude of subsequent responses.

exo- A prefix meaning outside, or outward.

exobiology The science concerned with the study of life on planets other than the earth.

exocytosis Expulsion of material from a cell. The reverse of endocytosis.

exopeptidase A proteolytic enzyme the action of which is limited to terminal peptide linkages.

exotoxin A toxic heat-stable protein produced and released into the surrounding medium by bacteria. Examples are the hemolysins of streptococci and the poisons of such clostridia as *Clostridium botulinum* and C. *tetani*.

explant 1. To take from the body and place in an artificial medium for growth. 2. Tissue taken from its original site and transferred to an artificial medium for growth.

extinction In behavioral science, the progressive decrease in the magnitude or frequency of a response.

    experimental e., the progressive decrement in the magnitude or frequency of a conditioned response resulting from the omission of reinforcement following or accompanying the occurrence of the response, while other variables are held constant.

    resistance to e., the strength of resistance as measured by the number of instances in which a conditioned response is given during experimental extinction before reaching some predetermined criterion of low response strength, such as a return to the rate of operant level.

extinguish In behavioral science, to omit reinforcement of a response sufficiently often that a decrement in response strength is observed.

eyeworm See *Thelazia*.

F

F_1 First filial generation; commonly used in referring to first generation offspring of experimental breeding. Subsequent generations are F_2, F_3, etc.

Fabricius See *bursa of Fabricius*, the structure first described by Hieronymus Fabricius of Aquapendente in 1604

factor F The fertility factor in bacterial conjugation. It appears to be DNA in nature, and promotes the formation of conjugation bridges, with the subsequent transfer of F or F-associated chromosomal material.

FAD Flavin adenine dinucleotide.

falconiform birds Members of the avian order Falconiformes, which includes the hawks, eagles, falcons, vultures, and secretary-bird.

fasciola A genus of trematodes, or flukes, which parasitizes the biliary passages of man and other animals. *F. hepatica* has recently been reported in guinea pigs. The eggs are ovoid, operculated, and yellowish-brown, and measure about 140μ in length and 65 to 85μ in width. See table of *Common Trematodes* accompanying *trematode*.

fast green An acid triphenylmethane dye.

Solubility at 15° C.: water 4 per cent, absolute alcohol 9 per cent, and glycerol 13.5 per cent. It is used in tissue for basic proteins, with magdala red as a differential stain for parasite and host in plant tissues, as one of the reagents for the Feulgen reaction for DNA, and in Harman's stain for mitochondria.[57, 153]

fatigue In behavioral science, habituation in which the response involves a considerable amount of physical work. See *habituation.*

FA virus See *Theiler's mouse encephalomyelitis,* under *encephalomyelitis.*

fawn variant See *schizochroism.*

fear In comparative psychology, the behavior and physiological changes produced either by sudden intense stimulation or by specific classes of stimuli, depending upon the species being studied. Responses include alterations of sphincter control, flight behavior, and the suppression of behavior which was occurring at the onset of stimulation.

Federation of American Scientists 1700 K Street, N.W., Washington, D.C. 20006.

Federation of American Societies for Experimental Biology 9650 Rockville Pike, Bethesda, Md. 20014.

feline respiratory disease See under *respiratory disease.*

Felis catus The domestic cat.

feral Wild; said especially of animals that have escaped domestication and become wild.

fer-de-lance See table accompanying *snake.*

ferritin The iron-apoferritin complex, which is one of the forms in which body iron is stored. Because of its electron-dense character, ferritin is frequently used as a label in electron microscopy.

Feulgen reaction A technique for demonstrating DNA, consisting of mild hydrolysis of a section in hydrochloric acid, followed by treatment with Schiff's reagent.

fibrinogenase An enzyme that influences coagulation of protein.

fibrinolysin Any enzyme that catalyzes the digestion of fibrin. See also *plasmin.*

fibro- A combining form denoting relationship to fibers.

fibroadenoma Adenoma containing fibrous tissue.

mammary f. R2737 (rat mammary fibroadenoma), a spontaneously arising fibroadenoma of the mammary gland found in an August line 28807 rat in the laboratory of W. F. Dunning at Wayne University, Detroit, in 1946. When inoculated subcutaneously it grows in 100 per cent of the recipients of the same strain, killing the host in six to ten months. The tumor may weigh more than the host itself. Spontaneous mammary fibroadenomas are the most common tumor of laboratory rats.[150]

fibroangioma An angioma containing much fibrous tissue.

fibroblastoma A tumor arising from the ordinary connective tissue cell or fibroblast. It includes fibroma and fibrosarcoma.

fibrocystic disease Cystic fibrosis.

fibroelastosis Overgrowth of fibroelastic elements.

endocardial f., a condition characterized by hypertrophy of the wall of the left ventricle and conversion of the endocardium into a thick fibroelastic coat, with reduction in the capacity of the ventricle. The leaflets of the aortic valve are often irregular in size or number, and thickened and covered with hyalinized verrucous overgrowths. An almost identical condition is seen occasionally in the cat, dog, and cow.

fibroma A tumor composed mainly of fibrous or fully developed connective tissue.

Shope f., a spontaneous poxvirus disease of wild cottontail rabbits (*Sylvilagus*) in the United States. The disease was first recognized in a wild cottontail by R. E. Shope of The Rockefeller Institute in which he observed the presence of prominent subcutaneous tumors. When inoculated into domestic laboratory rabbits (*Oryctolagus*), large tumors were produced, which regressed spontaneously after reaching a maximum size by the tenth or twelfth day after inoculation. Solid immunity was established not only to the fibroma virus, but also to a related viral disease, myxomatosis, of South American rabbits (*Sylvilagus*). A similar fibroma virus of squirrels is included in the same immunologic subgroup with the myxomatosis and Shope fibroma viruses.

The clinical picture of the Shope fibroma in *Oryctolagus* is prolonged, and in general the intratesticular and subcutaneous routes of infection are more successful than intracutaneous or other routes. The virus is cultivable in tissue culture and on the embryonating chick CAM.

Histologically, the lesion in wild or domestic rabbits is that of a proliferant fibroma with abundant cytoplasmic inclusion bodies. The inclusion bodies are present in tissue-culture infected cells, where they stain well with fluorescent antibody. This histologic picture is similar to that of myxomatosis, except that in the latter the cytotoxic and necrotizing effect of the virus is much more pronounced. The virus has been well characterized physically and chemically, and is widely used as a model on the frontier between viral oncology and inflammation.

The immunologic relationship is emphasized by the Berry-Dedrick transformation, an experiment utilizing heat-inactivated myxomatosis virus and live fibroma virus in which the myxomatosis virus was reactivated by incubation with the fibroma virus, thus establishing the concept of viral reactivation.[150]

fibromatosis A tendency to the development of fibromas; the formation of multiple fibromas.

fibropapilloma A papilloma containing much fibrous tissue.

fibroplasia The formation of fibrous tissue, as in the healing of wounds.

retrolental f. (RLF; Terry's syndrome), a condition characterized by the presence of opaque tissue behind the lens, leading to detachment of the retina and arrest of growth of the eye, generally attributed to use of high concentrations of oxygen in the care of premature infants.

fibrosarcoma   A sarcoma containing fibrous elements.

Earle L f. (Earle L sarcoma; L sarcoma; fibrosarcoma Earle L), a tumor developed by W. R. Earle, who explanted strips of mouse subcutaneous tissue into tissue culture flasks beginning in October 1940. These were maintained by continuous serial culture until November 1941, at which time methylcholanthrene was added to the culture, which was maintained for an additional three and a half months. Then, the L line of cells was transferred to a methylcholanthrene-free medium for 68 more days (June 1942). These cells were then injected into C3H mice (Andervont substrain), in which tumors grew at the inoculation site. Earle observed that control L cells (without carcinogen) also underwent neoplastic transformation when injected, and this has been subsequently confirmed many times. Subcutaneous transplants become palpable five to ten days after inoculation in C3H/An mice and grow progressively, to kill the host in about two months.[150]

filter-top cage   See *infantile diarrhea of mice.*

fishpox (carp pox; hyperplastic epidermal disease)   A chronic localized epidermal hyperplasia that results in superficial papillomatosis in a variety of fish species. Nuclear and cytoplasmic inclusions appear early in the disease. There are mitotic figures, but no necrosis. The disease is seldom life-limiting and is difficult to distinguish from a true neoplasm. It has not been experimentally transmitted, although virus particles are associated with the lesions.[114]

fixative   A chemical used for preparation of a specimen for histologic study, which preserves structure.[153]

fixed action pattern   A highly stereotyped response observable in most members of a species when there has been no experimental manipulation or conditioning. See *stereotyping,* and see *species-specific behavior,* under *behavior.*

flacherie   A flaccid condition seen in silkworm larvae suffering from dysentery. The affected larvae appear flabby, weak, withered, or loose-hanging. Death is rapidly followed by a darkening of the body and decomposition of the larval tissues. Many of the early pathologists used the word flacherie indiscriminately for various maladies of differing etiology, in different species of insects, implying "a diseased condition accompanied by diarrhea." In modern usage, the term should be accompanied by a modifier, to denote one type of flacherie as distinct from another of differing etiology, e.g., viral flacherie and touffe flacherie.

touffe f., a noninfectious form that occurs in silkworm-rearing establishments after sudden abnormal increases in environmental temperature and humidity (thus "touffe," meaning "whisps of heat"). Fifth-instar larvae are particularly affected by touffe flacherie.

viral f., an infectious form caused by a small nonoccluded virus.

flagellosis   Infection with a flagellate protozoon.

flamingo   See *ciconiiform birds.*

flavin adenine dinucleotide (FAD)   A flavoprotein that serves as the prosthetic group (coenzyme) in the catalyzing of cellular oxidation-reduction reactions.

flight   See under *behavior.*

Florida Academy of Sciences   University of Miami, Miami, Fla.

fluffy   Denoting a colony surface covered with a dense, deep pile of aerial hyphae.

fluke   Trematode.

fluorescein   The simplest of the fluorane dyes and the mother substance of eosin, $C_{20}H_{12}O_5$. It is used intravenously in tests to indicate by its fluorescence the adequacy of the circulation, and combined with radioactive iodine in localization of brain tumors, etc.

fluorescence   The property of reacting with light or ultraviolet light to increase wavelength so that visible light of lower wavelength is emitted.[153]

fluorescence microscopy   Technic for examining biological specimens stained with fluorochrome dyes under ultraviolet illumination. The methods designed for staining specific substances such as DNA, RNA, and amyloid have a high level of sensitivity. It is especially useful in localizing tissue sites of immunological reactions by the application of fluorescein-tagged antibodies.[153] See *immunofluorescence technic.*

5-fluoro-2′-deoxyuridine (FUDR)   A halogenated pyrimidine that blocks cellular and viral DNA synthesis by inhibition of thymidilic acid synthetase, but has no effect on riboviruses. It is also used as an immunosuppressant.

foot-and-mouth disease (epizootic aphthous fever)   An extremely contagious viral disease that occurs naturally in cloven-hoofed animals, particularly cattle, sheep, goats, and swine. It may also affect wild ruminants, such as deer, goats, and antelope and, under some conditions, these species act as reservoirs of the infection. The lesions consist of vesicular eruptions of the mucous membrane of the tongue, the skin of the lips and cheek, and the coronary band above the hoof. Localized skin lesions are occasionally seen in man.

Foot-and-mouth disease is prevalent throughout Europe, Africa, and Asia, and in some countries in South America. The disease has been prevented from reentering the United States since 1929, when a severe outbreak occurred in California. The agent can resist drying and other environmental stresses, so that it is extremely difficult to eradicate from contaminated premises. The accidental entry of this disease into the livestock population of the United States would be an economic disaster of tremendous proportions. The agent is classified in the picornavirus group and occurs in six antigenic types that do not cross-immunize.[16]

foot disease of oysters See *maladie du pied.*

Forssman antigen See under *antigen.*

foulbrood Any of several bacterial diseases affecting larval bees and giving rise to a foul odor.

American f. (black brood; ropy brood), a disease of larval honeybees caused by *Bacillus larvae.* Infection occurs in the youngest larvae, and death is most frequent when the insects are in the prepupal or pupal stage, after the cells have been capped. American foulbrood is found at any time of the year when brood is present in the temperate and subtropical regions throughout the world. No large beekeeping area is entirely free of the disease.

European f. (New York bee disease; melting brood), a disease of larval honeybees caused by *Streptococcus pluton.* Mortality is high among four- to five-day old larvae in typical epizootic outbreaks of the disease but, occasionally, sealed brood may die, too. Fairly common secondary invaders of the diseased larvae are *Streptococcus faecalis* and *Bacillus alvei,* both of which are responsible for the foul odors emanating from the dead larvae. The disease is usually enzootic throughout the beekeeping areas of the world, with well defined seasonal epizootics at the beginning of nectar flows.

fowl plague (fowl pest) An acute viral disease of all species of domestic fowl, characterized by high mortality.

fowl leukosis See *avian leukosis,* under *leukosis.*

fowlpox A pox disease affecting chickens and other birds and characterized by lesions on the comb, wattles, eyes, nostrils, and mouth which may ulcerate.[16]

fox encephalitis See under *encephalitis.*

freemartin A sexually underdeveloped female calf born as a twin to a male sibling with whom it shares an anastomotic placental circulation. A similar condition has been observed in sheep, goats, marmosets, and swine. See *blood group chimerism.*

freeze brand A mark made for identification of an animal by freezing the skin in a desired pattern, resulting in the production of a bald spot or white hair growth because of cryogenic melanocyte destruction. This method is less painful and in some instances may replace branding.

freeze-dry Lyophilization.

Friend leukemia virus A reticulum cell leukemia virus recovered by Friend from the spleen of an adult Swiss mouse that had been inoculated with the cell-free extract of an Ehrlich carcinoma. When injected into adult or young Swiss or DBA/2 mice, the virus induces reticulum cell leukemia and erythroblastosis with hepatosplenomegaly in as short a time as two weeks after inoculation. Rats are also susceptible. The virus may be maintained in mouse embryo cell cultures.[114]

fright disease Canine hysteria, a psychic disturbance in dogs marked by symptoms of fright and by hysterical barking and running. It is caused by intoxication with the bleaching agent nitrogen trichloride.

frounce See *avian trichomoniasis,* under *trichomoniasis.*

fructoaldolase An enzyme of the Embden-Meyerhof glycolytic pathway that catalyzes the conversion of D-fructose-1,6-phosphate to D-glyceraldehyde-3-phosphate, and D-fructose-1-phosphate to dihydroxyacetone phosphate.

fructose-1,6-diphosphatase An enzyme of the Embden-Meyerhof pathway that converts D-fructose-1,6-diphosphate to D-fructose-6-phosphate.

frugivorous A term applied to fruit-eating organisms.

fruit fly (pomace fly) Any fly of genus *Drosophila,* family Drosophilidae, order Diptera. These flies, particularly, *D. melanogaster,* are much used in genetic studies because the giant chromosomes in the salivary gland facilitate chromosome mapping and because of the low number of linkage groups, the short generation interval, the ease and economy of culturing them, the availability of interspecific hybrids, and the large numbers of species available (nearly 1000).[50, 157]

frustration The state produced in an animal by preventing it from making a response to a stimulus. This may be done by (1) withholding the stimulus, (2) mechanically preventing the response, or (3) placing the animal in a conflict situation.

fuchsin (basic) A basic triphenylmethane dye. Solubility at 15· C.: water all proportions, absolute alcohol 3 per cent, and glycerol 10 per cent. It is a mixture of rosaniline and pararosaniline hydrochlorides used to stain tubercle bacilli and *Treponema pallidum,* and as a topical germicide.[57, 153]

fuscidic acid (Fucidine) A steroid antibiotic produced by a species of fungus, *Fuscidium coccineum,* which has strong activity against gram-positive organisms and relatively little activity against gram-negative organisms. Its activity is through inhibition of protein synthesis by interference with the final polymerization of amino acids into peptide chains.[36, 49]

-fugal A word termination implying banishing, or driving away, affixed to a stem designating the object of banishment, as cucifugal, driving away mosquitoes and gnats (*Culex*), or febrifugal, relieving or dispelling fever. 2. A word termination implying traveling away from, affixed to a stem designating the object from which flight is made, as centrifugal, traveling away from a center, or cortifugal, directed away from the cortex.

fumarase An enzyme of the Krebs cycle that converts fumarate to L-malate.

Furth pituitary tumor See *pituitary tumor of Furth.*

G

g Abbreviation for the force of gravity, used in describing the intensity of sedimenting force in centrifugation. Easily calculated by comparing the speed of rotation to the radius of the centrifuge arm.

Gaboon viper. See table accompanying *snake.*

gaffkaemia (gaffkemia) A highly fatal disease of the American lobster, *Homarus americanus,* held in artificial ponds. The causative organism, *Gaffkya homari,* is a gram-positive micrococcus found in the hemolymph and hemocytes of the lobsters. The disease has been produced experimentally in certain crabs.

galactase A proteolytic enzyme that hydrolyzes caseinogen in the stomach.

galacto-, galact-, galacta- Combining form denoting relationship to milk.

galactose-4-epimerase An enzyme active in glycogenesis that converts uridine diphosphoglucose into uridine diphosphogalactose, using reduced NADP as a co-factor.

galactose uridyl transferase An enzyme active in glycogenesis that converts uridine diphosphogalactose to D-galactose-1-phosphate, using uridine diphosphoglucose (UDPG) as a co-factor.[17]

galactozymase A starch-liquefying enzyme.

galliform birds Members of the avian order Galliformes. Typically the birds in this order are ground-feeding, or partly arboreal in the wild. They may also be referred to as gallinaceous birds. One family, the Phasianidae, is of great agricultural importance because of the domesticated varieties, and is of great interest because some species are important in research and conservation.[154] See table.

gallinaceous birds See *galliform birds.*

Gallus gallus domestica Domestic poultry (chicken); see *galliform birds.*

gamete 1. A reproductive element, being one of two cells, male and female, whose union is necessary in sexual reproduction to initiate the development of a new individual. 2. The malarial parasite in its sexual form in the stomach of a mosquito, either male (microgamete), or female (macrogamete). The latter is fertilized by the former to develop into an ookinete.[31, 121]

gameto- A combining form denoting relationship to a gamete.

gammopathy A primary disturbance of the gamma-forming template in conditions characterized by abnormal gammaglobulin formation.

monoclonal g., a form in which a high level of one molecular type of immunoglobulin (i.e., a single clone of plasma cells) is produced at the expense of other types. Thus, even though there may be an increase in quantity of immunoglobulins, there is a decrease in the functional quality. The term includes all the homogeneous hypergammaglobulinemias. Some examples are (1) multiple myeloma, which may be of type IgG, IgA, IgD, IgE, IgM, or light chains; (2) primary IgM macroglobulinemia (Waldenstrom's syndrome); (3) heavy chain IgG (Franklin) or IgA (Seligman). In anomen, there is a transplantable plasmacytoma of mice and perhaps an IgA and IgM macroglobulinemia of dogs. Aleutian mink disease (q.v.) is sometimes associated with IgG gammopathy in advanced cases.

polyclonal g., a form in which there is proliferation of plasma cells from many clones. The term includes all the heterogeneous hypergammaglobulinemias.

gander See *anseriform birds.*

gangrene Death of tissue, usually in considerable mass and generally associated with loss of vascular supply and followed by bacterial invasion and putrefaction.

dry idiopathic g. of budgerigars, a disease of unknown etiology in caged parakeets, characterized by dry necrosis of one or both legs, beginning with the last phalanx of the digits· and gradually progressing up the foot, and most commonly terminating at the tarsometatarsal or tibiotarsal joint. There is

SOME IMPORTANT GALLIFORM BIRDS

DOMESTIC OR BREED NAME	SCIENTIFIC NAME	WILD DERIVATION
White leghorn chicken	*Gallus gallus*	Red jungleflow
Barred rock chicken	*G. gallus*	Red jungleflow
Rhode Island chicken	*G. gallus*	Red jungleflow
Bronze turkey	*Meleagris gallopavo*	Wild turkey
Beltsville turkey	*M. gallopavo*	Wild turkey
Peafowl	*Pavo cristatus*	– – –
Guinea fowl	*Numida meleagris*	– – –
Bobwhite quail	*Colinus virginianus*	– – –
Ringneck pheasant	*Phasianus colchicus*	– – –
Japanese quail	*Coturnix coturnix japonica*	– – –

no pain, but a fatal termination is most common.[112]

gannet See *pelecaniform birds.*

GAS General adaptation syndrome.

gastric adenocarcinoma See under *carcinoma.*

gastric carcinoma 342 See under *carcinoma.*

gastro, gastr- Combining form denoting relationship to the stomach or to the abdomen.

gastroenteritis See *transmissible gastroenteritis.*

gastropod See *mollusk.*

gattine A term used to describe a type of flacherie (q.v.) of silkworm larvae, said to be caused by concomitant infection by a virus and an enterococcus closely related to *Streptococcus faecalis.* However, the viral origin of gattine remains in doubt. Certain climatic and nutritional conditions are also known to act as predisposing factors necessary for the proliferation of the enterococci and production of overt disease. The cephalic end of affected silkworms frequently becomes swollen and almost translucent thus gattine is also known as disease of the clear heads.

gaviiform birds Members of the avian order Gaviiformes, typified by the loons and divers.

GDVII virus See *Theiler's mouse encephalomyelitis,* under *encephalomyelitis.*

gel diffusion (Ouchterlony technique) An antigen-antibody precipitation technic in which the reactants diffuse from slots or holes in agar toward each other. When the antigen meets its specific antibody, a precipitin line is formed. Many variations of this method have been developed, including immunoelectrophoresis.

gel filtration (exclusion chromatography) A method used for the separation of substances of different molecular size, employing gels such as Sephadex or cross-linked dextran, agar, agarose, or polyacrylamide beads. This technic is useful for the fractionation of serum proteins, enzymes, hormones, nucleic acids, etc., and for desalting or removing excess dyes from solutions.

-gen A word termination denoting an agent productive of the object or state indicated by the word stem to which it is affixed, as allergen (allergy), cryogen (cold), and pathogen (disease).

gene A locus on the chromosome responsible for directing the synthesis of a specific enzyme, protein, or peptide. Believed to be a discrete sequence of nucleotides in the chromosomal DNA which functions to provide, via messenger RNA, the information necessary for the polypeptide sequence of a particular protein. Studies of bacteria indicate that there are three interacting units referred to as the *structural gene,* responsible for production of the protein, the *operator gene* (or *operon*), which controls the structural gene, and the *regulator gene,* responsible for activating or switching on and off the operator gene.

This concept, which may or may not be valid for animal cells, is an attempt to explain the hypothesis that every fertilized ovum possesses sufficient information to produce all proteins or enzymes contained in the fully developed animal and passes this potential on to all somatic cells. Because of a remarkable degree of redundancy and the presence of repressor mechanisms in the regulator, these capabilities are only fractionally expressed by any given cell, resulting in specialized functions of cells or organs.

Patterns of inheritance in man, anomen, and plants are fundamentally similar. Genes controlling individual traits and their phenotypic expression are carried on each pair of homologous chromosomes. Genes for alternative characteristics within the individual occupy corresponding loci on homologous chromosomes and occur in pairs known as alleles. Only one of these alleles is expressed in the phenotype. If the genes on the paired chromosomes differ, the individual is referred to as heterozygous. In this circumstance, the trait expressed is referred to as dominant, and the one not expressed is referred to as recessive. If both chromosomes carry the same trait, the individual is referred to as homozygous. The homozygous state is a mechanism for expression of recessive traits.

There is considerable evidence that genetic loci of similar function exist in most species of animals, including man. Evidence of this is seen in the expression of certain genetic diseases of identical or similar patterns in several species, as in Chediak-Higashi syndrome of man, mink, cattle, and mice. If this hypothesis is borne out, it could provide the basis for very important studies of the mechanisms of the inherited diseases in man by searching out and studying analogous disease patterns in anomen.[31, 61, 90, 144]

complementary g's, nonallelic genes that complement each other. Such genes are typified by a trait that can only be expressed as a double recessive.

epistatic g., a gene that prevents the expression of another, e.g., a gene for lack of a limb precludes expression of any gene affecting the nature of the missing limb.

histocompatibility g's, the genes for antigens that play an important role in the acceptance or rejection of tissue grafts. See *histocompatibility loci.*

general adaptation syndrome (GAS) An integrated nonspecific response of the body to various kinds of stress which results in stimulation of the hypothalamus, increased release of adrenocorticotropic hormone (ACTH) from the anterior pituitary gland, and increased function of the adrenal cortex with release of glucocorticoid (cortisol). Effects on the body are increased breakdown of the lymphoid tissue with atrophy of lymph nodes and thymus gland, enlargement of the adrenal gland, and gastric erosions.[144]

generalization See under *stimulus*, and see *equivalence response*, under *response*.

genetic disease A disease for which there is evidence of inheritance.[142] See accompanying table; see *chromosomal aberrations;* see *inborn errors*, under *metabolism;* and see table of animal models (Addendum).

genetics The study of heredity.

Genetics Society of America, Inc. Department of Zoology, University of Texas, Austin, Tex. 78712.

genetotrophic disease An inborn error of metabolism; see under *metabolism*.

-genic A word termination meaning producing, or productive of.

geno- A combining form denoting relationship to reproduction or to sex.

genome The complete set of hereditary factors contained in the genetic constitution of an organism.

genopathy A genetic disease; any disease that involves or affects the genetic appara-

EXAMPLES OF GENETIC DISEASES OF DOMESTIC ANIMALS*†

DISEASE	MODE OF TRANSMISSION	BREED AND CLINICAL AND PATHOLOGIC FEATURES
CATTLE		
Achondroplasia (bull-dog calves)	Autosomal recessive	Dexter breed: heterozygous for gene; occurs also in other breeds; fetus aborted fourth to sixth month of gestation; anasarca, phocomelus, prognathia, domed skull, protruding tongue, achondroplasia.
Hypotrichosis congenita (hairless)	Autosomal recessive	Guernsey, Holstein: viable and nonviable forms may be different genes; complete atrichia.
Hereditary congenital ataxia, hypomyelinogenesis congenita (jittery)	Autosomal recessive	Jersey, Shorthorn, Angus (may occur in many breeds): calves 2 to 3 weeks of age —incoordination, microcephaly, leukodysplasia of cerebellum, midbrain, and medulla with loss of neurons and myelin.
Ichthyosis fetalis (fish skin)	Autosomal recessive	Norwegian red poll cattle, probably other breeds: (similar to "Harlequin fetus" in man) alopecia, scaly, fissured skin, hyperkeratosis-acanthosis, deep fissures.
Eptheliogenesis imperfecta (epithelial defects, skinless)	Autosomal recessive	Ayrshire, Holstein, Jersey breeds: calves born alive, absence of skin in patches over fettocks and knees, sometimes over ears and muzzle.
Hydrocephalus internus	Autosomal recessive	Hereford and Holstein-Friesian breeds: congenital hydrocephalus interna in newborn calves; symmetrical distention of lateral ventricles.
Hairlessness, streaked	Sex-linked dominant	Holstein-Friesian breed: vertical streaks of atrichia over hips in heterozygous females; hemizygous males presumed dead in utero.
Aphakia, microphakia, cataract, ectopia-lentis, iridermia, multiple eye defects	Autosomal recessive	Jersey breed: newborn calves blind due to congenital cataract, with iridermia, microphakia, and ectopia lentis.
Dwarfism "snorter dwarfs"	Autosomal recessive (may be more complex)	Hereford and Angus breeds: calves are short in stature and fail to grow; short bulging foreheads, malocclusion; nasal obstruction may cause dyspnea.
Acroteriasis congenita (adactyly) "amputated"	Autosomal recessive	Holstein-Friesian breed: forelegs terminate at elbow, hindlegs at hock; cleft palate, anodontia; prognathism and maxillar distortion; death near time of birth.
THE DOG		
Hemophilia A	Sex-linked recessive	Aberdeen terrier, greyhound, Irish setter, Scotch terrier: hemizygous males and homozygous females affected; deficiency of antihemophilic factor (factor VIII) results in failure of blood to clot, hemorrhage into joints, under skin, etc.; may result in death.
Hemophilia B; Christmas disease	Sex-linked recessive	Cairn terriers: deficiency of factor IX results in deficiency of plasma thromboplastin. *(Table continued)*

*Adapted from H. A. Smith and T. C. Jones: Veterinary Pathology, 3rd ed. Lea & Febiger, Philadelphia, 1966.

†Diseases listed are those in which (1) evidence indicates genetic determination and (2) pathologic manifestations have been described.

EXAMPLES OF GENETIC DISEASES OF DOMESTIC ANIMALS (*Continued*)

DISEASE	MODE OF TRANSMISSION	BREED AND CLINICAL AND PATHOLOGIC FEATURES
THE DOG (Continued)		
Atrichia; hairlessness	Autosomal dominant	Hairless breeds: heterozygous for this gene; homozygotes usually born dead; lack pinnae; may have stenotic esophagus.
Hereditary blindness and deafness, "dappling"	Autosomal dominant	Collies, Norwegian dunker hounds, Great Danes, bull terriers: Merle or harlequin hair coat in heterozygotes; white hair coat, microphthalmia, coloboma, often deaf
DOMESTIC FOWL		
Achondroplasia (creeper)	Autosomal dominant	Scots, Dumpies, Japanese Bantams, heterozygous breeds: assume crouching stance due to shortened extremities; achondoplasia; homozygotes usually die during first week of incubation.
Short limbs; Cornish lethal	Autosomal dominant	Shortened extremities in heterozygotes; homozygotes die during last week of incubation; note similarity to "creeper."
Featherless (naked) chicks	Sex-linked recessive	Many homozygous chicks die a few days before hatching; other featherless chicks die after hatching; more survive if kept warm; almost complete absence of feathers at hatching, but grow some plumage after 4 months; females hemizygous are affected.
THE CAT		
Manx, tailless	Autosomal dominant(?)	Manx cats: heterozygous dominance incompletely expressed, homozygotes die in utero, some presumed heterozygotes have imperforate anus, and defects in pelvic bones.
Deaf, white	Autosomal recessive	Deafness in dominant white cats with blue or yellow eyes; due to agenesis of organ of Corti, spiral ganglia, and cochlear nuclei.
Polydactyly	Autosomal dominant	Extra toes on front feet; sometimes hind feet affected also, but not without involvement of front feet; one to three extra digits.
THE MOUSE		
Yellow coat color	Autosomal dominant	All yellow mice are heterozygous; first lethal gene demonstrated (by Cuenot) in mammals.
SWINE		
Amelia, congenital	Autosomal recessive	All appendages missing; piglets are born alive.

tus, including chromosomal aberrations, hereditary disease, defects in the regulator gene system which lead to enzyme deficiencies, and hereditary anomalies. See table of *Genetic Diseases*, and see *inborn error*, under *metabolism*.

genophobia   Morbid dread of sex and sexuality.

gentian violet (crystal violet)   A basic triphenylmethane dye which has three methylated amino groups. Solubility at 15° C.: water 9 per cent, absolute alcohol 8.5 per cent, and glycerol 5 per cent. It is used to stain amyloid tissue, alpha cell granules of the pancreas, sections of the anterior pituitary gland, cartilage matrix, chondroitin sulfates, elastic fibers, mast cells, and bacterial cells in Gram's stain.[57, 153]

geobiology   The biology of terrestrial life.

geochronology   The study of time measurement in relation to evolution of the earth.

geologic time divisions   See diagram on page 84.

geopathology   The study of the peculiarities of disease in relation to topography, climate, food habits, etc., of various regions of the earth.

geophilic dermatophyte   See *dermatomycosis*.

gephyrophobia   Fear of walking on a bridge, river bank, or other structure near the water.

gerbil (sand rat; antelope rat; desert rat; jird)   A small rodent of which there are 12 genera and over 300 species. The commonest species used in American laboratories is the Mongolian gerbil (*Meriones varguiculatas*), which came to this country from a laboratory in Japan. Those used in other countries may be of several species, e.g., *M. libycus* and *M. shawi* in France and Britain, and *M. tristrami, M. erythrourus*, and *M. crassus* in Israel. They weigh 50 to 100 gm. and are

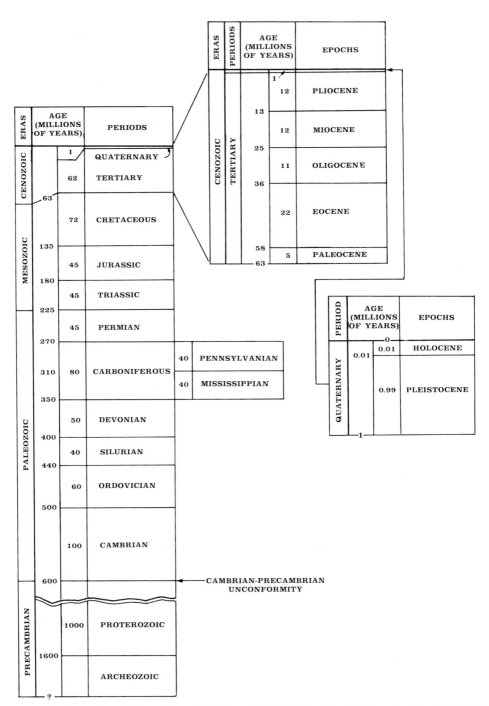

Figure 2. Geologic time divisions. (From L. L. Sloss and L. H. Nobles: Earth History: An Illustrated Syllabus in Historical Geology. Northwestern University Press, Evanston, Ill., 1964.)

well adapted to desert life. They are valuable for studies of cholesterol metabolism, renal function, and water metabolism, because they can survive without ingestion of free water (they get it from plants) and are susceptible to a wide range of biological pathogens. Another species, *Psammomys obesus*, is used to study diabetes mellitus.[85]

German measles Rubella.

germ-free See *axenic* and *gnotobiote*.

gero-, geronto- Combining form denoting relationship to old age or to the aged.

Gerontological Society, Inc. 660 S. Euclid Avenue, St. Louis, Mo. 63110.

gestalt In experimental behavior science, a complex set of stimuli not fully experimentally defined but which controls a response or set of responses. See also *gestaltism*.

gestaltism (gestalt theory) That theory in psychology which proposes that the objects of mind, as immediately presented to direct experience, come as complete unanalyzable wholes or forms (Gestalten) which cannot be split up into parts.

gestation period See table of *Mammalian Reproductive Data*, accompanying *mammal*.

giant cell pneumonia of monkeys See under *pneumonia*.

Giardia muris See *protozoan parasites*, under *rat*.

gibberellin One of a group of plant hormones that promote growth and seed germination.

gibbon One of the anthropoid apes, genus *Hylobates*. See *primate*.

giga- A combining form designating gigantic size; used in naming units of measurements to indicate a quantity one billion (10^9) times the unit designated by the root with which it is combined.

gill rakers Small projections on the gill arches of some fishes, which serve to strain food particles and prevent them from clogging the gills.

gingerbread disease (of oysters) See *maladie du pain d'épices*.

glabrous Smooth and bare, as a surface of a fungal colony without aerial hyphae, or an area of skin surface without hair, as between the toes, palms, etc.

glaucoma A condition of the eye characterized by increased intraocular pressure.

congenital g. (buphthalmia; buphthalmos; hydrophthalmia; hydrophthalmos), in the domestic rabbit, a well characterized model for heritable congenital glaucoma in man. The condition may be unilateral or bilateral and usually is manifested by the third or fourth month of life. It has usually been considered to be the expression of a single autosomal recessive allele.[123]

glio- A combining form denoting relationship to a gluey substance, or specifically to the neuroglia.

glioma A tumor composed of tissue which represents the neuroglia in any one of its stages of development.

Globidium besnoiti (*Besnoitia besnoiti*) A cyst-forming organism, probably protozoan, which can cause cutaneous and systemic lesions in cattle and horses. *Besnoitia jellisoni* is a similar organism which occurs in wild rodents.[142]

Globocephalus urosubulatus A hookworm that infects hogs. Its life cycle probably resembles that of other hookworms.[21]

glomangioma An extremely painful, small, firm, slightly elevated, rounded red-blue tumor, usually occurring on the distal portions of the fingers and toes, in the skin, or in deeper structures.

glomerulonephritis An inflammatory lesion of the kidney that affects many species. The pathogenesis of many forms is not well understood, but that of other clear-cut forms is known. These include nephritis caused by antiglomerular basement membrane antibody (Masugi nephritis), and nephritis caused by antigen-antibody complex deposition within the glomeruli. Much has been learned recently about glomerulonephritis by the use of fluorescence microscopy, electron microscopy, and immunological techniques. Valuable animal models for the study of glomerulonephritis occur in the mink, mouse, sheep, rabbit, and dog.[34, 47, 82, 93]

Glossina A genus of biting flies that are the vectors of various trypanosomiases of man and anomen.

glucagon A hormone secreted by alpha cells of the pancreas which causes hyperglycemia.

glucase An enzyme of plants and microorganisms that hydrolyzes starch into D-glucose.

gluco- A combining form denoting relationship to sweetness, or to glucose.

glucokinase An enzyme of the Embden-Meyerhof pathway that converts D-glucose or D-mannose into D-glucose-6-phosphate or D-mannose-6-phosphate, using ATP and Mg as co-factors.

gluconeogenesis The formation of carbohydrates from molecules that are not themselves carbohydrates, as protein or fat molecules. Also referred to as glyconeogenesis.

gluconolactonase An enzyme of the hexose-monophosphate shunt that catalyzes the conversion of 6-phosphogluconolactone to 6-phosphogluconate, using Mg^{++} as a co-factor.

glucose-6-phosphatase An enzyme of high concentration in the liver that catalyzes the hydrolysis of glucose-6-phosphate. Glycogen storage disease of von Gierke (type I) is due to hereditary deficiency of this enzyme.

glucose-6-phosphate dehydrogenase An enzyme of the hexose-monophosphate shunt that catalyzes the oxidation of glucose-6-phosphate to 6-phosphogluconolactone through the intermediary action of NADP as a co-factor. Hereditary deficiency of this enzyme is seen in man and sheep. See table accompanying *inborn errors*, under *metabolism*.

glucose-1-phosphate kinase An enzyme found in yeast and muscle that catalyzes phosphorylation of glucose-1-phosphate to glucose-1,6-diphosphate.

glucosidase An enzyme that splits a glucoside.

glucuronic acid A chemical formed from glucose through the oxidation of UDP-glucose. Complete breakdown of this acid leads to its conversion to L-gulonic acid, which serves as the source of ascorbic acid and ketopentose xylulose, which can be metabolized through the pentose-phosphate pathway. It is in this cycle of reactions that congenital absence of enzymes may lead to inborn errors of metabolism such as (1) pentosuria, (2) inability to synthesize ascorbic acid, as in the rat, (3) galactosemia, and (4) hyperbilirubinemia.

β-glucuronidase An enzyme contained within lysosomes of many organs, which catalyzes the splitting of glucuronides. It is frequently used along with other hydrolytic enzymes as a biochemical marker for lysosomes.

glutamic dehydrogenase One of the groups of enzymes that catalyze the passage of hydrogen from a substrate to a hydrogen acceptor. It is active in the change of glutamic acid into α-ketoglutarate. Increased activity of this enzyme may be an indication of damage to mitochondrial membranes.[90]

glutaminase An enzyme that catalyzes the splitting of glutamine into glutamic acid and ammonia.

glycase An enzyme that converts maltose and maltodextrin into dextrose.

glycerophosphatase An enzyme that catalyzes the dephosphorylation of glycerophosphates.

glycocalix A carbohydrate-rich external layer seen on many types of cells.

glycogenase An enzyme that hydrolyzes glycogen to lower saccharides.

glycogenesis 1. The formation or synthesis of glycogen. 2. The production of sugar.

glycogenolysis The splitting up of glycogen in the body tissues.

glycogenosis Any of the glycogen storage diseases caused by a genetically determined deficiency of certain enzymes. See table accompanying *inborn error*, under *metabolism*.

glycogen storage disease See *glycogenosis*.

glycopeptide (mucopeptide; murein; peptidoglycan) The primary component of the insoluble rigid matrix of the bacterial cell wall, which is composed of six compounds found in equimolar amounts and connected by polypeptide cross-links. These compounds are N-acetylglucosamine, N-acetylmuramic acid, and four amino acids: L-alanine, D-alanine, D-glutamic acid, a diamino acid.[32]

gnatho-, A combining form denoting relationship to the jaw.

gnathocephalus A fetal monster with all parts of the head missing except the jaws.

Gnathostoma A genus of nematodes of the family Gnathostomatidae, most species of which have been found in the stomach wall of mammals.

    G. histidium, a species found in the stomach wall of wild and domestic pigs, associated with tumorous growths. It may occasionally infect man.

    G. spinigerum, a species that parasitizes the cat, dog, and occasionally man. Fish or aquatic reptiles act as intermediate hosts.

gnosis Edinger's term for the arousal of associative mnemonic (memory) complexes by sensory pallial impulses; one of the functions of the cerebral cortex.

gnotobiology The study of organisms living by themselves or in association with other known species in the absence of all other demonstrable living organisms.[86]

gnotobiosis The condition of existence either with no other species, i.e., germ-free, or with only organisms known to the investigator.[86]

gnotobiota The specifically and entirely known microfauna and microflora of a specially reared laboratory animal.

gnotobiote A specially reared laboratory animal the microfauna and microflora of which are specifically known in their entirety.[86]

gnotophoresis The state of existence of an organism bearing one or more known species in intimate contact with it and no other demonstrable viable organism.[86] Cf. *axenobiosis*.

gnotophoric Designation of an organism that exists in intimate contact with one or more known species and no other demonstrable viable microorganisms or infestations with metazoans.[86] Cf. *gnotobiote*.

goal In behavioral science, the term applied to a reinforcing stimulus; also used loosely to refer to responses to reinforcing stimuli, to consummatory acts, and to the stimuli for or releasers of consummatory acts.

goal-gradient The functional relationship between the strength of a response and the distance in space or time from the reinforcing stimulus.

goal response See under *response*.

goat See *pygmy goat*.

goatpox A poxlike disease of goats that occurs in North Africa and the Middle East and produces generalized lesions of the mucous membranes and skin.[16]

Golgi apparatus (Golgi complex) A complex of juxtanuclear intracellular membranes distributed in characteristic parallel orientation, which appear as flat saccules piled one upon the other. Each cisternal unit is seen in section as a pair of parallel membranes of considerable length and continuous with one another at the ends. The function of this organelle is not well understood but it plays an important role in production and packaging of cell secretions.[38]

gon- A combining form denoting relation (1) to seed or to the semen, and (2) to the knee.

gonadotrophic activity unit The specific gonadotrophic activity of 0.1 mg. of the standard material preserved at and distributed from the National Institute for Medical Research, Hampstead, London. It is derived from pregnancy urine, and the unit is approximately the amount required to produce cornification of the vaginal epithelium of the immature rat.

Gongylonema neoplasticum A species of nematodes of the superfamily Spiruroidea which are commonly found on the tongue and in the esophagus and stomach of rodents. The intermediate host is the American or German cockroach. *G. pulchrum* is another member of this group, usually found in various ruminants, in the monkey, pig, bear, and hedgehog, and rarely in man.[21] See *helminth parasites,* under *rat.*

goose See *anseriform birds.*

gorilla An anthropoid ape, genus *Gorilla.* See *primate.*

gosling See *anseriform birds.*

gougerotin An antibiotic produced by species of *Streptomyces,* which has a broad spectrum of antibiotic activity but is highly toxic to mammalian cells. Its mode of action is the inhibition of protein synthesis, similar to that of puromycin.[30, 49]

gout A hereditary disease affecting uric acid metabolism, characterized by the presence of excessive levels of serum uric acid, attacks of acute arthritis, and formation of chalky deposits (tophi) in joints, bursae, and tendon sheaths. Except for visceral gout of birds, which is common, it is rarely seen in anomen.[142, 152]

gradient of approach See under *approach.*

gradient of avoidance See under *avoidance.*

Graffi leukemia virus A virus that induces myeloid leukemia in mice and rats following a latent period of three to thirteen months. It was isolated from several transplantable mouse tumors (including sarcoma I and II, sarcoma 37, SOV16, carcinoma 45) and an Ehrlich's carcinoma that had been carried in Agnes Blum mice. When the virus was injected into neonatal mice, myelogenous leukemia developed rather than the tumors from which it was derived. After a number of passages, both lymphosarcomas and reticulum cell sarcomas developed in certain individuals, in addition to myelogenous leukemia.[114]

graft-versus-host reaction A syndrome produced by injecting immunologically competent cells into genetically foreign hosts (allograft) which are unable to reject to these elements, resulting in abnormalities of the recipient. See also *runt disease.*

-gram A word termination meaning that which is written or recorded.

gramicidin An antibiotic produced by *Bacillus brevis,* which is active against gram-positive organisms. It affects mitochondrial and erythrocyte permeability. Its toxicity has precluded its use as a systemic drug. Gramicidin-S (Soviet) is more closely related to the tyrocidine group.[49]

gram-negative Denoting loss of stain or decolorization by alcohol in Gram's method of staining, a primary characteristic of certain microorganisms.

gramnivorous Denoting grain-eating organisms, also granivorous.

gram-positive Denoting retention of stain or resistance to decolorization by alcohol in Gram's method of staining, a primary characteristic of certain microorganisms.

granuloma Any of a group of lesions characterized by chronic inflammation and composed of a necrotic or calcified center surrounded by giant cells, macrophages, lymphocytes, and usually a peripheral fibrous capsule. In some, as in those of tuberculosis, the causative agent can be found. There are many variations of the characteristics of granulomata, depending on the stage, cause, and immunologic status of the host.[142]

granuloma pouch An experimental lesion developed by Selye. Into a pocket formed under the skin by the injection of air, an irritant such as croton oil is placed, causing a wall of granulation tissue to form around the cavity or pouch, which can then be used as an experimental chamber to study the effects of irritants, infectious agents, toxins, etc. Cf. *skin window.*

granulomatous disease An inherited defect of leukocytes that renders them unable to phagocytize and digest bacteria properly.

granulosa cell tumor XIV A tumor induced by whole-body x-irradiation in a 30-month-old RF × AK hybrid mouse in the laboratories of Jacob Furth at Oak Ridge National Laboratories in 1947. The tumor grows progressively in 50 to 75 per cent of RF × AK hybrid hosts, usually does not invade surrounding tissue, and does not metastasize. It is endocrinologically active, inducing a state of continuous estrus and endometrial hyperplasia in females, and atrophy of the testes and seminal vesicles in males. Hypervolemia is induced in both sexes.[150]

granulosis In certain insects, a viral disease characterized by the presence of minute granular inclusion capsules in infected cells. One may speak of a "granulosis virus," but the inclusion body itself is referred to as a "capsule."

grapho- A combining form denoting relationship to writing or to a record.

graphophobia Abnormal dread of writing.

graphology The study of handwriting.

grasserie (jaundice) Nucleopolyhedrosis of the silkworm, *Bombyx mori.*

gray collie disease A complex hereditary disease of collie dogs characterized by partial albinism, poor viability, and cyclic neutropenia (q.v.).

gray lung disease An inapparent infection, probably caused by a virus isolated from mice inoculated with materials from animals with calf pneumonia and infantile diarrhea of mice. It may occur as a latent agent of normal mice, but has never actually been recovered from them. The virus was readily transmissible, with low mortality, persistent viral presence without active immunity, and pulmonary lesions consisting only of complete red-gray consolidation of one or more lobes. Tetracycline suppressed development of the pulmonary lesions. It is not considered a significant entity in the epizootiology of murine respiratory disease.[27]

gray variant See *schizochroism.*

grebe See *podicipediform birds.*

green monkey (vervet) A monkey of the species *Cercopithecus aethiops.* See *primate* and *Marburg virus.*

green muscardine See under *muscardine.*

griesin See *sideromycin.*

griseofulvin An antibiotic produced by species of *Penicillium,* which has no effect on bacteria but inhibits the growth of mycelial fungi. Its mechanism of action is incompletely known. It does not inhibit synthesis of protein, it does inhibit mitosis in metaphase, and there are conflicting data concerning its effect on RNA and DNA metabolism.[36, 49] See *antimetabolite.*

Gross leukemia virus (GLV; passage A virus) A spontaneously occurring murine leukemia virus isolated by Gross from lymphoid tumors of AK mice. He found that the virus would, following an inoculation period of about six months, induce in C3H mice a lymphoid leukemia similar to that in the AK strain mice. Continued serial passage of the agent reduced the incubation period, increased the age at which mice were still susceptible to the agent, and increased the percentage of injected mice that developed lymphosarcoma. Rats injected with GLV also develop leukemia. It may be propagated in cell cultures prepared from C3H mice, especially those in which no CPE is observed. A great deal is known of its ultrastructure and cytopathology.[53, 114]

gruiform birds Members of the avian order Gruiformes, marsh birds which include the cranes, rails, and bustards.

guanase A deaminizing enzyme that catalyzes the change of guanine into xanthine and ammonia.

guanidase An enzyme formed by *Aspergillus niger,* which hydrolyzes guanidine into urea and ammonia.

guanidine HCl An imino derivative of urea that inhibits picornavirus by interference with the synthesis of viral RNA polymerase.

guanosine diphosphate phosphorylation enzyme An enzyme of the Krebs cycle that converts succinyl coenzyme A to succinate, using guanosine diphosphate (GDP), inosine diphosphate (IDP), and Mg^{++} as co-factors.

di Guglielmo's disease See under *D.*

guinea pig (cavy) A rodent of the genus *Cavia,* family Caviidae. *Cavia porcellus* was domesticated by the Indians of Peru, Ecuador, and Colombia. It weighs about 2 pounds, measures from 225 to 355 mm. in length, and may show a great variety of colors, including black and ochraceous, and has a banded or agouti pattern. Long-haired cavies originate in Peru. Domesticated varieties are Abyssinian (coarse-haired) and Bolivian or English (short-haired). They feed mainly on grass and may survive without water in captivity if provided with fresh vegetables. They also eat rabbit or rat food, but require supplementation with vitamin C.[80]

animal parasites of g.p., the guinea pig is singularly unafflicted with parasitic diseases. None of those listed in the accompanying table is important as a disease agent of laboratory guinea pigs, but the most common are indicated with an asterisk.[21]

bacterial diseases of g.p., with the elevation of standards for maintenance and supply of laboratory guinea pigs, many bacterial diseases occupy a position of diminished importance. Those still important as causes of clinical disease are indicated with an asterisk in the accompanying table.

soft tissue calcification of g.p., a disease of nutritional origin in laboratory guinea pigs (*Cavia porcellus*) characterized by calcification in various soft tissues, including the myocardium, stomach, aorta, kidneys, and, most strikingly, at the colonic flexure. The condition occurs when there is an imbalance in magnesium, calcium, and phosphorous interrelationships and is corrected by

COMMON PARASITES OF THE GUINEA PIG

SPECIES	DISEASE OR COMMON NAME	LOCATION IN HOST
Campylochirus caviae	Fur mite	Skin, hair
Chilomastix intestinalis	− − −	− − −
Cryptosporidium (parvum?)	Cryptosporidiosis	Small intestine
*Eimeria caviae**	Coccidiosis	Small intestine
Entamoeba caviae	− − −	− − −
*Gliricola porcelli**	Chewing louse	Skin, hair
*Gyropus ovalis**	Chewing louse	Skin, hair
*Paraspidodera uncinata**	Pinworm	Cecum, colon
Toxoplasma gondii	Toxoplasmosis	Reticuloendothelial system, central nervous system
Trichomonas caviae	− − −	− − −
Trimeropon jenningsi	Chewing louse	Skin, hair

*See discussion under *guinea pig.*

BACTERIAL DISEASES OF THE GUINEA PIG

ORGANISM	DISEASE	COMMENTS
Bordetella bronchiseptica	Pneumonia	Carriers important in maintaining an enzootic state
Klebsiella pneumoniae	Pnuemonia	– – –
Pasteurella multocida	Epizootic pasteurellosis	Rare, high mortality
P. pseudotuberculosis*	Pseudotuberculosis	Disease originates with mesenteric lymphadenitis, then hematogenous spread to liver and spleen
Pneumococcus pneumoniae	Pneumonia; peritonitis	Especially Type XIX
Salmonella enteriditis	Paratyphoid	Rare
S. typhimurium	Salmonellosis or paratyphoid	Rare
Spherophorus necrophorus*	Cervical lymphadenitis	Golf ball-sized swellings under the ramus of each mandible
Streptobacillus moniliformis	Cervical lymphadenitis	Golf ball-sized swellings under the ramus of each mandible
Streptococcus spp.*	Septicemia, lymphadenitis	Especially those of Lancefield Group C

*Still important causes of clinical disease.

providing an adequate amount of magnesium in the diet.[80]

guinea pig paralysis   See under *paralysis*.

guinea worm disease   Dracunculosis.

guppy   A small tropical fish, *Lebistes reticulatus*, that has been used extensively in genetics research.

gynandroblastoma   A rare ovarian tumor containing histological features of both arrhenoblastoma and granulosa cell tumor.

gynase   A hypothetical enzyme-like substance regarded as the material basis of femaleness in heredity. A yellow substance also known as I-M-kuriase.

gyneco-, gyn-, gyne-, gyno-   Combining form denoting relationship to woman or the female sex.

gynecology   That branch of medicine which treats of diseases of the genital tract in women.

gynephobia   Dread of or morbid aversion to the society of women.

H

habituation   In behavioral science, the decrement in response strength which occurs with repeated elicitation of that response.

habu viper   See table accompanying *snake*.

hadacidin   An antibiotic produced by several species of *Penicillium*, which was first noted to inhibit the growth of human adenocarcinoma cells growing in embryonated eggs. It appears to act by inhibition of adenylic acid synthesis.[36, 49]

Haemonchus contortus   (twisted stomach worm)   A blood-sucking nematode found in the abomasum of sheep and other ruminants. Heavy infestations may be fatal. It has been estimated that 4000 worms can suck about 60 ml. of blood a day, and it is not uncommon to find thousands of worms in a single host.[21]

half-life   1. The time in which the radioactivity originally associated with an isotope will be reduced by one half through radioactive decay.   2. The time required for the body to catabolize and eliminate one half of any substance, or the time for one half of a cell population to be replaced.

halo-   A combining form denoting relationship to a salt.

hamartoma   A tumor-like nodule of superfluous tissue.

hamartophobia   Morbid fear of error or sin.

hamster   A small rodent of the family Cricetidae, superfamily Muroidea. It is nocturnal, has burrowing habits, a stout body, short tail, large cheek pouches, and thick soft fur. There are three outstanding species. The most common, *Cricetus cricetus*, is a large, light brown hamster found in Europe and Asia. *Cricetulus larabensis* (Chinese hamster) is small and gray, and inhabits Asia and the southern parts of Europe. *Mesocricetus auratus*, the most common Syrian species, is of medium size and reddish brown in color. Also known as the golden hamster, it is native to Asia Minor and the Balkans. Hamsters are very prolific, and aggressive to other rodents. They are useful in biomedical research because of their marked susceptibility to neoplasms, their value as bioassay screens for teratogenic materials, and their short gestation period.[80, 84]

hamster "virus"   An agent of the *Chlamydia* (*Bedsonia*) group, isolated from the lungs of suckling hamsters inoculated with human throat washings. It may be related to the mouse pneumonitis agent.[114]

Hanson unit   A unit of parathyroid extract, being one one-hundredth of the amount required to increase by 1 mg. the amount of calcium in the blood serum of a parathyroidectomized dog weighing 15 kg.

haplo- A combining form meaning simple or single.

haploid Having a single set of chromosomes, as normally carried by the gamete.

haploid parthenogenesis Development of a haploid egg without fertilization.

haplomycosis An infection caused by the fungus *Emmonsia (Haplosporangium) pervum,* seen in many wild animals such as ground squirrels, pocket mice, white-footed mice, kangaroo rats, pine squirrels, muskrats, beavers, rock and cottontail rabbits, mink, martens, skunks, weasels, wood rats, and raccoons. The spores of the fungus are inhaled into the lungs and enlarge, but then become encysted, with little host reaction. Natural infection of domesticated animals has not been reported.

hapten, haptene A substance such as *p*-aminobenzenearsonate which is not by itself immunogenic, but when coupled to a protein molecule reacts with antibodies that bear the same specificity. See *diazo reaction.*

hapto-, hapt- Combining form denoting relationship to touch or to seizure.

haptor The disk or sucker of a trematode.

harderian gland A large horseshoe-shaped gland located within the orbit of the eye of animals having a nictitating membrane. A small superior arm is connected to a large inferior arm by a narrow band medial to the optic nerve. The color varies from pink to gray depending on the number of melanocytes in the capsule and interlobar septa. A single excretory duct opens at the base of the nictitating membrane. In addition, the gland is speckled with a porphyrin pigment that fluoresces under ultraviolet light. Histologically, the gland is of the tubulo-alveolar type, covered with a connective tissue capsule and divided into lobes and lobules by strands from the capsule. The epithelial secretory cells are pyramidal and of varying height depending on the secretory phase. The secretion in the lumina of the tubules is oily and reddish brown in color.[51]

Harding-Passey melanoma See under *melanoma.*

harem mating See *breeding system.*

Harvey Society, Inc. Columbia University College of Physicians and Surgeons, New York, N.Y. 10032.

hashish The stalks and leaves of *Cannabis indica.* See *Cannabis.*

Hawaiian Academy of Science Bishop Museum, Honolulu, Hawaii 96819.

heartwater A fatal disease of cattle, sheep, and goats, marked by fluid accumulation in the pleural and pericardial cavities. It is caused by *Cowdria ruminantium.*

hedonophobia Fear of pleasure.

Heidenreich's disease (histolytic disease) A lethal disease of larvae of rhinoceros beetles (*Oryctes*). The etiology is unknown, but many of the symptoms and signs are very similar to those of a viral disease (*watery disintegration* or *wassersucht*) of cockchafer grubs (*Melolontha*). The diseased larva fails to accumulate lipids, and its body, especially the abdomen, becomes translucent. The fat-body and muscles become atrophic and eventually necrotic. Necrosis can be observed also in the integument. As the disease progresses, the larva ceases to move.

HeLa cells A cell line isolated from human cervical carcinoma.

helio- A combining form denoting relationship to the sun.

heliotropism The tendency of an organism to orient itself in relation to the stimulus of light.

    negative h., the tendency of an organism to orient itself away from the source of the light stimulus.

    positive h., the tendency of an organism to orient itself toward the source of the light stimulus.

helminth A worm or wormlike parasite. Parasitic helminths are common in all species of animals, although many of them produce no serious damage to the host. Some, on the other hand, compete for food substances or are blood-suckers and may cause serious disease. The principal helminth parasites are the trematodes (flukes), the cestodes (tapeworms), the nematodes (roundworms), and Acanthocephala (thorny-headed worms). See individual parasites, and see under specific animal hosts, e.g., *rabbit, rat,* and *primate.*

helper virus One that assists a defective virus.[39] See *complementation.*

hemagglutination Agglutination of erythrocytes, which may be caused by antibodies (see *hemagglutinin*) or by certain virus particles (e.g., the viruses of influenza and mumps).

    passive h., the agglutination of erythrocytes on which antigen has been absorbed in the presence of antiserum to that antigen.

    viral h., the agglutination of erythrocytes (usually chicken) in the presence of hemagglutinating viruses, e.g., those of influenza, mumps, etc.

hemagglutinin An antibody that agglutinates erythrocytes, classified according to the cells which it agglutinates as autologous (cells of the same organism), heterologous (cells of individuals of other species), and homologous (cells of other individuals of the same species). Some hemagglutinins are effective with erythrocytes suspended in 0.85 per cent sodium chloride solution; others are ineffective unless hydrophilic colloids (e.g., albumin and fibrinogen) are added, or unless the erythrocytes have been treated with a proteolytic enzyme.

    cold h., one that acts only at temperatures near 4° C.

    warm h., one that acts only at temperatures near 37° C.

hemangioblastoma A capillary hemangioma of the brain consisting of proliferated blood vessel cells or angioblasts.

hemangioendothelioma A tumor formed

by malignant proliferation of the endothelium of the capillary vessels.

hemangioendothelioma H6221   A spontaneously arising tumor found at necropsy in the epididymis of an untreated male BALB/c mouse in the laboratory of K. Hummel at the Jackson Memorial Laboratory in 1951. The tumor grows progressively in 80 to 100 per cent of BALB/c hosts to which it is transplanted, killing the host in four to six weeks. It has a transplant interval of 30 days. No metastases have been observed.

hemangiopericytoma   A tumor composed of spindle cells with a rich vascular network, which apparently arises from pericytes. It is related to the glomus tumor but, unlike the latter, has no nerve elements.

hemangiosarcoma   A malignant tumor formed by proliferation of endothelial and fibroblastic tissue.

hematein   An acid dye prepared from hematoxylin. It is an amphoteric dye used to stain tissues; in combination with mordants it functions as a cationic dye.[57, 153]

hematoxylin   A crystalline stain extracted from logwood with ether. Solubility at 15° C.: water 1.5 per cent, absolute alcohol 1.5 per cent, and glycerol 18 per cent. It is used in Verhoeff's carbol-fuchsin acid-fast stain, in Harris', Heidenhain's, and Mallory's stains, and for quenching nuclear fluorescence and to stain amyloid. It is important as a counterstain for naphthal, and is used in the D-chloracetate technic for esterases and in Weigert's elastica stain. It is also used with alizarin S for staining hemoglobin, with Bismark brown for mast cells, in Mallory's phloxine for hyalin, in metal impregnation technics for the Golgi apparatus, with phosphotungstic acid for Negri bodies, and with acid fuchsin-methylene blue and Mallory's aniline blue for collagen.[57, 153]

hemi-   A prefix signifying one half.

hemimelia   A developmental anomaly characterized by absence of all or part of the distal half of a limb.

hemipenes   Paired male copulatory organs.

hemo-, haemo-, hem-, haem-, hema-, hemato-   Combining form denoting relationship to the blood.

Hemobartonella   A genus of organisms of the family Bartonellaceae. See *Bartonellaceae.*

hemocoel   The blood-containing body cavity of some animals, e.g., arthropods and mollusks.

hemoglobin   The oxygen-carrying pigment of red blood cells. Hemoglobin of man occurs in at least nine forms that have electrophoretic patterns different from the normal F (fetal) and A (adult) forms. These are S, C, D, E, G, H, I, J, and K. Hemoglobin types are inherited as mendelian traits and, in heterozygous individuals, two forms may be present, e.g., HgA (normal) and HgS (sickle cell trait). This type of inheritance suggests that the specific proteins are produced by the progeny of individual clones of cells.[76, 162] See also *sickling.*

hemoglobin levels   See *hemogram.*

hemogram   The blood picture; a written record or graphic representation of the differential blood count. See tables on pages 92 and 93 for hemograms of various animals.

hemolytic unit   The amount of inactivated immune serum which, in the presence of complement, will completely hemolyze 1 cc. of a 5 per cent emulsion of washed red blood corpuscles.

hemophilia   A defect of the clotting mechanism resulting in reduced ability of blood to coagulate, and characterized by hemarthroses and deep tissue bleeding. The disease is hereditary and is expressed when an abnormal X chromosome is passed from carrier mother to male offspring. The defective chromosome is incapable of producing the antihemophilic factor.

Parents: xX   XY
             carrier   normal

F_1:   XX   xX   XY   xY
        normal   carrier   normal   hemophiliac

The two major types of hemophilia are classical hemophilia (factor VIII deficiency) and Christmas disease (factor IX deficiency), which are indistinguishable in their clinical manifestations or hereditary patterns. Counterparts of both major types have been found in anomen: factor VIII deficiency has been studied in several breeds of dogs and in horses and swine, and factor IX deficiency has been observed in dogs. A less common type (factor VII deficiency) has also been found in dogs.[76, 147, 162]

Hemophilus   A genus of nonmotile gram-negative rods which leads a strictly parasitic existence and requires phosphopyridine nucleotide (V factor) or biotin (X factor), or both, to grow. It is usually involved in infections of the upper respiratory tract, meningitis, or conjunctivitis, and also appears in chancroid.[36] See table on page 94.

hemorrhagic enterocolitis   See *mucoid enteritis of rabbits,* under *enteritis.*

hemorrhagic typhlitis   See *mucoid enteritis of rabbits,* under *enteritis.*

hen   Postpubertal female of various avian species, especially gallinaceous birds.

heparin   An acid mucopolysaccharide occurring in many tissues, especially the liver and mast cell granules. See table accompanying *allergy.*

hepatitis   Inflammation of the liver.

  canine infectious h. (hepatitis contagiosa canis; Rubarth's disease), a viral disease of foxes, dogs, wolves, and coyotes, characterized by apathetic appearance and loss of appetite. The temperature may reach 105° F. or higher. A stable DNA-containing member of the adenovirus group is the causative agent. Canine infectious hepatitis is unrelated to the human forms of the disease.[16]

  mouse h., infection with mouse hepatitis viruses (MHV). Such infections usually occur as latent or silent infections which may

NORMAL BLOOD VALUES: RED BLOOD CELLS*

SPECIES	RBC (cells/mm.^{3} × 10^6)	HB (g/100 mL.)	PCV (%)	MCV (μ^3)	MCH ($\mu\mu g.$)	MCHC (%)	RBC DIAM. (μ)	TOTAL PROTEIN (PLASMA) (g./100 mL.)	ICTERUS INDEX UNITS
Cow	5.0-10.0	8-15	24-46	40-60	11-71	30-36	4.5-8.0	6-8	2-15
	7.0	11	35	52	14	33	5.8		5-10
Sheep	8-16.0	8-16	24-50	23-48	9-12	31-38	3.2-6.0	6-7.5	<5
	12.0	12	38	33	10.7	33	4.5		
Goat	8.0-18.0	8-14	19-38	15-30	10-12.6	35-42	2.5-3.9	5-7.5	2-5
	13.0	11	28	23	Derived Value	38	3.2		
Swine	5.0-8.0	10-16	32-50	50-68	17-23	30-34			
	6.5	13	42	63	20	32			
Dog	5.5-8.5	12-18	37-55	60-77	19.5-24.5	32-36	6.7-7.2	6-7.5	<5
	6.8	15	45	70	22.8	34	7.0		2-5
Horse Cold-blooded	5.5-9.5	8-14	24-44	34-58		31-37	4.0-8.0		7.5-20
	7.5	11.5	35	46		35	5.9-5.8		
Hot-blooded (thoroughbred)	6.5-12.5	11-19	32-52					6-8	7.5-20
	9.5	15	42						
Cat	5.0-10.0	8-15	24-45	39-55	13-17	30-36	30-36	6-7.5	2-5
	7.5	12	37	45	15	33	33.2		
Chicken	2-4	7-13	25-45					3.6 (2)	
	3	10	35						
Monkey, *Macaca mulatta*	5.57 ± .73	11.72 ± 3.02	37 ± 6.75				6.1-6.9		7 (101)
							6.4 (12)		
Rabbit	4-7	8-15	30-50				6.7	6.2 (2)	
	6	12	40						
Guinea pig	4-7	11-17	33-45				7.5	4.7 (2)	
	6	14	40						
Hamster	7.5 ± .5	17.6 ± 1.0	47.4 ± 2.4				6.2-7.0		
							6.6		
Rat	7-10	12-18	35-45	60.4 ± 3.0 (47)	19.1 ± 0.8 (47)	31.8 ± 1.6 (47)	6.3	6.0 (2)	
	9	15	40						
Mouse	7-11	10-20	35-45				7.8		
	9	15	40				6.1		
Mink ♂	8.9-10.4	9.5-15.6	41-57	56.4-82	18.3	27.8-35	6-9.5		
	9.68	11.9	(53)	68	20	29	7.8		
Chinchilla	5.6-8.4	11.8-14.6					7.8		
	6.93	13.2							

*From W. Medway, J. E. Prier, and J. S. Wilkinson: Textbook of Veterinary Clinical Pathology. The Williams & Wilkins Co., Baltimore, Md. 21202, U.S.A.© 1969. Additional data and hemograms for other species can be found in Schalm[123] and Altman and Dittmer.[1]

Normal Blood Values: White Blood Cells*

Species	Thrombocytes $\times 10^5$	WBC $\times 10^3$	Segmented Neutrophil cell/mm³	Segmented Neutrophil %	Band Neutrophils cells/mm³	Band Neutrophils %	Eosinophil cells/mm³	Eosinophil %	Monocyte† cells/mm³	Monocyte† %	Lymphocyte† cells/mm³	Lymphocyte† %	Osmotic Fragility % NaCl min	Osmotic Fragility % NaCl max
Cow	1-8 / 5.0	4-12 / 8	600-4000 / 1200	15-45 / 28	0-120 / 20	0-2	0-2400 / 700	2-20 / 9	25-840 / 400	2-7 / 4	2500-7500 / 4500	45-75 / 58	0.52-0.60	0.44-0.52
Sheep	2.5-7.5 / 4.0	4.0-12.0 / 8.0	700-6000 / 2400	10-50 / 30	rare		0-1000 / 400	0-10 / 5	0-750 / 200	0-6 / 2.5	2000-4000	40-75 / 62	0.58-0.76	0.40-0.55
Goat	0.5 (43.86)	4.0-13.0 / 9.0	1200-7200 / 3250	10-50 / 30	rare		50-650 / 450	0-10 / 5	0-550 / 250	0-6 / 2.5	2000-9000	40-75 / 62	0.74	0.44
Swine	3.25-7.15	11.0-22.0 / 16.0	3200-10,000 / 5500	28-47 / 37	0-800 / 150	0-4 / 1	50-2000 / 500	1-11 / 3	250-2000 / 800	2-10 / 5	4500-13,000 / 8000	39-62 / 53	0.70	0.45
Dog	2.0-9.0	6.0-7.0 / 11.5	3000-11,500 / 7000	60-77 / 70	0-300 / 300	0-3 / 0.8	100-1250 / 550	2-10 / 4	150-1350 / 750	3-10 / 5	1000-4800 / 2800	12-30 / 20	0.4-.5 / 0.46	0.32-0.42 / 0.33
Chicken	2.54 ♂ / 2.65 ♀ (72)	15-45 / 30	Heterophils 3000-17,000 / 10,000				0-500 / 50		0-5000 / 1000	5	10,000-30,000 / 20,000	20	0.46	0.33
Monkey, Macaca mulatta		15.15±5.98		35.79±16.70				7±2.63 / 2.37	0.717±0.379			60.52±17.26		
Rabbit	7.43±2.18 (77)	6-12 / 9	Amphophil 2000-6000 / 4000				0-500 / 200		100-1000 / 500		200-500 / 300		0.3	0.5
Guinea pig	2-9 (86)	7-14 / 10	2000-6000 / 4000				200-2000 / 500		200-2000 / 500		3000-8000 / 5000		(76) / 0.30	0.52
Hamster	2.97-9.52 / 3.38±.89(86)	8.56±1.54 / 8.38±.58(47)		2±11.0				0.68		2.43	5000	67.0±11.9	0.40(87)	0.30
Rat	5-23 / 14	5-23 / 14	1-5000 / 3000		0-100 / 20	0-2 / 0.5	0-1000 / 200	0-11 / 4	0-1000 / 500	1-7 / 4	7000-13,000 / 10,000		0.50	0.30(76)
Mouse	2.46-3.39 (18)	4-12 / 8	500-4000 / 2000		0-300 / 100	0-3 / 0.5	0-500 / 200	2-12 / 2	0-1000 / 500	1-4 / 3	3000-9000 / 6000		0.50	0.30
Mink	1.94-3.80 / 2.50 (53)	3.8-10.2 / 6.38		18.5-69.0 / 41.7				2.5-16.0 / 7.2		0-5.5 / 1.1		22.5-57.5 / 43.5		
Chinchilla		5.4-15.6 / 9.3		39-54 / 45				0-5 / 2		0-5 / 1		45-60 / 51		
Horse Cold blooded		6-12 / 8.5		35-75 / 54										
Hot blooded (Thoroughbred)		5.5-12.5 / 9.0	2700-6700 / 4700	30-65 / 49	0-100 / 20	0-2 / 0.5		2-12 / 5		2-10 / 5	1500-5500 / 3500	15-50 / 35	0.34-0.56	0.45
Cat	3-7 / 4-5	5.5-19.5 / 12.5	2500-12,500 / 7500	35-75 / 59	0-300 / 100	0-3 / 0.5	0-1500 / 650	2-12 / 5	0-850 / 350	1-4 / 3	1500-7000 / 4000	25-70 / 44 ; 20-55 / 32	0.66-0.72 / 0.69	0.46-0.54 / 0.50

*Adapted from W. Medway, J. E. Prier, and J. S. Wilkinson: Textbook of Veterinary Clinical Pathology. The Williams & Wilkins Co., Baltimore, Md. 21202, U.S.A.© 1969.

Diseases Caused by *Hemophilus*

Agent	Host	Disease
H. agri	Lamb	Contagious disease of lambs
H. bovis	Cow	Infectious keratitis of cattle
H. ovis	Sheep	Mastitis
H. suis	Swine	Secondary invader in swine influenza

be activated by experimental stressors, or rarely, with no known source of provocation. The first isolated member of the group was the JHM virus (so-called for J. H. Mueller, by Cheever), which was found in the central nervous system of a paralyzed mouse. This agent, when passed in other mice, induced demyelinating encephalitis and occasionally focal necrosis of the liver. In contrast to the original isolate, later many MHV isolates were found to be more hepatotropic and came from adult animals.

Three types of stresses have been most commonly associated with hepatitis induction in JHM infected mice: (a) infection with *Eperythrozoon coccoides*, (b) inoculation with murine leukemia viruses, and (c) neonatal thymectomy. More recently, isolates of MHV have occurred as neurotropic agents with limited hepatotropism. In addition to the JHM (=MHV4) strain, other antigenically related variants are MHV-1, MHV-3, H-747, A-59, Nelson(PR) (=MHV2), EHF 120, and the MHV (SR) series. The infection is basically enteric, and entry of virus into other tissues is generally inhibited by maternal antibody in those colonies with endemic infection. Spontaneous or induced infections of suckling mice are seen usually in susceptible nurslings from nonimmune dams.[27, 63]

vibrionic h. of fowl (vibriosis of fowl), an infectious disease of chickens characterized by degenerative changes in the liver and, less frequently, in the heart and other organs. Bile is the source of the infective agent, which can be isolated in artificial media by means of chick embryos. A vibrio-shaped organism has been found by direct phase-contrast microscopy.

viral h. of ducklings, an acute viral disease of ducklings characterized by a short incubation period and high mortality rate. There is no serological relationship with viral hepatitis of the dog and man.[16]

viral h. of turkeys, a highly contagious disease of turkeys that produces a high death rate in poults under two weeks of age.

hepato-, hepat- Combining form denoting relationship to the liver.

Hepatocystis kochi A protozoan malarial parasite of the class Sporozoa, which infects Old World nonhuman primates. The life cycle differs from that of *Plasmodium* in that the entire cycle of schizogony (but not gametogenesis) occurs in the liver without an erythrocytic stage. The infection is generally asymptomatic in monkey hosts; the numerous raised opaque cysts (1 to 3 mm.) in the liver are usually encountered as incidental postmortem findings. No human cases are known. *H. kochi* is important because it led to the discovery of the exoerythrocytic stage of human malaria. The vector is believed to be midges of the genus *Culicoides*.[21, 41, 128, 159]

hepatoma 98/15 A spontaneous tumor of the liver found at necropsy in a 17-month-old C3H mouse in the laboratory of H. B. Andervont at the National Cancer Institute in 1940. The tumor grows without metastases in C3H mice and subcutaneous transplants kill the host in four to six months.[150]

Hepatozoon muris See *protozoan parasites,* under *rat.*

herbivorous Plant-eating.

hermaphroditic Having both male and female reproductive organs, a normal state in many invertebrate forms, as the parasitic tapeworms, which are capable of self-fertilization.

heron See *ciconiiform birds.*

herpesvirus A group of DNA viruses which includes some of the important animal viruses such as the viruses of canine herpes, simian herpes, pseudorabies, malignant catarrhal fever, feline and bovine viral rhinotracheitis, equine rhinopneumonitis, infectious laryngotracheitis of chickens and infectious pustular vulvovaginitis.[16, 39] See also *classification,* under *virus.*

h. B (B virus, *Herpesvirus simiae*), a virus antigenically related to the virus of herpes simplex that is the cause of an important zoonosis. The first two cases in man (in 1934 and 1949) were reported by Sabin, and the virus named by him for the physician infected (Dr. B.) in the first encounter. The disease is important not only because of its role as a zoonotic hazard, but also because it exemplifies a benign clinical disease in homotypic infection, which is expressed with much greater severity in the uncommon heterotypic relationship.

Spontaneous herpesvirus B infections of nonhuman primates have so far been limited to Asian species, particularly *Macaca mulatta, M. irus,* and *Cercopithecus aethiops,* although all primate species are known to be susceptible. In these natural hosts, the infection behaves as does herpes simplex of man; i.e., it causes benign herpetic vesicles and ulcers of the oral and perioral tissues, particularly the lips and tongue. Typical herpetic intranuclear inclusion bodies may be seen at the borders of the lesions. The clinical course, which runs approximately two to six weeks, appears to cause little discomfort to the host. A rising titer of neutralizing antibody can be demonstrated. The diagnosis is established by demonstration of inclusion bodies, a virus neutralization test, and production of herpes B encephalitis in susceptible rabbits.

The disease is transmitted to man by bites, scratches, accidental contact of broken skin with B-virus infected tissues, or laboratory accidents involving virus-contaminated fomites. Of the approximately twenty known human infections, most have followed bites or scratches, and of them there have been only two known survivors. The agent causes an ascending encephalomyelitis or encephalitis in man, the heterotypic host.

The question of whether nonhuman primates can carry the agent in latent infections (without lesions) is not clear, although rising antibody titers have been demonstrated. Similar relationships exist in herpesvirus T and Aujesky's virus infections, in which primates (tamarins and owl monkeys) and cattle occupy the heterotypic host role (with encephalitis) and squirrel monkeys and pigs, respectively, occupy the homotypic host role (with benign clinical disease).[41, 68, 114, 128]

h. T (*Herpesvirus tamarinus*) A herpesvirus that infects nonhuman primates of the New World. The disease was originally described by Hunt in tamarins (*Saguinus nigricollis*) and owl monkeys (*Aotus trivirgatus*), in which the infection is invariably fulminant and fatal without prodromal signs. In these species, the lesions include focal necrosis of the liver, bilateral adrenal hemorrhage, pneumonitis, and necrotic enteritis. Eosinophilic intranuclear inclusions are observed in cells bordering the necrotic areas, especially in the liver. Recently it has been observed that the squirrel monkey (*Saimiri sciureus*) is the probable natural host for the virus and may carry latent infections. The tamarin and owl monkey infections are aberrant and occupy an unnatural host status, similar to the situation in herpesvirus B infections of man, and Aujeszky's virus (*Herpesvirus suis*) infections of cattle. Old World primates are not susceptible to herpesvirus T.[126] See also *herpesvirus B*.

Herpesvirus simiae See *herpesvirus B*.

Herpetamonas A genus of flagellated parasites that closely resembles one of the stages of the life cycle of Trypanosomes and that completes its life cycle in a single invertebrate host. *H. muscarum* is a species found in the gut of house flies and blow flies. Its life cycle has leishmanial, leptomonal, crithidial, and trypanosomal stages. Infection occurs through cysts.[109]

Herpetologists League 900 Veteran Avenue, Los Angeles, Calif. 90024.

Heterakis spumosa See *helminth parasites*, under *rat*.

heterauxesis Growth of an organ or part at a different rate than that of the whole. It is known as tachyauxesis when the growth of the part is more rapid; bradyauxesis if slower. Cf. *isauxesis*.

hetero-, heter- Combining form meaning other, or denoting relationship to another.

heteroantibody An antibody combining with antigens originating from a species foreign to the antibody producer.

heteroantigen An antigen originating from a species foreign to the antibody producer.

heterocercal Denoting a tail of a fish in which the vertebral column runs into the larger, dorsal lobe. See also *diphycercal* and *homocercal*.

heterochromatin A genetically inert chromatin fraction that consists of histone, deoxyribonucleic acid, and ribonucleic acid. Cf. *euchromatin*.

heterodont Having teeth of various shapes and functions in different parts of the mouth, e.g., incisors and molars.

heteroecious Denoting a parasite requiring two or more hosts in its life cycle, as the trematodes.

heterogametic Characterized by the production of gametes bearing different kinds of sex chromosomes such as XY in the male. In some species the female is heterogametic. See also *W chromosome*, under *chromosome*.

heterograft Former name for xenograft.

heterokaryon (hybrid cell) A cell that results from the mixing of chromosomal material from two cells. Cells of this type provide important tools to study control mechanisms, because of the ability of cells from different organs and even unrelated species to fuse and read instructions from each other so that ordinarily repressed genes may become active. Such cells can be produced by exposure to certain viruses, e.g., myxoviruses and herpesviruses, in cell culture systems and may also play an important role in pathogenesis of disease.[59]

heteromorphosis Regeneration of an organ or structure different from the one that was lost.

heterophile antigen See under *antigen*.

heteroploidy The state of having an abnormal number of chromosomes.

heterosis (hybrid vigor) The increase in vigor as measured by growth, survival, and fertility that results from outcrossing of inbred lines. It is said to occur when the mean of the character in the F_1 falls outside the range of the mean of the two parental strains. Heterosis is the converse of inbreeding depression (q.v.) and is considered to be the result of the dominance (or interaction) of favorable alleles not common to both parental populations.

heterothallic Requiring copulation between the mycelia of two strains (of fungi) for the production of ascospores.

heterotopia 1. Displacement or misplacement of parts or organs; the presence of a tissue in an abnormal location. 2. A jumbling of sounds in words.

heterotopic graft A graft transferred from a given site of the donor to an anatomically different site in the recipient, i.e., to a position formerly occupied by tissue of a different kind.

heteroxenous Requiring more than one host in order to complete the life cycle; said of parasitic organisms. Cf. *monoxenous.*

hexa-, hex- Combining form meaning six.

Hexamita muris See *hexamitiasis,* and see *protozoan parasites,* under *rat.*

hexamitiasis A disease caused by species of *Hexamita,* well known as pathogens of wild fowl. Certain *Hexamita* have been indicted as the cause of death in several species of oysters, but some authors consider *Hexamita* to be only a fortuitous secondary invader in dead or dying oysters.

hexokinase An enzyme that catalyzes the transfer of a high-energy phosphate group of a donor to D-glucose, producing D-glucose-6-phosphate.

hexosephosphatase An enzyme that catalyzes the oxidation of hexose-phosphate.

hexoxidase An enzyme that catalyzes the oxidation of hexuronic (ascorbic) acid.

hibernation A dormant state accompanied by narcosis and physiological reduction of energy expenditure in various animal species during the winter. Several levels of hibernation are recognized. Cf. *estivation, torpor,* and *dormancy.*

  deep h., a form that is usually seasonally linked, and characterized by reduction of many processes of the body, e.g., reduction of deep body temperature to levels approximating the ambient, and reduction of metabolic heart and respiratory rates. Representatives of only three mammalian orders show deep hibernation: Insectivora, Chiroptera (bats), and Rodentia.

hibernoma A rare tumor made up of large polyhedral cells with a coarsely granular cytoplasm, occurring on the back or around the hips. So called because it is considered by some to be a manifestation of a vestigial fat storage organ and comparable to the dorsal fat pads of hibernating animals.

hierarchy In behavioral science, the classification of a series of responses by rank or order.

hiero-, hier- Combining form denoting relationship to the sacrum, or to religion.

hieromania Religious insanity or frenzy.

hierophobia Fear of sacred or religious things.

high altitude disease Brisket disease.

hip dysplasia See *dysplasia.*

hippanthropia A condition in which the patient believes himself to be, and makes movements in imitation of, a horse.

hippuricase An enzyme that catalyzes the hydrolysis of hippuric acid to benzoic acid and glycine.

Hirschsprung's disease (megacolon) Massive enlargement of the colon in man, resulting from obstruction caused by an aganglionic segment of bowel. A similar condition is sometimes seen in dogs.

histamine An amine occurring in many animal and vegetable tissues which is a powerful dilator of capillaries and a stimulator of gastric secretion. See table accompanying *allergy.*

histaminase An enzyme that has the power of oxidizing the alpha amino group of histamines.

histidinase An enzyme of the liver that acts specifically on histidine, splitting it into ammonia, glutamic acid, and formic acid.

histio-, histo- Combining form denoting relationship to tissue.

histocompatible (isohistogenic) Capable of being accepted and remaining functional; applied to cells or tissues showing these characteristics when grafted into another organism.

histocompatibility That quality of genetic characters which governs the antigenic structure and ability of an individual to accept or reject tissue grafts. See *histocompatibility loci.*

histocompatibility loci Loci on chromosomes that contain the genes controlling the acceptance or rejection of tissue grafts. In the mouse, it has been shown that the compatibility of tissue grafts is governed by 15 or more loci. These loci are widely distributed throughout the chromosomes. Histocompatibility genes have so far been identified on the X and Y chromosomes and in linkage groups I, V, and IX. Histocompatibility genes act as such because their end-products are alloantigens possessing the property of antigenicity when grafted to an individual lacking them. Although it is probably true that all histocompatibility genes determine alloantigens, the reverse, i.e., that all alloantigens determine histocompatibility, is not true. Histocompatibility loci differ in their immunogenicity or "strength." In the mouse, the histocompatibility 2 (H-2) locus possesses the most potent alloantigens, with 20 or more alleles, and is unique in that species because the histocompatibility determinants are identical to the blood group material borne in the erythrocytes.[51]

histolytic disease See *Heidenreich's disease.*

histone A basic protein soluble in water and insoluble in dilute ammonia. The globin of hemoglobin is a histone. The protein material that surrounds the nucleic acid of chromosomes is made up of histone.

History of Science Society Department of Medical History, UCLA, Los Angeles, Calif. 90024.

Hjarre's disease A granulomatous disease of chickens caused by *Escherichia coli.*

H-2 locus See *histocompatibility loci.*

H-melanosis See *melanosis.*

Hodgkin's disease A painless, progressive, and fatal enlargement of the lymph nodes, spleen, and general lymphoid tissues, which often begins in the neck and spreads over the body. Called also infectious granuloma, malignant granuloma, malignant lymphoma, lymphomatosis granulomatosa, lymphadenoma, lymphogranulomatosis, granulomatosis maligna, lymphosarcoma, anemia lymphatica, and pseudoleukemia. Similar but not identical lesions have been reported in the cat.

hog cholera (swine fever) A highly contagious viral disease of swine caused by an agent related to the bovine diarrhea virus. The swine lungworm may serve as a reservoir and intermediate host for the hog cholera virus.[16]

hog flu Swine influenza.

holandric Denoting a trait inherited through the male; transmitted by the Y chromosome.

holarctic Having a distribution which includes Europe, northern Asia, and North America.

holo- A combining form meaning entire, or denoting relationship to the whole.

holoenzyme The functional compound formed by the combination of an apoenzyme and its appropriate coenzyme.[90, 118]

hologynic Inherited exclusively through the female; transmitted through genes located on the X chromosome.

holophytic Requiring only inorganic chemicals for nutrition, as photosynthetic plants.

homeo- A combining form denoting sameness, similarity, or a constant, unchanging state.

homeopathy A system of therapeutics founded by Samuel Hahnemann (1755-1843), in which diseases are treated by drugs which are capable of producing in healthy persons symptoms like those of the disease to be treated, the drug being administered in minute doses.

homo- 1. Combining form meaning the same. 2. A prefix in chemical names indicating the addition of one CH_2 group to the main compound.

homocercal Denoting a tail of a fish in which the dorsal and ventral lobes are the same size. Cf. *heterocercal* and *diphycercal*.

homogametic Having but one class of gametes, as the female XX chromosomes.

homograft Former name for allograft.

homoiotherm (homotherm) An animal with the ability to regulate its body temperature at a constant level despite changes in the environment; warm-blooded animal.

homologous 1. Denoting organs which are similar in origin and structure but not in function. 2. Allogeneic.

homology The similarity of given structures in different organisms that have descended from common ancestors. In biochemistry, the degree of similarity of the base sequences of two DNA molecules.

homotransplant Former name for allograft.

homunculus A miniature animal thought by early biologists to be contained in the sperm. In psychiatry, a little man created by the imagination.

hookworm A worm of the family Strongylidae, parasitic in the intestine of man and anomen.

Hoplopleura enomydis See *arthropod parasites*, under *rat*.

hormone A chemical substance, produced in the body, that has a specific effect on the activity of a certain organ; originally applied to substances secreted by various endocrine glands and transported in the blood stream to the target organ on which their effect was produced, the term was later applied to various substances not produced by special glands but having similar action.

    juvenile h., see *corpora allata*.

horned rabbit See *Shope papilloma*, under *papilloma*.

horotelic See *evolutionary rate*.

horsehair worm A of the genus *Gardius*. See *Nematomorpha*.

horsepox (contagious pustular stomatitis; grease-heel) A disease of horses, resembling vaccinia.[16]

horseshoe crab See *merostome*.

host 1. An animal or plant that harbors another organism. 2. The recipient of an organ or other tissue transplanted from another organism.

    definitive h., the animal in which a parasite passes its adult and sexual existence.

    intermediate h., the animal in which a parasite passes its larval or nonsexual existence.

    reservoir h., an animal that serves as a host for organisms that are also parasitic for man or other animals.

Houston Animal Science Association (formerly Laboratory Animal Technician Association) Texas Research Institute of Mental Science, 1300 Moursund Avenue, Houston, Tex. 77025.

howler monkey A member of the genus *Alouatta*. See *primate*.

hutch burn A type of superficial dermatosis in caged rabbits that results from prolonged contact of delicate skin, especially mucocutaneous borders or skin near the genital organs, with urine-soaked bedding. Yellowish or brownish crusts form which may be invaded by pathogens. It is similar to ammonia burn in the corneas of domestic poultry, which is associated with poor husbandry conditions and inadequate ventilation. It is necessary to differentiate this condition from spirochetosis.

hyalo-, hyal- Combining form denoting resemblance to glass.

hyaluronidase (Duran-Reynals factor; spreading factor) An enzyme that catalyzes the hydrolysis of hyaluronic acid, the cement substance of the tissues. It is found in leeches, in snake and spider venom, and in the testes and malignant tissues, and is produced by a variety of pathogenic bacteria.

hybrid An animal or plant produced from parents different in kind, such as parents belonging to two different species.

hybrid cell See *heterokaryon*.

hybridization The production of hybrids by crossing parents that are genetically unlike, especially when they are of different species. In biochemistry, a method of measuring the homology of nucleic acid molecules.[90]

hybrid vigor See *heterosis*.

hydatid disease An infection caused by larval forms of certain cestodes, e.g., *Echinococcus*, and characterized by the development of expanding cysts. See *Taenia*.

Hydra (hydroid) See *coelenterate*.

hydrase An enzyme that catalyzes the addition of water to a compound without producing hydrolysis.

hydrencephalocele Hernial protrusion through a cranial defect of brain substance containing cerebrospinal fluid.

hydro-, hydr- Combining form denoting relationship to water or to hydrogen.

hydrocephalus A condition characterized by abnormal accumulation of fluid in the cranial vault, accompanied by enlargement of the head and atrophy of the brain, often as a result of blockage of the cerebral aqueduct. It is seen in many species of anomen and may be hereditary or acquired.

hydrogenase An enzyme that catalyzes the reduction of various substances by means of molecular hydrogen.

hydrogenlyase An adaptive enzyme formed by many strains of *Escherichia coli* that catalyzes the breakdown of formic acid to carbon dioxide and hydrogen.

hydrolase An enzyme that catalyzes the hydrolytic cleavage of compounds such as esters, peptides, glycosides, and amides.

hydromania A mental disorder marked by a tendency to commit suicide by drowning.

Hydrophidae See table accompanying *snake*.

hydrophobia Rabies.

hydrophthalmia See *congenital glaucoma*, under *glaucoma*.

2-α-(hydroxybenzyl)-benzimidazol (HBB) An aromatic carbanol that inhibits picornavirus replication by interference with synthesis of viral RNA polymerase.

hydroxyurea A hydroxylamine derivative used as an antitumor drug because of its ability to interfere with DNA synthesis.

hylo- A combining form denoting relationship to matter (material or substance).

hylology The study of elementary or crude materials.

Hymenolepis A genus of cestodes of the family Hymenolepidae.

   H. diminuata, a species commonly parasitizing rodents, less frequently man. See table of Common Cestode Parasites, accompanying *cestode,* and see *helminth parasites,* under *rat*.

   H. nana (dwarf tapeworm), a species that infects the mouse, rat, hamster, and man. See table of Common Cestode Parasites, accompanying *cestode,* and see *helminth parasites,* under *rat*.

hyper- A prefix signifying above, beyond, or excessive.

hyperaminoacidemia Presence of amino acids in the blood or hemolymph in excess of the normal amount. Silk retention in silkworms produces a lethal increase of amino acids in the hemolymph of the insect larvae. See *silk toxicity*.

hyperergy Reactivity to a substance, usually an antigen, of greater intensity than that observed in normal individuals exposed to the same substance. Cf. *hypoergy, anergy,* and *pathergy*.

hypergammaglobulinemia An excess of gamma globulin in the blood; seen in myeloma, Aleutian mink disease, and various diseases characterized by excessive immunologic reactions.[93, 129]

hyperhedonia Morbid increase of the feeling of pleasure in agreeable acts.

hypernephroma A tumor of the kidney whose structure resembles that of the cortical tissue of the adrenal gland.

hyperphosphatasia Abnormal elevation of the level of phosphatase in the body.

hyperplasia A cellular abnormality characterized by increase in size and number of cells, which still retain their functional ability and resemble normal tissue arrangement more than neoplasia. Cf. *hypertrophy*.

hyperplastic epidermal disease See *fishpox*.

hyperpsychosis Exaggeration of mental activity with abnormal rapidity of the flow of thought.

hypersensitivity A state of altered reactivity in which the body reacts to a foreign body more strongly than normal. See also *allergy* and *anaphylaxis*.

hypertrophy The enlargement of an organ because of an increase in the size of its constituent cells. Cf. *hyperplasia*.

hypervolemia Abnormal increase in the volume of circulating fluid (plasma) in the body.

hypha (pl. hyphae) A filamentous element or strand of fungal mycelium.

hypno- A combining form denoting a relationship to sleep.

hypnosis An artificially induced passive state in which there is increased amenability and responsiveness to suggestions and commands, provided that these do not conflict seriously with the subject's own conscious or unconscious wishes.

hypnosophy The study of sleep and its phenomena.

hypo- A prefix signifying beneath, under, or deficient. In chemistry, it denotes that the principal element in the compound is combined in its lowest state of valence.

hypoamylasemia (neonatal) See *mucoid enteritis*, under *enteritis*.

hypochromy (hypochromic effect) An increase in the intensity of absorption of a dye.[57, 153]

hypoergy Reactivity to a substance, usually an antigen, of less intensity than that observed in normal individuals exposed to the same substance. Cf. *anergy* and *hyperergy*.

hypogammaglobulinemia An abnormally low level of gamma globulin in the blood.

hypophosphatasia An inborn error of metabolism with a genetic basis, characterized by lowered phosphatase activity of the serum, apparently due to lack of alkaline phosphatase in the cells, and resulting in defective rebuilding and mineralization of bone.

hypoplasia Defective or incomplete development. Cf. *aplasia* and *atrophy*.

hypoproteinemia Abnormal decrease in the

amount of protein in the blood, sometimes associated with starvation. It may result in abnormal accumulation of fluid in the peritoneal cavity because of lowered blood osmotic pressure.

hypso-   A combining form denoting relationship to height.

hypsochromy (hypsochromic effect)   A shift in the absorption curve of a dye in solution toward shorter wavelength. Colors of metachromatic dyes may be arranged in order of increasing hypsochromic effect.[57, 153]

hypsophobia   Morbid fear of great heights.

I

-iasis   A word termination meaning a process or the condition resulting therefrom, particularly a morbid condition.

iatro-   A combing form denoting relationship to a physician or to medicine.

iatrogenic   Resulting from the activity of physicians. Originally applied to disorders induced in the patient by autosuggestion based on the physician's examination, manner, or discussion, the term is now applied to any condition in a patient occurring as the result of treatment by a physician or surgeon.

Ibis   See *ciconiiform birds*.

ichthyo-   A combining form denoting relationship to fish.

ichthyosis (fish skin disease; xeroderma)   A disease characterized by dryness, roughness, and scaliness of the skin, due to hypertrophy of the horny layer.

-id   A word termination meaning having the shape of or resembling; also used in combination with a root representing the causative factor, as dermatophytid.

Idaho Academy of Science   Department of Physical Science, University of Idaho, Moscow, Idaho 83843.

ideology   1. The science of the development of ideas.   2. The body of ideas characteristic of an individual or of a social unit.

idiogram   Diagrammatic representation of chromosomes usually prepared by cutouts of phase contrast photomicrographs of metaphase chromosomes arranged in paired sequence. Cf. *karyotype*.

ileitis   Inflammation of the ileum, the distal portion of the small intestine.

  regional i. (regional enteritis; Crohn's disease), an asymmetrical thickening of the mucosa and submucosa of the lower portion of the small intestine, consisting of fibrosis and proliferation of endothelial tissue and many bizarre multinucleated giant cells. An entirely comparable disease has been reported in dogs and may be of significance in the pathogenetic studies of the disease in man.

  terminal i. of hamsters (regional ileitis; wet-tail, enzootic intestinal adenocarcinoma), a disease of uncertain etiology in laboratory-reared hamsters, characterized clinically by profuse, watery diarrhea (hence "wet-tail"), prostration, and death. The gross lesions usually include thickening and enlargement of the terminal ileum, with exten-

sion occasionally toward both the colon and the jejunum. Necrotic foci appear as white spots on the serosal surface of the ileum. No method of treatment or prevention is known. Although there appears to be common agreement among workers that the disease is infectious, there is intense disagreement as to whether the essential lesion is basically inflammatory or neoplastic (i.e., carcinoma in situ).

Illinois State Academy of Science   State Geological Survey, Urbana, Ill. 61801.

imitation   See *imitative* and *mimetic behavior,* under *behavior.*

imitation courtship feeding   A neurosis of psittacine birds, especially the budgerigar (parakeet), in which the bird repeatedly fills its crop with seeds only to regurgitate them on its owner or on its reflection in shiny objects such as a mirror in its cage. Such birds will often lose weight through starvation. Treatment consists of removing shiny objects and providing a mate.[112]

immune response   See *phylogeny of immunoglobulins,* under *immunoglobulin.*

immunity   The condition of being immune; security against any particular disease or poison, specifically the power which an individual sometimes acquires to resist and/or overcome an infection to which most or many of its species are susceptible.

immunoblast   A large cell with highly pyroninophilic cytoplasm found in lymph-draining areas where antigen has been injected and antibody synthesis is in progress. Also seen in cell cultures exposed to transforming substances such as phytohemagglutinin. Immunoblasts are thought to be precursors of lymphocytes or plasma cells. See *plasmablast.*

immunoelectrophoresis   A method combining electrophoresis and double diffusion for distinguishing between proteins and other materials by means of differences in their electrophoretic mobility and antigenic specificities. The supporting medium may be agar gel, cellulose acetate film, or other material. In general the antigen is placed in a central well and subjected to electrophoresis. The antibody is then placed in rectangular wells, which are parallel to the direction of the electrophoresis. Double diffusion occurs between the antibody in the rectangular wells and the antigen.[129]

immunofluorescence technic   Localization

and study of antigens in tissues by application of specific antibodies against the substances in question. Antibodies are labeled with various fluorescing dyes, which can then be visualized under the microscope with ultraviolet illumination.[153] See *fluorescence microscopy*.

immunogen A substance capable of stimulating the formation of corresponding antibodies. See *antigen*.

  insect i., the stimulus to the immune response in insects. Immune responses in insects are probably not the consequence of antigen-antibody-globulin reactions as in vertebrates, but more likely the result of the production of some other principle in insect hemolymph. Thus the term "immunogen" may be used to replace "antigen" when describing the stimulus to immune response in insects. Many insect immunogens may be conventional antigens.

immunogenetics The study of genetic phenomena with immunologic technics and theories, e.g., studies of inheritance of tolerance, blood chimerism, histocompatibility loci, etc.

immunoglobulin Any of several classes of macromolecules possessing antibody activity. They are composed of multiple polypeptide chains, each under separate genetic control. They also contain a variable percentage of carbohydrate. The humoral or circulating antibodies are found in these macromolecules.[32, 36] See table, and see *antibody* and *gammopathy*.

  phylogeny of i., the evolution of the immune response. The evolutionary history of antibody-forming ability remains one of the most intriguing and important questions of biology. Implicit in the immune process is the ability of an individual to recognize and accept as friendly all of his own complex chemicals, to know that those of his species are friendly to a lesser degree, and to understand that the rest of his environment contains a multiplicity of materials which may be acceptable or unacceptable for incorporation into his physiological machine. Survival of the individual, and collective survival of the species, depend on this ability to read, record, and recall the myriad of environmental challenges encountered in the day-to-day experiences of the living organism.

  Invertebrates possess an active immune system and, although they do not have gamma globulins, they do produce natural agglutinins and lysins. The horseshoe crab, *Limulus polyphemus*, produces a hemagglutinating protein resembling beta globulin, with a molecular weight of 390,000 and subunits of about the same size as vertebrate light chains, i.e., 20,000.

  Humoral antibodies have been demonstrated in cyclostomes, the lowest living subclass of vertebrates, although one order, Myximoidea (hagfish), has been reported unable to produce humoral immunity but capable of graft rejection. Elasmobranchs (sharks and rays) produce gamma globulins of both 17 to 19S and 7S size. Thus, even though many details remain to be discovered, there appears to be a strong thread of unity in mechanisms of antibody structure and function in the vertebrates.[34, 47, 108]

immunohematology That branch of medicine dealing with diseases of the blood in which the cause, the pathogenesis, or the clinical manifestations have been shown to be determined by an antigen-antibody reaction.

immunological drift A term used to refer to changes in antigenic characteristics of strains of viruses in which they evolve, slowly changing the degree of, their cross-activity. Changes in human influenza virus provide excellent examples.[39]

immunologic competence The condition (of a cell) of being capable of producing antibody.

immunology The biological discipline that concerns itself with the study of the interaction between antigens and antibodies. This science originally was devoted to the study of immunity against disease but has broadened during the past several decades, to be much more inclusive. Cf. *immunopathology*.

immunopathology That branch of biomedical science which concerns itself with the study and interpretation of immunological phenomena as they relate to the mechanisms of disease.

immunoproliferative A name created by Dameshek to describe diseases characterized by excessive proliferation of the lymphoreticuloendothelial tissues, sometimes with production of abnormal globulins and autoantibodies. There is some disagreement as to whether this group should include only malignant conditions such as leukemia, leukosis, lymphosarcoma, myeloma, and perhaps Hodgkin's disease, or whether it should also embrace such immunological disorders as lupus erythematosus, rheumatoid arthritis, Aleutian mink disease, equine infectious anemia, and lymphocytic choriomeningitis.

immunosuppressant Any substance that can depress immunological reactions by in-

CLASSIFICATION OF IMMUNOGLOBULINS

GLOBULIN	SEDIMENTATION COEFFICIENT	MOLECULAR WEIGHT
IgG (γG)	7	160,000
IgA (γA)	7 to 15.5	150,000 to 500,000
IgM (γM)	19	1,000,000
IgD (γD)	7	160,000
IgE (γE)	7 to 9	200,000

terference with cellular or humoral antibody synthesis. Many immunosuppressants are also useful as oncolytic agents. See *antimetabolite*.

impaternate   Pertaining to parthenogenesis, i.e., reproduction in which no male parent takes part.

imperforate anus   See *atresia ani*.

imprinting   A rapid learning process, seen usually in early development, especially in birds, whereby an animal forms a strong social attachment to an object. Thus, newly hatched birds, in the absence of the mother, will follow almost any moving object, and will then persist in showing specific behavior patterns to that object which it would normally show to the rest of the species if the initial moving object had been its mother.

Imuran   Trademark for *azathioprine*.

inborn   Formed or implanted during intrauterine life. See also *innate behavior*, under *innate*, and *inborn error*, under *metabolism*.

inbred-derived   See *breeding system*.

inbred strain   A population produced by inbreeding. The practice of inbreeding strains of various species is undertaken in order to provide research animals of isogenic background. A strain is regarded as inbred when brothers and sisters have been mated for twenty or more consecutive generations. Parent and offspring matings may be substituted for brother and sister matings provided that, in the case of consecutive parent and offspring matings, each mating is to the younger of the two parents. Any strain separated after eight to nineteen generations of brother and sister inbreeding and maintained thereafter in the same laboratory without intercrossing for a further twelve or more generations is regarded as a substrain. Substrains are also constituted when (a) pairs from the parent strain or substrain are transferred to another laboratory or (b) detectable genetic differences become established.[51, 146] See *breeding system*, see *coisogenic* and *congenic*, and see under *mouse*.

inbreeding   See *breeding system*.

inbreeding depression   A term introduced by Sewall Wright to characterize the overall decrease in fitness associated with increasing degrees of inbreeding. The fitness characters so affected include litter size, body weight, disease resistance, and life-span. The most probable explanation for inbreeding depression is the gradual fixation of deleterious recessive alleles normally masked and rendered ineffective by dominant alleles in a genetically heterogeneous population.[51] Cf. *heterosis*.

inclusion blennorhea of guinea pigs   See *inclusion body conjunctivitis of guinea pigs*.

inclusion body conjunctivitis of guinea pigs (inclusion blennorhea)   A *Chlamydia* infection of guinea pigs manifested clinically by mild conjunctivitis. The agent is involved in both enzootic and epizootic infections in which the key histologic lesion is inclusion bodies in the cytoplasm of conjunctival epithelial cells. Most commonly affected are four- to eight-week-old weanlings. Partial immunity is believed to develop following clinical infection. The relationship of this agent (described originally by Murray) to the agent of the *Chlamydia* disease of guinea pigs described by Storz is uncertain. The latter disease is characterized by fever, peritonitis, splenomegaly, and focal necrosis of the liver, while inclusion body conjunctivitis is clinically mild.[114]

incross   Breeding of individuals homozygous for the same gene. See also *breeding system*.

index case   See *propositus*.

Indiana Academy of Science   State Library, 140 North Senate, Indianapolis, Ind. 42604.

indigocarmine   An acid dye of the indigoid series. Solubility at 15° C.: water 1.3 per cent and glycerol 5 per cent; insoluble in absolute alcohol. It is used with eosin and hematoxylin as a differential stain for keratin in vaginal smears.[57]

inducer   A compound that causes an increase in the net quantity of a specific (adaptive, or inducible) enzyme. In some cases, inducers are known to increase the rate of synthesis of an enzyme, e.g., the β-galactoside-induced synthesis of β-galactosidase in *Escherichia coli*, or the glucocorticoid-induced synthesis of tyrosine transaminase in the rat liver. However, since the level of an enzyme is determined by the rate of degradation as well as the rate of synthesis, and since these processes can be independently varied, the specific degree of action of an inducer cannot be generalized.

inducible enzyme   See under *enzyme*.

industrial melanism   See *Biston betularia*.

infantile diarrhea of mice (epidemic [epizootic] diarrhea of infant mice)   Descriptive name given to two distinct viral disease entities of nursling mice. *Epidemic diarrhea of infant mice* (EDIM) is characterized by peak morbidity in the twelve- to thirteen-day-old age group, low mortality, and unthrifty, diarrhea-stained nursling mice. There is usually a pot-belly resulting from a milk-filled stomach, and a distended but nonedematous colon that is filled with mustard-yellow, mucoid fecal material. Inclusion bodies in the intestinal epithelium may be demonstrable. The growth of survivors is so retarded that they are unsuitable for research purposes. It is extremely contagious and may occur as a colony-wide epizootic. The infection rate in first litters is usually higher than in subsequent litters. The virus may be transmitted vertically (parents to offspring) or horizontally (cage to cage).

In contrast, *lethal intestinal virus of infant mice* (LIVIM) is associated with lower morbidity, peak incidence in the sixteen- to twenty-day-old age group, and high mortality. The intestine, unlike the case in EDIM, is empty and gas filled. Microscopically there are distinctive lesions which include enteritis and multinucleated giant cells ("balloon cells"). It is not as common as EDIM.

Two approaches are used to control and prevent infantile diarrhea (of either form) in production colonies. The first of these, employed in conventional colonies, consists of the use of filter tops, which are applied to single-pair mating boxes (filter-top cages). The incoming (and outgoing) filtered gas prevents the ingress of virus to susceptible nurslings. The cages are opened for changing only under a negative pressure (or laminar flow) hood. The second approach is more radical, consisting of delivery of neonates by hysterectomy, which are then reared and maintained behind a virus-excluding barrier.[27, 63]

infaunate To introduce a commensal or mutualistic microfauna into an organism that is capable of serving as a host. The introduction of certain flagellates or ciliates in a defaunated (q.v.) termite constitutes an infaunation.

infectious bovine rhinotracheitis See under *rhinotracheitis.*

infectious canine hepatitis See under *hepatitis.*

infectious feline peritonitis A transmissible disease of domestic cats caused by an RNA-containing virus that replicates by budding from cytoplasmic vacuoles. The lesions consist of serofibrinous peritonitis, focal necrotic areas that resemble small granulomata, meningitis, uveitis, and arteritis.

infectious kidney swelling See *Egtved virus.*

infectious pancreatic necrosis An acute and highly contagious viral disease of trout, especially young brook trout (*Salvelinus fontinalis*). Little is known of its epizootiology, but outbreaks with mortality rate as high as 80 per cent have been observed in hatcheries. Affected fish exhibit whirling or corkscrew type of swimming. Gross lesions consist of petechiae of the pyloric ceca, a digestive tract empty of ingesta but filled with mucus, flaccid hindgut, and pale liver and spleen. Microscopic lesions consist of destruction of pancreatic tissue and necrosis of surrounding adipose tissue. Round or oval cytoplasmic inclusion bodies with a clear halo are seen in pancreatic cells. The agent is cultivable in fish cell cultures, and is classified as a picornavirus.[114]

infectious pustular vulvovaginitis (IPU) An acute viral disease of cattle characterized by swelling of the vulva, sticky exudate, frequent urination, and fever. Males may show lesions of the penis and prepuce. The causative agent appears to be a member of the herpesvirus group.[16]

influenza See *porcine influenza.*

infra- A prefix meaning situated, formed, or occurring beneath the element indicated by the word stem to which it is affixed.

infrared Denoting rays of energy beyond the red end of the spectrum, between the red waves and the radio waves, having wavelengths between 7700 and 120,000 angstroms.

inhibition 1. Arrest or restraint of a process. 2. In behavioral science, used to account for decrements in response magnitude or habit strength. 3. In biochemistry, interference with a chemical reaction by a variety of chemical agents (inhibitors). Cf. *enzyme repression.*

competitive i., inhibition (as of enzyme action) which occurs in the presence of an inactive compound that is similar to and tends to replace an essential metabolite, and which can be reversed by increasing the concentration of substrate.

external i., in classical conditioning, a decrease in the magnitude of a conditioned response when an extraneous stimulus is presented with the conditioned stimulus.

irreversible i., the reaction in which the EI (enzyme concentration-inhibitor concentration) complex does not show reversible dissociation.

noncompetitive i., inhibition in which the addition of more substrate does not affect the inhibition. Cf. *competitive i.*

innate 1. Inborn, hereditary; congenital. 2. In behavioral science, a term sometimes used to refer to species-specific or unlearned behavior, which are more exact terms and are preferred to the word innate.

innate releasing mechanism (IRM) A hypothetical neurosensory mechanism thought to explain the action of sign stimuli.

insect Any member of the class Insecta (Hexapoda), subphylum Mandibulata, phylum Arthropoda. Characteristically insects have a distinct head, thorax, and abdomen; one pair of antennae; mouth parts adapted for chewing, sucking, or lapping; and a thorax with, typically, three pairs of jointed legs and two pairs of wings that may be variously modified, reduced, or absent. The heart and aorta are mid-dorsal, respiration is by branched tracheal tubes conveying air from spiracles directly to tissues, and excretion by malpighian tubules jointed to hindgut. The brain comprises fused ganglia, there is double ventral nerve cord with segmental ganglia, and the eyes are both simple and compound. The sexes are distinct, and females are usually oviparous. Development after hatching takes the form of gradual or abrupt metamorphosis. At least 675,000 species known. See table.

insect-borne diseases Diseases caused by insect-transmitted microorganisms. The principal ones are dengue, encephalitis lethargica, filariasis, infantile paralysis, Japanese river fever, kala-azar, leishmaniasis, malaria, nagana, pappataci fever, plague, relapsing fever, Rocky Mountain spotted fever, surra, Texas fever, trypanosomiasis, tularemia, typhus fever, and yellow fever.[66] See arbovirus and table accompanying *zoonosis.*

insecticide See *biotic* and *microbial insecticide.*

insect immunogen See under *immunogen.*

A CLASSIFICATION OF INSECTA

SUBCLASS	METAMORPHOSIS	ORDER	EXAMPLES
Apterygota (wingless)	Ametabola (no metamorphosis)	Protura	Springtails
		Collembola	
		Diplura	Japygids
		Thysanura	Bristletails
Pterygota (winged, but reduced or absent in some)	Hemitetabola (young are nymphs with compound eyes, metamorphosis gradual)	Orthoptera	Roaches, grasshoppers
		Dermaptera	Earwigs
		Plecoptera	Stone flies
		Isoptera	Termites
		Embioptera	Embiids
		Odonata	Dragonflies
		Ephemeroptera	May flies
		Mallophaga	Biting lice
		Anoplura	Sucking lice
		Corrodentia	Book lice
		Hemiptera	True bugs
		Homoptera	Aphids
		Thysanoptera	Thrips
	Holometabola (young are larvae without compound eyes, metamorphosis complex)	Mecoptera	Scorpion flies
		Neuroptera	Dobson flies
		Trichoptera	Caddis flies
		Lepidoptera	Moths, butterflies
		Diptera	True flies
		Siphonaptera	Fleas
		Coleoptera	Beetles, weevils
		Strepsiptera	Stylops
		Hymenoptera	Ants, wasps, bees

insectivorous Insect-eating; many insectivores also consume other invertebrates in addition to insects.

insightful learning See under *learning*.

instar The stage between two molts during the larval development of an insect.

instinct A class of sets of responses that are unlearned and shown by most members of a species.

instinctive movement See *fixed action pattern*.

Institute for Comparative Biology Zoological Society of San Diego, P.O. Box 551, San Diego, Calif. 92112.

Institute of Laboratory Animal Resources 2101 Constitution Avenue, N.W., Washington, D.C. 20418.

insulinase An enzyme in body tissues that destroys or inactivates insulin.

insulin unit One twenty-second of a milligram of the pure crystalline insulin now adopted as the standard.

integrated control The integration of the activities of natural enemies of pest organisms with cultural, physical, and/or chemical control measures; pest control that combines and integrates biological control and chemical control.

intention movement A behavioral pattern that usually occurs in a behavior chain in association with other portions of the same chain; e.g., a certain species of bird may proceed through an ordered series of movements before becoming airborne and from these behavior patterns flight can be predicted.

intercross See *breeding system*.

interference Depression of virus yield because of mixed infection of a single cell. Several types of interference have been described: viral-attachment, intracellular, heterologous, and homologous.[39] Cf. *complementation* and *interferon*.

interferon An antiviral substance produced by the cells of many vertebrates in response to virus infection. It appears to be protein or polypeptide in nature, is antigenically distinct from virus, and acts by conferring on cells resistance to the multiplication of a number of different viruses.[32, 39]

intermediate host One that harbors the larval or asexual stage of a parasite.

International Committee on Laboratory Animals National Institute of Public Health, Geitmyrsveien 75, Oslo 1, Norway.

International Primatological Society Anatomisches Institut der Universitat, Ludwig-Rehn-Strasse 14, 6 Frankfurt a.M., Germany.

International Union for Conservation of Nature and Natural Resources International Commission of National Parks, 2000 P Street, N.W., Washington, D.C. 20036.

interphase The period during which a cell is not dividing; the interval between production of a new cell and its mitosis.

Intersociety Committee on Pathology Information 1501 New Hampshire Avenue, N.W., Washington, D.C. 20036.

interstitialoma A tumor or mass of interstitial tissue.

intrahemocoelic Within the hemocoel or perivisceral cavity of an invertebrate, as an intrahemocoelic injection.

intro- A prefix meaning into or within.

invertase Invertin.

invertin (invertase; saccharase; sucrase) An enzyme produced by yeasts and the intestinal mucosa, which catalyzes the hydrolysis of cane sugar to invert sugar.

Iodamoeba butschlii See *protozoan parasites*, under *rat*.

iodine agglutination test A test using a mixture of potassium iodide and serum from a patient or experimental animal. When mixed in equal parts, agglutination indicates a rise in circulating gamma globulin. It is a screening test for diseases characterized by hypergammaglobulinemia, including Aleutian disease of mink.

5-iodo-2′ deoxyuridine (IUDR) A halogenated pyrimidine that interferes with synthesis of viral DNA; it is also used as an immunosuppressant.

iridescent virus disease A disease of Diptera, Lepidoptera, and Coleoptera, caused by large icosahedral viruses. The larval fat body appears to be the principal site of replication, although the virus multiplies in the cytoplasm of other tissues. Diseased larvae show a marked opalescence, which is particularly intense in the fat body. The pellets of virus purified by centrifugation reflect strongly iridescent light. The virions are about 130 mμ in diameter.

isabelline An adjective applied to the light brown coloration of some desert-dwelling organisms.

isatin-β-semicarbazone An antimetabolite that inhibits poxvirus replication by interference with synthesis of virus specific proteins.

isauxesis Growth of a part or parts at the same rate as the growth of the whole. Cf. *heterauxesis*.

ischio- A combining form denoting relationship to the ischium, or to the hip.

Isle of Wight disease Under this name were included several maladies of adult honeybees having analogous symptoms and said to have reached epizootic proportions in the British Isles between 1905 and 1919. Some authors believe that acarine disease was the principal, if not the only, constituent of the Isle of Wight disease. Other authors believe that Isle of Wight disease might have been a type of dysentery or some other malady of the digestive system caused by poisoning or malnutrition. See also *acarine disease*.

isoantibody An antibody formed in response to immunization with tissue constituents from individuals of the same species.

isoantigen A constituent of tissue cells or fluids (e.g., a blood group antigen) that is capable of eliciting specific antibody formation in some other (genetically different) animal of the same species, but not in the animal itself (or in animals of the same inbred strain). A better term, alloantigen, has been suggested, which is more logical and etymologically appropriate.

isocitric enzyme An enzyme of the Krebs cycle that converts *d*-isocitrate to oxalosuccinate, using NADP as a co-factor, and oxalosuccinate to α-ketoglutarate, using Mn^{++} as a co-factor.

isoenzyme (isozyme) Any enzyme that possesses the same substrate specificity as another but differs in polypeptide sequence. Isoenzymes are often detected by electrophoresis and are not necessarily immunologically distinct.

isogeneic (syngeneic) Of the same origin; used, in contrast to allogeneic, to denote the immunologic relationship between individuals of the same genotype. The term isologous is sometimes used in this context. See *isograft*.

isogenic Denoting a condition of genetic identity.

isograft (isogenic or isogeneic graft; syngeneic graft) A graft of tissue between genetically identical individuals, e.g., a graft within inbred strains, between identical twins, or between F$_1$ hybrids produced by crossing inbred strains.

isohemagglutination Agglutination of erythrocytes caused by a hemagglutinin from another individual of the same species.

isohistogenic See *histocompatible*.

isoimmunization Development of antibodies against an antigen derived from an individual of the same species.

isomerase Any enzyme of the class that catalyzes the process of isomerization, such as interconversion of aldoses and ketoses.[90, 118]

isoniazid (INH; isonicotinic acid hydrazide) A drug used for both prophylaxis and treatment of tuberculosis. In subhuman primates it is used at a dose rate of 5 mg. per day for prophylaxis. There is some evidence to indicate it is not entirely successful in preventing infection by isoniazid-resistant mycobacteria, and also that the drug itself has central nervous system side effects that may impair the value, for purposes of neurophysiologic experimentation, of monkeys which have received isoniazid.[155]

N-isopropyl-α-(2-methylhydrazino)-p-toluamide (MIH) An antimetabolite with considerable antineoplastic activity in experimental trials.

isoproterenol A sympathomimetic agent used clinically in man as a bronchodilator and experimentally in animals (rats) to induce necrotizing (noncalcifying) cardiopathy.

isopycnic Having the same density; used to refer to cell organelles with similar buoyant densities. See *density gradient*, under *centrifugation*.

isotope An element with the same atomic number as another, but with a different atomic mass.

isotopology The scientific study of isotopes, and of their uses and application.

-itis A word termination denoting inflammation of a part indicated by the word stem to which it is attached, as hepatitis (inflammation of the liver), gastritis (inflammation of the stomach).

-ize A word termination denoting subjection to the specific action or treatment indicated by the stem to which it is affixed, as adrenalectomize, thyroidectomize, etc.

J

jaagsiekte A respiratory disease of sheep derived from the Dutch words meaning drive (jaagt) and sickness (siekte). The disease runs a chronic afebrile course of several months or even years, and results in pronounced thickening of the alveolar walls and partial obliteration of the alveolar spaces. It may be related to maedi and pulmonary adenomatosis (q.v.). There is some indication that it may be caused by a viral agent, which would place it in the group of slow virus diseases.

Janus green B A basic mono-azo dye. Solubility at 15° C.: water 5 per cent and glycerol 8 per cent. It is used for counting bacterial colonies and staining oocysts of coccidia and, in combination with neutral red, for supravital staining of blood.[57, 153]

Japanese gypsy-moth disease A disease of larvae of *Porthetria dispar*, presumably caused by the bacterium *Streptococcus disparis*. The affected larvae cease to eat, and develop diarrhea. In the late stages of the disease, the streptococcus is found in the hemocoel, and the insect's muscle tissue gradually disintegrates in a rather characteristic fashion.

Japanese quail A small bird, *Coturnix coturnix japonica*, used in laboratories for studying the effects of light and dark cycles, genetic defects, and infectious diseases.[137]

jaundice In addition to its meaning in mammalian pathology, this term refers particularly to nucleopolyhedrosis (q.v.) of the silkworm, *Bombyx mori*.

jellyfish See *coelenterate*.

JHM See *mouse hepatitis*, under *hepatitis*.

Johne's disease See *paratuberculosis*.

joint dysplasia See *dysplasia*.

juvenile hormone See *corpora allata*.

K

kallidin A kinin liberated by the action of kallikrein on a globulin of blood plasma. See *kinin*, and see table of Mediators of Allergic Reactions, accompanying *allergy*.

kallikrein An enzyme present in the pancreas, saliva, urine, blood plasma, etc., which liberates kallidin from a globulin of blood plasma and has vasodilator and whealing actions. See *kinin*.

kallikreinogen The inactive precursor of kallikrein; it is normally present in blood; its conversion into kallikrein may be triggered by a variety of physical or chemical changes. See *kinin*.

kangaroo See *marsupial*.

Kansas Academy of Science Department of Biology, Fort Hays Kansas State College, Hays, Kansas 67601.

Kaplan leukemia virus Lymphoid leukemia virus isolated by Kaplan from a lymphosarcoma in C57B1 mice that was induced by x-irradiation. Repeated passage of the agent in C57B1 mice and their hybrids resulted in a decrease in the incubation period prior to tumor formation and an increase in the incidence.[114]

karyo- A combining form denoting relationship to a nucleus.

karyosome A small mass of chromatin present in the nucleus of a cell.

karyotype A systematized arrangement of the chromosomes of a single cell. Cf. *idiogram*.

Kentucky Academy of Science College of Arts and Sciences, University of Kentucky, Lexington, Ky. 40506.

keratinase A proteolytic enzyme that enables the clothes moth to digest wool keratin.

kerato- A combining form denoting relationship to the cornea, or to horny tissue.

keratoacanthoma A rapidly growing papular lesion with a superficial crater filled with a keratin plug, usually on the face, which reaches maximum size and then resolves spontaneously within four to six months from onset. It is sometimes confused with squamous cell carcinoma.

kethoxal bis (thiosemicarbazone; KTS) An antimetabolite used as an antitumor drug because of its ability to interfere with DNA synthesis.

kidney tumor agent (of fish) An infectious agent isolated originally from an aquarium species, *Pristella riddlei*, but subsequently shown to be infectious also for the guppy (*Lebistes reticulatus*) and zebra fish (*Brachydanio rerio*). The original specimen had tumors of the musculature and coelom, but all experimentally infected fish had tumors of the kidney, which subsequently metastasized to various locations. Inclusions were not observed.[114]

kidney worm A nematode that parasitizes the kidney. There are two distinct species: *Dioctophyma renale* (q.v.) is found in the adult form in the renal pelvis of the dog and mink and rarely of man. They are extremely large roundworms reaching a length of over 100 cm. The other species is the swine kidney worm, *Stephanurus dentatus*, a large parasite about 40 mm. in length, found principally in the perirenal tissues. Its ova are discharged into the urine through the lumen of the ureter. It is especially common in the southern part of the United States.

kilo- A combining form used in naming units of measurement to indicate a quantity one thousand (10^3) times the unit designated by the root to which it is affixed.

Kikuth's disease Canary pox.

kinase 1. An enzyme that catalyzes the transfer of a high-energy group of a donor, usually adenosine triphosphate (ATP), to some acceptor, and is variously named, according to the acceptor, as creatine kinase, fructokinase, galactokinase, hexokinase, and phosphoglycerate kinase. Called also *phostransferase* and *transphosphorylase*. 2. An enzyme that activates a zymogen, variously named according to its source, as enterokinase, staphylokinase, and streptokinase.

kinin One of a group of endogenous peptides, of which bradykinin is the prototype, found in the bloodstream. Of particular interest in experimental pathology is the kallikrein-kinin-kininase system (see diagram). Kinins are formed from kininogen by the action of kallikrein, which is found in plasma, various exocrine glands, and granulocytes. Hageman factor is often necessary for the activation of kallikrein. Activation is inhibited in some systems by several antiinflammatory agents, metabolic inhibitors, and EDTA. Kinins can produce the cardinal signs of inflammation, but some of these effects are altered by salicylates or phenothiazines. Kinin is rapidly destroyed by a variety of kininases, which can be inhibited by several chelating agents. The split products resulting from kininase action are biologically inactive.

kiwi See *apterygiform birds*.

Klebsiella A genus of short, gram-negative, encapsulated bacilli that produce a profuse, mucoid, and tenacious growth on solid media. Capsular antigens are used for immunologic typing of members of this group (Quelling reaction).[16, 36] *K. pneumoniae* causes Friedlander's pneumonia in man. *K. pneumoniae* var. *genitalium* causes metritis in mares.

kleptomania An uncontrollable impulse to steal, the objects taken usually having a symbolic value of which the subject is unconscious, rather than a monetary value.

kleptophobia Insane dread of becoming a thief or of being stolen.

Klinefelter's syndrome A disease of males characterized by gynecomastia, aspermatogenesis, and increased levels of folliclestimulating hormone, and by an abnormal karyogram (q.v.), consisting of excessive numbers of X chromosomes, XXY, XXXY, or XXXXY. In anomen, the counterpart of this disease is the tricolored male calico cat which occurs occasionally. This color pattern is a recessive trait carried on the X chromosome, and male cats with this color pattern must of necessity have two X chromosomes.

Klossiella muris See *protozoan parasites*, under *rat*.

koala See *marsupial*.

koinoniphobia Morbid fear of a room filled with people.

krait See table accompanying *snake*.

krebiozen An unidentified substance isolated from the blood of horses injected with *Actinomyces bovis*, claimed to be effective in the treatment of cancer.

krebspest A disease of the European freshwater crayfish, *Astacus fluviatilis*. In the 1800's a prolonged epizootic of krebspest virtually wiped out commercial use of *Astacus*. It is caused by a fungus, *Aphanomyces astaci*, which has a predilection for nervous tissue.

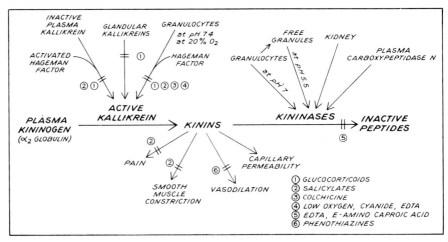

Figure 3. The Kallikrein-kinin-kininase system. See *kinin* for further details. (From A. S. Nies and K. L. Melmon: Kinins and arthritis. Bull. Rheum. Dis., 19:512–517, 1968.)

Krebs 2 tumor (Krebs 2 carcinoma)　A rapidly growing, undifferentiated neoplasm that originated spontaneously as a carcinoma, probably of the mammary gland, in a non-inbred stock mouse. It was found at necropsy in the laboratory of Krebs, in Copenhagen in 1932, and was considered to be the rare finding of a mammary tumor in a male mouse. The solid variant grows in 100 per cent of transplant hosts, killing the animal in about four weeks. It grows progressively in most mouse strains. In 1950, G. Klein and E. Klein developed an ascites form of the tumor by successively transplanting it to strain A inbred and non-inbred Swiss mice. They designated this variant as the Krebs 2 ascites tumor, which kills Swiss female hosts six to eleven days after intraperitoneal injection.[150]

krill　See *cetacean*.

Kurloff body　An intracytoplasmic structure found in peripheral blood leukocytes of guinea pigs, probably of the lymphoid or mononuclear series. It was previously thought to be a developmental stage of a protozoon, but it probably consists of some internal cellular degenerative component such as a residual body.

kuru　A chronic, progressive, degenerative disorder of the central nervous system characterized by tremor, ataxia, dysarthria, strabismus, terminal dysphagia, and death in less than a year in most patients. The condition has been restricted to Melanesian natives of one region in the Eastern Highlands of the Australian Trust Territory of New Guinea, where in past years it was a major cause of death, especially in young adult women. Recent research has indicated that it may be caused by a transmissible agent (perhaps a virus) with a strong genetic predilection for certain families and that it may be related to the agent of scrapie of sheep. Elimination of some cannibalistic practices in this tribe has markedly reduced the incidence of kuru. Resemblance of the lesions of kuru to scrapie (q.v.) stimulated exhaustive efforts to determine whether an infectious agent was its cause, and it has been serially transmitted in primates by intracerebral inoculation of brain material which originated from a person with kuru.[14, 44]

K virus　A virus of conventionally maintained mouse stocks, first isolated by Kilham from C3H inbred mice carrying the Bittner mammary tumor agent. It is a papovavirus and, when inoculated into suckling mice less than ten days of age, induces fatal pneumonia distinguished by swelling and proliferation of endothelial cells lining the small vessels. Feulgen-positive inclusion bodies have been observed in the nuclei of infected cells. No known disease is associated with natural infection with K virus. Diagnosis is established by serologic evidence of infection.[27, 63]

L

Laboratory Animal Breeders Association　Lakeview Hamster Colony, Newfield, N.J. 03844.

lacmoid　An acid dye of the oxazine group. Solubility at 15° C.: water 10 per cent, absolute alcohol 10 per cent, and glycerol 5 per cent. It is used with Martius yellow for staining callose in pollen tubes and with tannic acid and ferrous chloride for phloem and contiguous tissue.[57]

lactase　An intestinal enzyme that splits lactose into glucose and galactose.

lactic dehydrogenase virus (LDV; Riley's LDH virus; LDH elevating virus)　A virus first recognized and isolated in 1960 as the cause of a rise in plasma LDH in mice with tumors, a finding that laid to rest earlier conclusions that the tumors were responsible for elevated LDH levels. LDV is a small (40 mμ) RNA virus not yet grouped with other viruses and not known to infect animals other than mice. In addition to its effect on LDH, viral activity also increases the levels of isocitric dehydrogenase, SGOT, and glutathione reductase. Viremia is believed to persist for the entire life-time of infected individuals; there are circulating antigen-antibody complexes present in the bloodstream. (Cf. *Aleutian disease* and *lymphocytic choriomeningitis*.) Although there are usually no morphologic abnormalities, certain individuals exhibit splenomegaly and lymphadenopathy.

Diagnosis is based on the rise in plasma LDH in susceptible mice inoculated with suspect plasma. It is believed that wild house mouse stocks are the primary infective reservoir (WMI virus). The virus will cross the placenta to cause fetal infection in dams inoculated when pregnant, but not in those chronically infected prior to pregnancy. The virus is shed in urine, saliva, and milk.[27]

lagomorph　A herbivorous mammal of the order Lagomorpha, which includes pikas, hares, and rabbits.

Lamarckism　The theory proposed by Lamarck that acquired characteristics could be transmitted to offspring.

laminitis　An inflammatory disease of the sensitive laminae of the hoof, especially of the horse. These are folded, vascular structures which nourish the horny hoof. When they become inflamed and congested, stasis and eventually tissue necrosis can result. The pathogenesis of the disease is not understood, although in some cases it appears to be of allergic origin and is responsive to treatment with antihistamines.

lampbrush chromosome See under *chromosome.*

lamprey See *cyclostome.*

lancamycin See *macrolide.*

Lancefield classification A system of classification of streptococci based on group-specific antigens in the cell wall. Examples of these are as follows: group A, pathogenic for man; group B, present in most cases of bovine mastitis; group C, from pathologic conditions of anomen; group D, isolated from cheese; group E, isolated from milk; group F, isolated from throat cultures of man; group G, isolated from man, dogs, and monkeys; groups H and K, nonpathogenic, isolated from throat and nose cultures.[36]

langur A long-tailed monkey of the genus *Presbytis.* See *primate.*

lapinization Passage of a virus through rabbits as a means of modifying its characteristics.

lappets See *wattles.*

larva (pl. *larvae*) An immature but self-supporting form of an organism, which differs significantly from that of an adult.

larva migrans See *visceral larva migrans.*

laryngotracheitis (roup) A viral disease of the respiratory tract of chickens and occasionally pheasants. Other birds are wholly immune.

laser An acronym (*l*ight *a*mplification by *s*timulated *e*mission of *r*adiation) for a device that produces an extremely intense and nearly nondivergent beam of monochromatic radiation with all waves in phase. It can be used in surgery, in microdissection technics, and for detecting very small objects which interrupt the beam when directed through a microscope.

late-replicating X chromosome See under *chromosome.*

lathyrism An intoxication from ingestion of seeds of the plants of genus *Lathyrus.* There are two forms of the disease: one is characterized by spastic paraplegia, hyperesthesia, and paraesthesia, and the other by improper development of connective tissues, especially in the walls of arteries. When ingested by certain animals, especially turkeys and swine, the seeds may cause dissecting aortic aneurysms (see *osteolathyrism*).

L cell A cell from strain of mouse fibroblasts grown in culture for many years. They are very useful because of their ability to support replication of many types of viruses.

LDH elevating virus Lactic dehydrogenase virus.

LDV Lactic dehydrogenase virus.

leaf monkey A member of genus *Presbytis.* See *primate.*

learning In behavioral science, a mental process or a group of such processes inferred from the observation that animals learn and that their behavior in a given situation is consequently modified from that which occurred in the same situation on previous occasions. Thus learning is a generic term for conditioning of various types.

insightful l., a term used to account for a relatively large and not easily reversible change in behavior which appears between two successive occasions in a given environmental situation.

latent l., the acquisition in the absence of obvious reinforcement of a rather marked change in the magnitude or relative frequency of a response.

place l., learning in which an animal is given reinforcement for approaching a certain place, rather than for performing specific movements as in response learning. For example, an animal is rewarded for always entering the white goal box in a T-maze whether it is presented on the left or right of the choice point.

response l., learning in which an animal receives the reinforcing stimulus when it exhibits certain movements rather than approaching a certain location as in place learning. For example, an animal is rewarded for turning left at the choice point in a T-maze.

serial l., the acquisition of a progressively stereotyped behavior chain contingent upon the occurrence of a series of different responses as the number of reinforcements increases.

trial-and-error l., conditioning as it is observed to occur in the absence of precise experimental controls. In this process the course of learning is slow and characterized by many irrelevant responses.

lecithinase An enzyme that catalyzes the splitting of lecithin.

leech See *annelid.*

LE factor An antinuclear antibody seen in the sera of those affected with systemic lupus erythematosus

leio- A combining form meaning smooth.

leiomyofibroma A tumor with leiomatous, myomatous, and fibromatous elements.

leiomyoma A benign tumor derived from smooth muscle.

leiomyosarcoma A sarcoma containing large spindle cells of unstriped muscle.

Leishmania A genus of hemoflagellate protozoa of class Mastigophora which are characterized by a two-stage life cycle, leishmanial and leptomonad. The leishmanial stage is an oval organism that measures 2μ in diameter and has no flagellum, but has a nucleus, an axoneme, a blepharoplast, and a kinetoplast. The leishmanial stage is found in man in the reticuloendothelial cells of the spleen, liver, and bone marrow and in the circulating monocytes. The leptomonad form is seen in insect hosts.[21, 109, 159] See table.

lemming A small rodent of the family Cricetidae, which is widely distributed throughout the world. The American species include the black-footed (*Lemmus nigripes*) and the brown lemming (*L. trimucronatus*) of the northwestern areas of Canada and of Alaska. The European species contain the Arctic collared or pied lemmings (*Dicrostonyx groencandicus*), which are the only rodents that turn white during the winter season.

DISEASES CAUSED BY *Leishmania* [142, 159]

SPECIES	DEFINITIVE HOST	INTERMEDIATE HOST	GEOGRAPHIC DISTRIBUTIONS	DISEASE
L. braziliensis	– – –	– – –	South America	Mucocutaneous leishmaniasis
L. donovani	Man, dog, cat, squirrel, cow, horse, sheep, laboratory animals	Sand fly (*Phlebotomus*)	Mediterranean area, Africa, Asia, South America	Visceral leishmaniasis, kala azar
L. tropica	Man, (occasionally the dog, cat, monkey, squirrel)	Sand fly (*Phlebotomus*)	Southern Europe, Africa	Cutaneous leishmaniasis

lemur Any member of several genera of arboreal mammals of the family Lemuridae. See *primate*.

lepraphobia Morbid dread of leprosy.

leprosy A chronic infective granuloma caused by organisms of the genus *Mycobacterium*. The lymph nodes, particularly those of the axillary and inguinal regions, may be affected. In other cases, the skin and subcutaneous tissue may be involved. *M. leprae* causes leprosy in man, *M. lepraemurium* in the rat. Other species of *Mycobacterium* cause skin lesion tuberculosis in the cow, leprosy in the buffalo, and amphibian tuberculosis in the frog, tadpole, snake, turtle, and fish.

    rat l., disease of wild rats caused by *Mycobacterium lepraemurium*, which has been seen in Europe, England, Australia, and the United States, but not in laboratory rats. It has a chronic course characterized by lymphadenopathy, swelling and ulceration of the skin, focal alopecia, and cachexia. The lymph nodes contain epithelioid cells with intracellular organisms. These aggregates of epithelioid cells are also seen in affected skin and in pulmonary and hepatic granulomata. The mycobacteria of the rat share many of the physiologic and physical characteristics of the human agent, *Mycobacterium leprae*, e.g., inability to grow on artificial media, but they are antigenically unrelated. The agent is susceptible to passage in rats, chicks, and pigeons. It appears to hold excellent promise as a model for human leprosy.[32, 92]

lepto- A combining form meaning slender, thin, or delicate.

Leptomonas ctenocephali The simple flagellated stage of the protozoa *Leishmania;* it is found in the gut of dog fleas. See *Leishmania*.

Leptopsylla segnis See *arthropod parasites*, under *rat*.

Leptospira A genus of microorganisms of the family Treponemataceae, order Spirochaetales, made up of finely coiled organisms 6 to 20μ long. They have a wide species range of infectivity (see table).

leptotene See *meiosis*.

lesion Any pathological or traumatic discontinuity of tissue or loss of function of a part. It may be visible or invisible, as a biochemical lesion.

lethal intestinal virus of infant mice See *infantile diarrhea of mice*.

leucism An abnormal loss of plumage pigmentation in birds. All white plumage accompanied by dark eyes, or otherwise normal plumage with patches of white, should be called leucism rather than partial or incomplete albinism. *Complete leucism* is the loss of all pigments (melanic and carotenoid) in the plumage but not in soft tissues. *Partial leucism* is a localized, often symmetrical loss of all pigments in the plumage. *Melanic leucism* refers to the loss of melanic but not carotenoid pigmentation, and *carot-*

DISEASES CAUSED BY *Leptospira*

AGENT	HOST	DISEASE
L. australis	Man, horse	Canefield fever in man, ophthalmia in the horse
L. autumnalis	Man	Akiyama, Hasami-Netsu fever, Fort Bragg fever
L. canicola	Dog, man	Stuttgart disease (canine typhus), canicola fever in man
L. grippo-typhosa	Horse	Periodic ophthalmia
L. icterohemoglobinuria vitrelorum	Young calves	Spirochetal jaundice
L. icterohemorrhagiae	Man, dog	Leptospiral jaundice, Weil's disease (the organism is harbored by wild rats)
L. pomona	Swine, man, horse, cow	Swineherd's disease in man, periodic ophthalmia in the horse, mastitis and sometimes fulminating disease and death in the cow

enoid leucism refers to the loss of carotenoid but not melanin pigments (also called carotenoid leucino). Leucism is often genetically dominant to wild-type coloration.[112] See also *schizochrosim.*

leukemia A fatal proliferative disease of the hematopoietic or reticuloendothelial tissues, some forms of which are characterized by an increase in the number of leukocytes and their precursors in the blood, together with enlargement and proliferation of the lymphoid tissue of the spleen, lymph nodes, and bone marrow. The disease is usually accompanied by progressive anemia, internal hemorrhage, and increasing exhaustion. Leukemia is classified clinically on the basis of (1) the duration and character of the disease—acute or chronic, and (2) the type of cell involved—myeloid (myelogenous), lymphoid (lymphogenous), or monocytic.

The term leukemia has been controversial since first used by Virchow, who intended it as a strictly descriptive appellation applied to the distinctive buffy coat of leukocytes in the blood of certain patients—"Weiss Blut" or white blood. Since then the argument has raged as to whether leukemia should refer only to the "manifestation" of increased circulating white blood cells or should be used to describe a complex of diseases of the hematopoietic or reticuloendothelial tissues, which sometimes exhibit increased numbers of peripheral blood leukocytes. The latter use of the word has resulted in such awkward expressions as "aleukemic leukemia." But who is to say this is worse than atelectasis for collapse, or nondisjunction for failure to separate? The trend seems to be away from strictness and toward liberalism, and in this book the broader use of the word will be followed.

The question of a name need not be settled before the problems of etiology, or whether leukemia is of multicentric or unicentric (clonal) origin, or whether indeed it should be considered "cancer of the blood," as it is often referred to by laymen. We can be certain it is one of the most devastating and widespread diseases of the animal kingdom, and provides scientists with some of nature's most important and complex scientific conundrums.[5, 11, 30, 39, 53, 120, 127, 133, 150, 162]

In anomen, many types of leukemia resemble those seen in man. Some are viral in origin, some are transplantable, and some appear to be hereditary, or at least vertically transmitted. Attempts to extrapolate these facts to analysis of human leukemia have resulted in a morass of speculation, theory, and misconception. But some of the facts known about leukemia in anomen can be stated as follows:

Transmissibility: Ellerman and Bang first proved in 1908 that chicken leukemia could be transmitted by a bacteria-free filtrate, later shown to be a virus. The first demonstration of viral leukemia in mammals was by Gross in 1951 by the inoculation into disease-free mice of a filtrate from leukemic AK strain mice, which show a high incidence of the disease. This virus also proved to be transmitted from parents to offspring. Virus particles can be seen in tissues and in concentrated serum. Cf. *oncogenic viruses,* and see *leukovirus* under *virus.*

Hereditary predisposition: Certain inbred strains of chickens are far more vulnerable to leukemia than others, and certain strains of mice are more susceptible to specific types of leukemia than others. Thus the interplay of host susceptibility and agent variation indicates the importance of genetic factors in leukemogenesis.

Ionizing radiation: Extensive epidemiologic studies of human leukemia have shown that exposure to radiation vastly increases its occurrence. Thus, there was a direct relationship between incidence of leukemia in survivors and proximity to the holocaustic epicenter at Hiroshima. In mice, does of 400 to 600 R of x-radiation increase susceptibility to leukemia. Mice kept germ-free for several generations will develop the disease when subjected to x-irradiation because of activation of virus.

The characteristics of leukemia in various species are as follows:

The cow: The disease is mainly of the lymphocytic type. Usually parenchymatous organs and lymph nodes are more involved than peripheral blood, resulting in the use of the term lymphoma or lymphosarcoma. Rare cases of granulocytic leukemia have been reported. The disease occurs with much greater frequency in some regions and in some herds than in others, leading to speculation about the possibility of vertical or horizontal transmission, or both. This also suggests genetic susceptibility.

The dog: Leukemia is common in all breeds of dogs from the age of five years upward. Lesions usually involve all palpable lymph nodes, and peripheral blood abnormalities occur late in the disease if at all. Transplantation experiments have been successful in immunosuppressed recipients or when injected in the fetus in utero.

The cat: The disease is most common in old cats, although it may occur at any age. There is generalized visceral lymphadenopathy and frequent invasion of the kidney, liver, or intestine. The mediastinal lymph nodes and the thymus are common sites of localization. Transmission with cell-free filtered material has been successful. Inoculated animals exhibit type C virus particles in bone marrow. Considerable evidence of horizontal transmission in cats derives from the occurrence of "clusters" of clinical cases.

Fowl: Lymphoid tumors of the chicken are properly referred to as the "leukosis complex" because of the many-faceted manifestations they are capable of exhibiting. These include neurolymphomatosis, osteopetrosis, and leukemic expressions of the lymphoid, myeloid, or erythroid form. It is not clear whether these are all caused by the same agent, but careful studies have shown that viral agents are responsible for some and perhaps all of the types. See *leukosis*.

The mouse: Of the many virus-induced leukemias, the common naturally occurring type is that caused by the Gross virus. Other agents include Rauscher, Friend, and Maloney viruses. Some strains of mice such as AKR, C58, DBA, and F show a high incidence, and others very low. The disease is probably of low incidence in natural populations of mice. It was the development of inbred strains which provided experimenters with adequate material to allow use of mouse leukemia as the important study model it is now known to be.

The guinea pig: A virus has recently been found in one type of guinea pig leukemia.

Other species: There have been occasional reports of leukemia in the horse, goat, pig, rabbit, rat, hamster, nonhuman primate, fish, and other animals. Leukemic proliferations of other types, such as myelogenous, monocytic, and basophilic, are also seen.

leukemia line 1 (MacDowell leukemia) A transplantable line of lymphocytic leukemia arising spontaneously in C58 inbred mice in 1926 in the laboratory of Richter and Mac-Dowell at Cold Spring Harbor.[150]

leuko- A combining form meaning white, or denoting relationship to a white corpuscle or leukocyte.

leukocyte count See *hemogram*.

leukoprotease A protein-splitting enzyme found in polymorphonuclear leukocytes.

leukosis Proliferation of leukocyte-forming tissue, including myelosis and lymphadenosis. Such proliferation forms the basis of leukemia.

    avian l. (fowl l.), a complex of diseases induced by closely related leukoviruses (oncornaviruses), involving proliferation of lymphoid cells (lymphomatosis), erythroblasts (erythroblastosis), myeloblasts (myeloblastosis), osteoblasts (osteoblastosis), fibroblasts (Rous sarcoma), and endothelial cells (endothelioma). Myelo- and erythroblastosis are typical leukemias. The others are solid tumors. See *leukemia*.

leukotaxis The cytotaxis of leukocytes; the tendency of leukocytes to collect in regions of injury and inflammation.

leukovirus See under *classification*, under *virus*.

levo- 1. A combining form meaning left, to the left. 2. A chemical prefix, for which the symbol (−) is frequently substituted, used to emphasize that the substance is the levorotatory enantiomorph, whether the configurational family is known or not. This practice avoids possible confusion with the occasional erroneous use of *l-* standing alone to designate the configurational family to which the substance belongs. Opposed to *dextro-*.

levophobia Dread of objects on the left side of the body.

Leydig-cell tumor (Furth tumor; interstitial cell testicular tumor of the mouse) A spontaneous malignant neoplasm found at necropsy in a 17-month-old RF/Fu strain mouse in the laboratory of Jacob Furth at Oak Ridge National Laboratory in 1951. The tumor grows successfully in approximately 75 per cent of RF mice inoculated, killing the host in about 120 to 200 days. It is transplanted at intervals of two months. The tumor is endocrinologically active, inducing obesity, adrenal atrophy, formation of uterine deciduomas in females, and exsanguinating hemorrhage of unknown cause from the cardiac atria and aorta.[150]

L-form A phenomenon of bacterial growth first discovered by Klieneberger-Nobel in *Streptobacillus moniliformis* culture and named after the Lister Institute. It is described as an osmotically fragile, filterable form which lacks a cell wall and mesosomes, but may be induced to grow and multiply under the influence of penicillin in a high salt medium. Some forms are stable, do not revert, and become indistinguishable from mycoplasmas.[32, 36]

life-span See table for recorded life-span of some vertebrates. For data on invertebrates, see Altman and Dittmer.[1]

LIFE-SPAN OF VERTEBRATES*

Species	Common Name	Life-Span
Mammalia		
Homo sapiens	Man	♂66.5 yr, ♀73 yr[1]
Balaenoptera physalus	Finback whale	36 yr
Bos taurus	Cow	30 yr
Camelus bactrianus	Bactrian camel	>25 yr 5 mo
Canis familiaris	Dog	34 yr
Capra hircus	Goat	18 yr
Cavia porcellus	Guinea pig	>6 yr
Didelphis marsupialis virginiana	Virginia opossum	>7 yr
Elaphas maximus	Asiatic elephant	57 yr
Equus caballus	Horse	50 yr
Erinaceus europaeus	European hedgehog	>3 yr 11 mo
Euphractus villosus	Six-banded armadillo	18 yr
Felis catus	Cat	21 yr
Macaca mulatta	Rhesus monkey	29 yr
Mesocricetus auratus	Golden hamster	1 yr 9 mo
Mus musculus	House mouse	>3 yr
Mustela vison	Mink	10 yr
Myotis lucifugus	Little brown bat	22 yr 10 mo[2]
Ondatra zibethica	Muskrat	6 yr 3 mo
Ornithorhynchus anatinus	Platypus	14 yr
Oryctolagus cuniculus	European rabbit	>13 yr
Ovis aries	Sheep	20 yr
Phoca vitulina	Harbor seal	19 yr
Procyon lotor	Raccoon	>13 yr 9 mo
Rattus norvegicus	Rat (albino)	>3 yr 4 mo
Sciurus carolinensis	Gray squirrel	14–15 yr
Sorex palustris	Water shrew	1 yr 6 mo
Sus scrofa	Swine	27 yr
Tamias striatus	Eastern chipmunk	7 yr 6 mo

(Table continued)

*From P. L. Altman and D. S. Dittmer: Biology Data Book. Federation of American Societies for Experimental Biology, Washington, D.C., 1964.
    Key: 1. Values are for average life span. 2. In natural habitat. 3. Still alive at time of report.

LIFE-SPAN OF VERTEBRATES (*Continued*)

SPECIES	COMMON NAME	LIFE-SPAN
	Aves	
Anas platyrhynchos	Mallard duck	19 yr[3]
		20 yr 6 mo[2]
Anser domesticus	Common goose	31 yr
Aptenodytes patagonica	King penguin	26 yr
Columbia leucocephala	White-crowned pigeon	8 yr 3 mo[2]
C. livia	Street pigeon	35 yr
Corvus brachyrhynchos	American crow	13 yr 9 mo[2]
C. corax	Raven	69 yr
Cygnus buccinator	Trumpeter swan	>29 yr 5 mo
Gallus domesticus	Chicken	30 yr
Gyps fulvus	Griffon vulture	>41 yr 5 mo
Larus argentatus	Herring gull	>44 yr
		19 yr[2]
Meleagris gallopavo	Turkey	12 yr 4 mo
Passer italiae	Italian sparrow	20 yr
Perdix perdix	European partridge	>5 yr
Phasianus colchicus	Ring-necked pheasant	27 yr
Serinus canarius	Canary	24 yr
Struthio camelus	African ostrich	50 yr
Sturnus vulgaris	Starling	>15 yr 10 mo
		8 yr[2]
Turdus migratorius	American robin	12 yr 10 mo
		12 yr 6 mo[2]
	Reptilia	
Alligator mississipiensis	American alligator	>56 yr[3]
Ancistrodon contortrix mokeson	Northern U.S. copperhead	18 yr 6 mo[3]
Anguis fragilis	Slowworm	32 yr
Anolis equestris	Giant Cuban "chameleon"	3 yr 5 mo
Caretta caretta	Loggerhead turtle	33 yr
Chalcides ocellatus	Sand skink	9 yr 6 mo
Chelydra serpentina	Snapping turtle	20 yr
Coluber constrictor	American black snake	5 yr 4 mo[3]
Crotalus viridis helleri	Southern Pacific rattlesnake	19 yr 5 mo
Heloderma suspectum	Gila monster	24 yr 7 mo
Malaclemys terrapin centrata	Southern diamond-back terrapin	>21 yr[3]
Naja naja	Indian cobra	12 yr 4 mo
Natrix sipedon	North American water snake	7 yr
Pseudemys scripta elegans	Red-eared-turtle	7 yr 1 mo
Sceloporus graciosus	Sagebrush lizard	8 yr
Sphenodon punctatus	Tuatara	>28 yr[3]
Sternotherus odoratus	Musk turtle	53 yr 3 mo[3]
Terrapene carolina	Box turtle	83–88 yr
Thamnophis sirtalis	Common garter snake	6 yr
	Amphibia	
Ambystoma maculatum	Spotted salamander	>24 yr
A. tigrinum	Tiger salamander	11 yr
Amphiuma means	Two-toed amphiuma	>26 yr 9 mo
Bufo americanus	American toad	10–15 yr
B. arenarum	Sand toad	>7 yr 5 mo
Cryptobranchus alleganiensis	Hellbender	>28 yr 7 mo
Hyla arborea	Tree frog	>14 yr 1 mo
Necturus maculosus	Mud puppy	>8 yr 10 mo
Pipa pipa	Surinam toad	7 yr 10 mo[3]
Rana catesbeiana	American bullfrog	>15 yr 8 mo
R. pipiens	Leopard frog	>5 yr 11 mo
Triturus cristatus	Crested newt	>4 yr 1 mo
T. viridescens	Common newt	>2 yr 11 mo
Xenopus laevis	Clawed toad	15 yr

LIFE-SPAN OF VERTEBRATES (*Continued*)

SPECIES	COMMON NAME	LIFE-SPAN
	Pisces	
Acipenser fulvescens	Lake sturgeon	152 yr[2]
A. ruthenus	Sterlet	>46 yr 1 mo
Amia calva	Bowfin	24 yr
		30 yr[2]
Anguilla anguilla	European freshwater eel	15 yr[2]
A. rostrata	American freshwater eel	50 yr
Carassius auratus	Goldfish	30 yr
Clupea harengus	Atlantic herring	19 yr[2]
Coregonus clupeaformis	North American lake whitefish	12 yr
		26 yr[2]
Cyprinus carpio	Carp	47 yr
Electrophorus electricus	Electric eel	>11 yr 6 mo
Esox lucius	Northern pike	10 yr
		24 yr[2]
Gadus morhua	Atlantic cod	16 yr[2]
Hippocampus hudsonius	Atlantic sea horse	>4 yr 7 mo
Hippoglossus hippoglossus	Atlantic halibut	40 yr[2]
Ictalurus catus	White catfish	>8 yr 1 mo
I. punctatus	Channel catfish	13 yr[2]
Lepidosiren paradoxa	South American lungfish	>8 yr 3 mo
Lepisosteus osseus	Longnose gar	24 yr
		30 yr[2]
Lepomis cyanellus	Green sunfish	>7 yr 6 mo[3]
		9 yr[2]
Melanogrammus aeglefinus	Haddock	15 yr[2]
Micropterus salmoides	Largemouth black bass	>11 yr[3]
		16 yr[2]
Osmerus mordax	American smelt	6 yr[2]
Perca fluviatilis	European perch	>10 yr 8 mo
		10 yr[2]
Pleuronectes platessa	European plaice	<30 yr[2]
Polyodon spathula	Paddlefish	24 yr[2]
Pomoxis annularis	White crappie	9 yr[2]
P. nigromaculatus	Black crappie	12 yr
Protopterus annectans	West African lungfish	18 yr
Salmo salar	Atlantic salmon	13 yr[2]
S. trutta	Brown trout	10 yr
Salvelinus namaycush	Lake trout	12 yr
		41 yr[2]
Scomber scombrus	Atlantic mackerel	3–4 yr
		15 yr[2]
Thunnus thynnus	Bluefin tuna	7 yr[2]
	Chondrichthyes	
Dasyatis pastinaca	Stingray	>21 yr
Raja maculata	Skate	>5 yr 10 mo
	Agnatha	
Lampetra fluviatilis	River lamprey	<1 yr
Petromyzon marinus	Sea lamprey	7 yr[2]

ligand A term used to refer to substrate or coenzyme in the case of enzymes, and to antigen and hapten in the case of antibodies.[32]

ligase (synthetase) An enzyme that catalyzes the joining together of two molecules, coupled with the breakdown of a pyrophosphate bond of ATP.[90, 118]

light green SF An acid triphenylmethane dye. Solubility at 15° C.: water 20 per cent, absolute alcohol 4 per cent, and glycerol 10 per cent. It is used with hematoxylin as a general purpose stain, with Kernechtrot and

Victoria blue to stain viral elementary bodies, and with safranin for plant tissues and spirochetes.[57]

lignin pink An acid non-azo dye. Solubility at 15° C.: water 12 per cent and glycerol 8.5 per cent. Insoluble in absolute alcohol. It is used with chlorazol black for lignin.[57]

Limulus polyphemus A species of merostomes, commonly called the "horseshoe" or "king crab" which inhabits the quiet shallow waters of the eastern coast of North America, from Nova Scotia to the Yucatan. Its entire body (up to 18 inches in length) is covered by a shiny brown carapace, and it has five pairs of legs. These animals have lateral compound eyes which are coarsely faceted with each segment connected to the brain by long individual optic nerves. This characteristic of eye structure has been extremely valuable in studies of the interaction of visual receptors, including the method whereby stimulation and inhibition contribute to the pattern of image formation.

lincomycin An antibiotic produced by a species of *Streptomyces* which is more active against gram-positive than gram-negative bacteria. It interferes with protein synthesis at the ribosomal level.[36, 49]

linkage The tendency for two or more nonallelic genes to be associated more frequently than would be expected from independent assortment. They are said to be linked in coupling when they are carried on the same chromosome, and in repulsion when on homologous chromosomes.

linkage group A linear group of genes on the same chromosome.

linkage map A chromosome map showing loci of known genes on a chromosome.

Linthal bees See *white head.*

lipase An enzyme that catalyzes the hydrolysis of ester linkages between the fatty acids and glycerol of the triglycerides and phospholipids.

lipo- A combining form denoting relationship to fat.

lipoblastoma A tumor made up of lipoblasts or embryonic fat cells.

lipochrome (carotenoid) Any one of a group of fat-soluble hydrocarbon pigments, such as carotene, xanthophyll, lutein, chromophane, and the natural coloring material of butter, egg yolk, and yellow corn.

lipofuscin Any one of a class of fatty pigments formed by the solution of a pigment in fat. As seen within cells, these pigments probably represent accumulations of fatty materials associated with autophagy or cell degeneration. They are similar to "wear and tear" pigments seen with advancing age.[153] Cf. *autophagic vacuole.*

lipoma A fatty tumor; a tumor made up of fat cells. Lipomas are painless and benign, but may become the seat of gangrene or fat necrosis.

liposarcoma A tumor made up of lipoblasts or embryonic fat cells.

liposarcoma D4888 A sarcoma induced experimentally in the laboratory of W. E. Heston at the National Cancer Institute in 1945.

A single subcutaneous injection of 20-methylcholanthrene in a family-2 guinea pig was found to have produced lipomas at the injection site when the animal was necropsied some 18 months later. It has since been transplanted at 30-day intervals in family-2 guinea pigs, is metastatic, and from the time of onset kills the host in approximately five weeks.[150]

liquid scintillation counter An electronic instrument that utilizes emission of light from fluorescent compounds when they are struck by an ionizing particle to measure the concentration of radioactive isotopes in a sample.

Listeria monocytogenes See *listeriosis.*

listeriosis A disease caused by *Listeria monocytogenes*, a species of the family Corynebacteriaceae, order Eubacteriales, made up of coccoid to bacillary, gram-positive microorganisms. It was first isolated from a spontaneous rabbit epizootic in England and has been found to be associated with a number of diseases of man and animen. The most important disease in anomen is encephalomyelitis or abortion of cattle, sheep, and goats. It is occasionally seen in young swine and can cause epizootic systemic disease in chinchillas.

In rabbits, the infection is associated with pregnancy resulting in abortion, pyometra, and retained fetuses most frequently, but it also may cause meningocephalitis. The gross lesions usually include an enlarged friable liver with focal necrosis. Microscopically the small abscesses are characterized by infiltration with a mixture of polymorphonuclear and mononuclear cells. Gram-stained sections show the typical gram-positive rods. Difficulty may be encountered in culturing the organism from clinical material.

litho- A combining form denoting relationship to stone or to a calculus.

Litomosoides carinii A filarial nematode that parasitizes the pleural cavity of the cotton rat. Insects are the vectors, and mites the intermediate hosts.[21]

littoral Pertaining to the shore.

LIVIM virus See *infantile diarrhea of mice.*

Loa loa A member of the superfamily Filaroidea, also known as the eye worm, found in the baboon and man in Central and West Africa. This is the only filarioid parasite of man to demonstrate diurnal periodicity. Daylight tabanid flies act as vectors.[21]

locus (pl. *loci*) In genetics, the specific site on a chromosome of a gene or group of genes. See also *histocompatibility loci.*

-logy A word termination meaning the science or study of, or a treatise on, the subject designated by the stem to which it is affixed.

loon See *gaviiform birds.*

lophodont Having cheek teeth with ridged surfaces.

loris Any of the primates comprising the genera *Loris* and *Nycticebus*. See *primate.*

Lorsch disease A rickettsial disease of the

larvae of May beetles and June beetles (species of *Melolontha* and *Amphimallon*), as well as other related scarab larvae. The causative agent is *Rickettsiella melolonthae.*

Louisiana Academy of Sciences Department of Entomology, Louisiana State University, Baton Rouge, La. 70803.

louping ill See *ovine encephalomyelitis,* under *encephalomyelitis.*

LSD See *lysergic acid diethylamide.*

luciferase An enzyme that catalyzes the bioluminescent reaction in certain animals.

luciferin A compound, of which there are many forms, which is present in certain animals capable of bioluminescence and which, when acted upon by luciferase, produces light.

Lucke renal adenocarcinoma See *renal adenocarcinoma,* under *adenocarcinoma.*

luminescence The property of emitting light without a corresponding production of heat.

lumpy skin disease A viral disease of cattle characterized by the appearance of multiple nodules in the skin. The etiologic agent may be a member of the herpesvirus group.[16]

lupus Originally a name given to a destructive local skin lesion, with a modifier attached to indicate the type, e.g., lupus vulgaris and lupus tuberculosis; now most commonly used to refer to systemic lupus erythematosus.

    systemic l. erythematosus (SLE), a disease affecting mainly young women in which nephritis occurs in 70 to 75 per cent of the cases. The disease is also characterized by immunological aberrations, including the production of autoantibodies directed against several components of host cells, such as nucleoprotein antibody (LE factor) and antibodies against DNA and histone. There are also anti-red cell antibodies present, as shown by a positive Coombs reaction. Animal counterparts of human SLE are seen in the dog and in the NZB mouse (q.y.).[93, 105, 129, 144]

luteoma IX (ovarian tumor IX, lutein-cell type) A tumor observed in an RF × AKR hybrid mouse one year after the injection of 20-methylcholanthrene and whole-body x-irradiation in the laboratory of J. Furth and M. C. Boon at Cornell University Medical College in 1945. The luteoma transplants grow successfully in 50 to 75 per cent of hybrids, do not metastasize from subcutaneous locations, and are endocrinologically active, causing polycythemic hypervolemia, obesity, involution of the thymus, and atrophy of the adrenal cortex. The tumor secretes progesterone.[150]

lymphangioma A tumor composed of newly formed lymph spaces and channels.

lymphoblast A lymphocyte in its germinative stage; a developing lymphocyte. Such cells are found in the blood in acute lymphatic leukemia. Cf. *immunoblast.*

lymphocystic virus A viral agent associated with lymphocystic disease of centrarchid fishes. The disease is characterized by distinctive tumor-like lesions in which the hypertrophied "lymphocystic cells" attain a size of 2000 to 5000μ. The disease is chronic; the cells mature slowly and in time may slough, or the lesion may regress. Mortality is low. Characteristic cytoplasmic inclusion bodies are seen.[114]

lymphocytic choriomeningitis (LCM) A viral disease principally of mice, but which may also affect many other species, including man, monkey, dog, guinea pig, rabbit, chicken, hamster, and horse. It is therefore a hazard to health as well as to experimental results. Diagnosis is based on isolation of the virus, demonstration of complement-fixing antibodies, and activation of latent infections by intracerebral inoculation of broth or by inoculation of suspect tissue samples into susceptible mice.

    The disease in mice exists as a persistent infection causing lesions in the brain, kidney, liver, and lymphoid and other tissues. Circulating antigen-antibody complexes are seen. There are complement-fixing and cell-bound antibodies but no neutralizing antibodies. (See also *slow virus.*) The agent is an RNA virus about 120 μ in size which buds from the plasma membrane of infected cells.

lymphoma (malignant lymphoma) A general term applied to any neoplastic disorder of the lymphoid tissue, including, with others, Hodgkin's disease and reticulum cell sarcoma.

lymphosarcoma A general term applied to malignant neoplastic disorders of lymphoid tissue, but not including Hodgkin's disease. Cf. *leukemia.*

    Murphy-Sturm l., a tumor that arose following subcutaneous injections of 1,2,5,6-dibenzanthracene in Wistar rats in the laboratory of Murphy and Sturm at The Rockefeller Institute in 1938. It is manifested as both lymphocytic leukemia and lymphosarcoma, but the preponderance of either form is dependent on the strain, age, route of inoculation, and adrenal integrity.[150]

Lyon hypothesis The hypothesis that in female mammals one X chromosome is inactivated in embryonic somatic cells and their descendants. The chromosome which remains active is randomly selected and females are thus X-chromosome mosaics. See *Barr body* and *drumstick,* and see *late-replicating X chromosome,* under *chromosome.*

lyophilization The creation of a stable preparation of a biological substance (blood plasma, serum, viruses, bacteria, etc.) by rapid freezing and dehydration of the frozen product under high vacuum.

lyophobic Not having an affinity for solution; designating a colloid system in which no attraction exists between the solvent and the dispersed particles and which is unstable.

lyrate Lyre-shaped.

Lysenkoism A theory of inheritance of

acquired characteristics which was followed in the Soviet Union for the period 1932 to 1965.

lysergic acid diethylamide (LSD)   A hallucinogenic drug which probably functions as a serotonin antagonist and is reputed to cause chromosomal abnormalities.

lyso-   A combining form denoting lysis or dissolution.

lysochrome   A compound which stains lipids by dissolving them.

lysogenic conversion   The change caused in a bacterial genome by the presence of a prophage.[64] See *temperate bacteriophage,* under *bacteriophage.*

lysogeny   A hereditary trait in a bacterial cell established by the presence of genetic material of a bacteriophage.[64]

lysosome   A cytoplasmic organelle found in most vertebrate cells, consisting of saclike structures surrounded by a single unit membrane. The organelles contain a variable complement of acid hydrolases, including acid phosphatase, β-glucuronidase, and cathepsin. They are visible under phase-contrast microscopy as dense granules and fluoresce a bright orange-red after acridine orange stain.[33, 165] A *primary lysosome* is one whose enzymes have never engaged in a digestive event. A *secondary lysosome* is one that is the site of present or past digestive activity.

lysotype   1. A type of microorganism as determined by its reaction to specific phages. 2. A taxonomic subdivision of bacteria based on their reactions to specific phages or a formula expressing the reactions on which such a subdivision is based.

lysozyme   An enzyme classified as an aminopolysaccharidase that dissolves the bacterial cell wall by hydrolyzing its structural linkage. Its action differs from that of penicillin, which inhibits cell wall biosynthesis and acts only on actively growing bacteria. Lysozyme is found in saliva, tears, egg white, and leukocyte granules. It is active against a limited range of bacterial species, of which *Micrococcus lysodeikticus* is most sensitive.[32, 165]

M

M 99   An oripavine derivative used for sedation of wild animals.

Macaca   A genus of Old World monkeys. See *primate.*

macaque   A monkey of any of several species of genus *Macaca.* See *primate.*

macro-   A combining form meaning large or of abnormal size or length.

macroglobulin   A globulin of high molecular weight, in the 1,000,000 range, with high sedimentation constants as determined by ultracentrifugation; observed in the blood in a number of diseases, but mainly in various proliferative disturbances affecting the lymphoid plasma cell and reticuloendothelial systems. See *immunoglobulin.*

macroglobulinemia   A condition characterized by increase in macroglobulins in the blood. See *monoclonal gammopathy,* under *gammopathy.*

macroevolution   A broad pattern of evolution measured in geologic time. One of the best records of macroevolution is found in the horse. Cf. *microevolution.*

macrolide   A name applied to a group of structurally related antibiotics produced by species of *streptomyces.* Included in the group are spiramycin, carbomycin, angolamycin, methymycin, and lancamycin, which are considered as a group, and erythromycin and oleandomycin, which are considered separately. The macrolides are mainly active against gram-positive bacteria. Of the five considered as a group, only spiramycin has antibacterial activity in vivo. They inhibit protein synthesis in bacteria by binding to ribosomes, and interfere either with growth of peptide chains or with release of peptides.[36, 49]

macrophage   Metchnikoff's name for the large mononuclear phagocytic cell that originates in the tissues and probably takes an active part in the formation of antibody. Their role in the immune process is not clear, but it appears to involve ingestion and processing of antigen so that lymphocytes can initiate the process of antibody formation.[39, 93, 165]

macrophage inhibition   A test for delayed hypersensitivity based on the fact that sensitized lymphoid cells in the presence of specific antigen release a substance that inhibits the migration of macrophages from normal as well as hypersensitive individuals. Release of the substance requires protein synthesis, as the reaction can be blocked with puromycin.

macula adherens   See *desmosome.*

maedi   A chronic progressive pulmonary disease of sheep in Iceland, caused by a viral agent. There is marked proliferation of reticuloendothelial cells and of the broncheolar alveolar epithelium. Of the several chronic pulmonary diseases in this general group which affect sheep, this is the only one from which a virus has been isolated and grown in tissue culture. The disease is of importance in comparative pathology because of its possible relationship to chronic pulmonary diseases of man.

malachite green   A basic triphenylmethane dye. Solubility at 15° C.: water 10 per cent, absolute alcohol 8.5 per cent, and glycerol 9 per cent. It is used with fuchsin and acid Martius yellow for staining parasite and host in plant tissue and for fibers in paper, with basic fuchsin for staining yeasts and bacteria, with crystal violet for staining gonococci, and with safranin for staining bacterial spores.[57]

maladie du pain d'épice (gingerbread disease of oysters) A disease of oysters which involves the shell, caused by species of *Cliona*, the boring sponges.

maladie du pied A disease of European oysters, *Ostrea edulis Linneaue*. The etiologic agent, apparently a boring fungus, causes formation of rubbery spots on the shell, pathological changes in the tissues, and calcareous deposits on the adductor muscle scar. Death is caused by improper shell closure.

malaria Infection by members of the genus *Plasmodium* (phylum Protozoa, class Sporozoa). Although plasmodial parasites are well distributed phylogenetically with representative species in all land-dwelling vertebrate phyla, the description here relates to plasmodia of the order Primates because of the great interest in them in comparative medicine. The malarial parasites and anopheline vectors of the order Primates have diverged, as have their hosts, to the extent that each host is naturally affected by a different spectrum of plasmodial species. The divergence is less complete in certain geographical areas, particularly Southeast Asia and South America. In some cases the human strain can infect monkeys, and vice versa.

The bionomics and ecology of plasmodial vectors is crucial in establishing the role of nonhuman primates as reservoir hosts of human parasites, because the vector must be capable of supporting plasmodial growth and also of attacking both hosts. These conditions have apparently been met for *P. knowlesi*, *P. cynomologi*, *P. bastianellii*, *P. simium*, and *P. brasilianum*, although there is no evidence yet that cross-infection from nonhuman primates to man is an important link in the chain of human infection. These recent findings may have an adverse effect on the success of malaria eradication programs but, on the other hand, are of great research importance in the provision of adequate models for chemotherapy.

Simian malaria typically has a benign course, many cases becoming clinically significant only under experimental stress. In many cases of cross-infection to more distantly related hosts, however, the classical signs of anemia, hyperpyrexia, depression, lesions of splanchnic pigmentation, and hepatosplenomegaly may be apparent. When the susceptible host is bitten by an infected mosquito, the infective sporozoites first localize in hepatocytes, in which schizogony (asexual multiplication) takes place. After this phase the schizonts enter erythrocytes and commence a phase of erythrocytic schizogony, following which sexual forms (gametes) develop and then undergo further development within the vector.

The classical cyclic fevers of malaria occur during the erythrocytic stages, when the maturing plasmodia rupture the cells. The length of time between fever cycles is determined by the length of the erythrocytic phase; this period is 24 hours in the case of plasmodia causing quotidian malaria, 48 hours for those causing tertian malaria, and 72 hours for those causing quartan malaria.[21, 41, 128, 159] See table of plasmodial parasites accompanying *primate*.

Malaya disease A lethal disease of larvae of the Indian rhinoceros beetle, *Oryctes rhinoceros*, caused by a virus. The diseased larvae cease to feed, and appear shiny and turgid, with enlarged, waxen abdomens. Rectal prolapse may occur. In the last stages of the disease, just before death, the larvae are totally lethargic. Virus multiplication occurs chiefly in the nuclei of the fat-body. The rod-shaped virions measure approximately 70 by 200 mμ.

malignant catarrhal fever (malignant head catarrh of cattle; bovine epitheliosis) A viral disease of cattle characterized by a short febrile period, inflammation of the mucous membrane of the mouth, encephalitis, and a high death rate. Sheep may harbor the disease and act as infectious carriers without exhibiting any signs of illness themselves. Rabbits can be infected experimentally. The etiologic agent is a virus, probably of the herpes group.[16, 142]

malocclusion The most common dental disease of laboratory rodents, lagomorphs, Dachshund dogs, and certain sheep families. Most mammalian species share a genetic locus involved with brachygnathia or prognathism, and thus, a class of malocclusion based on unequal jaw length. Syndromes of this type are well characterized in domestic sheep and Dachshund dogs, and have been recognized in laboratory rodents. The latter, in addition, are characterized by a well delineated malocclusion of both incisors and molars in normognathic animals, particularly the rabbit.

In both lagomorphs and rodents, the teeth are of the type that grow continuously throughout the life of the animal and, if the teeth escape from occlusal pressure (inhibition), not only is normal occlusive attrition prevented, but also, the rate of tooth growth is increased by a factor of 2 over the normal rate. The maloccluded teeth therefore become quite long, are responsible for the colorful synonyms (buck-toothed, walrus-toothed, wolf-toothed), often interfere with prehension and deglutition, and must be periodically clipped to prolong the life of the animal. In nature it is a life-limiting condition. Breeders, in the absence of comprehensive records, believe the disease to have a familial distribution. It is of unknown pathogenesis.

Malpeque disease A poorly understood but highly fatal disease of the American oyster, *Crassostrea virginica*. It occurs in the maritime provinces of Canada and was first observed in Malpeque Bay. Infected oysters

A COMPARATIVE SUMMARY OF REPRODUCTION IN MAMMALS

SPECIES	COMMON NAME	AGE AT PUBERTY	BREEDING SEASON	ESTRUS† Type†	ESTRUS† Cycle (days)	GESTATION PERIOD (days)	YOUNG PER LITTER
Homo sapiens	Man	♀13, 5 (11–16) yr	All year	P	28.4 (24–33)	278[1] (253–303)	1[2]
Balaenoptera physalus	Finback whale	3 yr	Nov–Mar[3], June–Aug[4]	...	....	360	1
Bos taurus	Cow	6–10 mo	All year	P	(14–23)	284(210–335)	Usually 1
Camelus bactrianus	Bactrian camel	....	All year	P	(10–20)	(389–410)	1
Canis familiaris	Dog	6–8 mo	Spring–autumn	M	9	63(53–71)	7(1–22)
Capra hircus	Goat	8 mo	Sept–winter	P	21	151(135–160)	(1–5)
Cavia porcellus	Guinea pig	55–70 da	All year	P	(16–19)	68(58–75)	3(1–8)
Dasypus novemcinctus	Nine-banded armadillo	1 yr	June–Aug	...	....	(210–240)	4
Didelphis marsupialis virginiana	Virginia opossum	♂ 8 mo, ♀ 6 mo	Jan–Oct	P	28	(12.5–13.0)	9(5–13)
Elephas maximus	Asiatic elephant	8–16 yr	....	P	....	624(510–730)	Usually 1
Equus caballus	Horse	1 yr	All year	P	(10–37)	336(264–420)	Usually 1
Erinaceus europaeus	European hedgehog	2nd yr	Mar–Sept	M	(35–49)	5(3–7)
Felis catus	Cat	6–15 mo	Feb–July	P[6]	(15–28)	63(52–69)	4
Macaca mulatta	Rhesus monkey	♂ 3–4 yr, ♀ 1.5–2.5 yr	All year	P	28	168(144–194)	1
Mesocricetus auratus	Golden hamster	5–8 wk	All year	P	4	16(15–18)	(1–12)
Mus musculus	House mouse	35 da	All year	P	4	(19–31)	6(1–12)
Mustela vison	Mink	1 yr	Mar–Apr	P[6]	(8–9)	53(39–76)	(4–10)
Myotis lucifugus	Little brown bat	♂, 2nd summer; ♀, end 1st summer	Autumn, spring	M[7]	....	(50–60)	1
Ondatra zibethica	Muskrat	1 yr	Apr–Oct	P	(3–5)	30(19–42)	7(1–11)
Ornithorhynchus anatinus	Platypus	1–2 yr	July–Oct	M	60	12 (incubation)	Usually 2
Oryctolagus cuniculus	European rabbit	5.5–8.5 mo	All year	P[6]	....	31(30–35)	8(1–13)
Ovis aries	Sheep	7–8 mo	Sept–late winter[8]	P	(14–20)	151(144–152)	(1–4)
Phoca vitulina	Harbor seal	5–6 yr	June–Aug[9], Sept[10]	M	....	270	1
Phocaena phocaena	Harbor porpoise	14 mo	July–Aug	...	....	(300–330)	1
Procyon lotor	Raccoon	♂ 2 yr, ♀ 1 yr	Jan–June	P	....	63(60–73)	4(1–6)
Rattus norvegicus	Norway rat	40–60 da	All year	P	(4–5)	21	(6–9)
Sciurus carolinensis	Gray squirrel	1–2 yr	Dec–Aug	...	....	44	4(1–6)
Sorex araneus	European shrew	2nd yr	Mar–Sept	P	....	(13–19)	7
Sus scrofa	Swine	7(5–8) mo	All year	P	(18–24)	114(101–130)	9(6–15)
Tamias striatus	Eastern chipmunk	2.5–3.0 mo	Mar–July	P	....	31	(3–6)

*From P. L. Altman and D. S. Dittmer: Biology Data Book. Federation of American Societies for Experimental Biology, Washington, D.C., 1964.

†Type of Estrus: P = polyestrous; M = monoestrous. Values in parenthesis are ranges.

Key: 1. From first day of last menses; 268(250–285) days after rise in basal body temperature. 2. Multiple pregnancies (mainly twins) = 1.0–1.5% of total births 3. Northern Hemisphere. 4. Southern Hemisphere. 5. Mainly spring-autumn. 6. Induced ovulation. 7. Ovulation in spring. 8. Coarse-wooled breeds only; fine-wooled breeds, all year. 9. Atlantic. 10. Pacific.

are thin and have yellow pustules in the tissues.

maltase An enzyme, widely distributed in the animal and vegetable world, which catalyzes the hydrolysis of maltose into dextrose.

Malthusianism The theory, named for its author and becoming more and more imminently substantiated, that the world's population will increase faster than the food supply, resulting in devastating famines. The only likely deterrent to proof of this theory is termination of the experiment by an explosion.

mamba See table accompanying *snake*.

mammal Any member of Mammalia, the division of vertebrates that includes all that possess hair and suckle their young. For a comparison of reproduction data about various mammals, see table. See also table accompanying *life-span*.

mammary adenocarcinoma See under *adenocarcinoma*.

mammary fibroadenoma R2737 See under *fibroadenoma*.

mammary tumor Neoplasm of the mammary glands. Among anomen, the dog and mouse have the highest incidence of mammary neoplasms, the Bittner tumor of mice being well known. The dog exhibits several types of mammary neoplasms, including adenocarcinoma, squamous cell carcinoma, adenoma, myoepithelioma, mixed tumors, fibroma, fibrosarcoma, lipoma, leiomyosarcoma, and hemangioma. The most common are adenocarcinomas, often of ductal cell origin, and mixed mammary tumors, composed of both connective tissue and epithelial portions. These also contain metaplastic cartilage and bone. Carcinoma of the bovine mammary gland is virtually unknown in spite of the fact that it is the most actively cycling and continuously traumatized breast in the animal kingdom.[142]

mammary tumor agent A milk-borne virus that induces mammary carcinoma in mice of certain genotype. See *murine mammary carcinoma* in table of *Oncogenic RNA Viruses*.

Manaker leukemia virus (C60 virus) A lymphoid leukemia virus isolated by Manaker from mouse cell cultures previously inoculated with Schwartz leukemia virus. Fluids from these cultures have induced generalized lymphocytic tumors in various strains of mice and in rats. Large quantities of virus were present in leukemia tissues.[114]

mandrill A baboon, *Papio sphinx*. See *primate*.

mania 1. A phase of mental disorder characterized by an expansive emotional state, elation, hyperirritability, overtalkativeness, or flight of ideas, and increased motor activity; specifically, the manic type of manic-depressive psychosis. 2. As a combining form, it signifies obsessive preoccupation with something, as in dipsomania, erotomania, oniomania, etc.

maniaphobia Fear of insanity.

mantle 1. An enveloping structure or layer. 2. The fold of skin covering part of the body of mollusks and some other invertebrates. The mantle usually secretes the mollusk shell and may also protect the organs which are situated in the cavity beneath.

MAP test An acronym for the *mouse antibody production* test, in which material suspected of viral content is inoculated into a mouse known to be immunologically naive. If antibody specifically directed against known viral determinants is later detected, it is assumed that the specific virus was in the inoculum.[63]

Marburg virus An agent isolated from animal caretakers who contracted a febrile disease (vervet monkey disease; green monkey disease) by exposure to vervets (green monkeys) imported from Africa. It causes hepatic necrosis, widespread hemorrhage and death, and may be transmitted by contact to other vervets and to rhesus monkeys.

Marek's disease (neurolymphomatosis) A lymphoproliferative disease of chickens caused by a herpesvirus (DNA). See *virus*. Lesions include lymphocytic cuffing of arteries in the white matter of the brain and spinal cord, infiltration of peripheral nerve trunks, and widespread diffuse infiltration of all visceral organs as well as the musculature and dermis. Originally included in the avian leukoses (q.v.), it is now known to be a separate entity. At present, Marek's disease is the most important cause of poultry losses and condemnations in the world and is important as a model for the study of such human diseases as Burkitt's lymphoma and infectious mononucleosis.

marihuana, marijuana The leaves and flowering tops of *Cannabis sativa*, usually employed in cigarets to produce a psychodelic effect.

mark disease An early synonym for muscardine (q.v.) of the silkworm. From *Del Mal Del Segno, Calcinaccio o Moscardino*, the title of a famous treatise written by Agostino Bassi and published in 1835.

Marmosa mitis See *mouse opossum*.

marmoset A small diurnal South American monkey of the family Callithricidae. It has a characteristic high-pitched voice, eats insects, spiders, and fruit, is docile, and adapts well to captivity. *Callithrix*, noted for its large ear plumes and ringed tail, is the most common genus. The young are nearly always the result of twin births, are either identical or chimeric twins, and exhibit tolerance to each other. Some species are *Callithrix argentata, Leontideus rosalia*, or the lionheaded marmoset, and *C. penicillata*. The tamarin (q.v.), *Saguinus*, is also called a marmoset by some.

marmot A small rodent of the genus *Marmota*, family Sciuridae. There are sixteen species which range from the Alps through Asia, north of the Himalayas, and are also found in North America. The common North American species (*M. monax*), also known as woodchuck, has a stout body, is brownish black, and has no cheek pouches. Marmots inhabit open country, either on mountains or in the plains, and hibernate during the winter. They eat raw crops, grasses, and legumes.

marsupial Any member of the mammalian order Marsupialia. They are primitive pouch-bearing mammals limited in distribution to Australasia and South America, except for one species in the United States. The use of marsupials as experimental animals in problem-oriented research has almost always been directly connected with their unique developmental processes. The young are born, after a variable period of nonplacental uterine gestation, into a pouch (the marsupium), where the young undergo additional development, each offspring being attached orally to a mamma. Investigators make use of the access to the incompletely developed fetuses in the pouch in studying particularly

A CLASSIFICATION OF MARSUPIALIA

SUBORDER	FAMILY	SPECIES	COMMON NAME
Polyprodontia	Didelphidae	*Didelphis virginiana*	Virginian opossum
		Marmosa mitis	Murine opossum
	Dasyuridae	*Dasyurus quoll*	Native cats, devils
	Myrmecobiidae	*Mymecobius fasciatus*	Banded anteater (numbat)
	Notoryctidae	*Notoryctes typhlops*	Marsupial mole
	Peramelidae	– – –	Bandicoots
Diprodontia	Phalangeridae	– – –	Phalangers
	Phascolarctidae	*Phascolarctus cinereus*	Koala
	Phascolomidae	– – –	Wombats
	Macropodidae	– – –	Kangaroo

problems in experimental embryology, immunology, transplantation biology, and neurophysiology. Marsupials are divided into two suborders based on numbers of incisor teeth.[4] See table.

marsupium See *marsupial.*

Martius yellow An acid dye of the nitro group. Solubility at 15° C.: water 1.25 per cent, absolute alcohol nil, and glycerol 1 per cent. It is used with malachite green and fuchsin as a differential stain for parasite and host in plant tissues and for callose in pollen tubes.[37]

Maryland Academy of Sciences 7 W. Mulberry Street, Baltimore, Md. 21201.

masochism A form of sexual perversion in which cruel treatment gives sexual gratification to the recipient.

mast cell tumor (mastocytoma) A subcutaneous neoplasm that is locally invasive and frequently metastasizes. It is seen with considerable frequency in middle-aged or old dogs, occasionally in the cat, and rarely in man (urticaria pigmentosa). The cells possess a round centrally located nucleus. Special stains such as Giemsa or toluidine blue reveal metachromatic cytoplasmic granules.[142]

masto- A combining form denoting relationship to the breast.

mastocytoma Mast cell tumor.

Masurenko leukemia virus A lymphoid leukemia virus of mice of interest because the incidence of this leukemia in CC57Br mice is potentiated by the inoculation of vaccinia or influenza viruses.[114]

mating system See *breeding system.*

matrocliny Inheritance in which the offspring resemble the female parent more than the male.

May disease A complex of diseases consisting of a group of maladies of adult honeybees characterized by similar syndromes but different etiologies. *Saccharomyces apiculatus,* for instance, has been found in bees afflicted with constipation and has been considered as the cause of one form of May disease. Collection of buttercup pollen may be the cause of another malady called Bettlach May disease (q.v.).

Maya's disease A lethal disease of unknown cause affecting larvae, pupae, and adults of rhinoceros beetles (*Oryctes*) and other scarabs. It is characterized by many spheroid vacuolated inclusions in the fat body, pericardial cells, tracheal matrix, and thoracic muscles.

measles (rubeola) 1. A contagious eruptive fever with coryza and catarrhal symptoms due to a virus. Measles tends to lead to complications, the chief of which are pneumonia, bronchitis, tuberculosis, and otitis media, and has recently been incriminated in chronic encephalitides.[14, 44] 2. A cysticercal disease of domestic animals. See *cysticercosis.*

  bastard m., rubella.

  German m., rubella.

  m. of monkeys, see *giant cell pneumonia of monkeys,* under *pneumonia.*

  pork m., a condition in which pork is infected with the *Cysticercus cellulosae.*

meat spot See *blood spot.*

Medical Library Association, Inc. National Library of Medicine, Bethesda, Md. 20014.

Medical Mycological Society of the Americas National Communicable Disease Center, Mycology and Parasitology Section, Atlanta, Ga. 30333.

medulloblastoma A cerebellar tumor composed of undifferentiated preneuroglial cells.

mega- A combining form designating great size; used in naming units of measurement to indicate a quantity one million (10^6) times the unit designated by the root with which it is combined.

megacin A bacteriocin (q.v.) produced by *Bacillus megaterium.*[49]

megacolon Hirschsprung's disease.

megalo- A combining form designating great size. See also words beginning mega-.

megalomania Delusion of grandeur; unreasonable conviction of one's own extreme greatness, goodness, or power.

megaspore Sabouraud's term for the large spores seen in ectothrix infection of hair by dermatophytes, e.g., *Trichophyton verrucosum.*

megoxyphil An eosinophil leukocyte containing large granules.

meio- A combining form denoting relation to decrease in size or number.

meiosis A special method of cell division, occurring in maturation of the sex cells, by means of which each daughter nucleus receives half the number of chromosomes characteristic of the somatic cells of the species. Cf. *mitosis.* The prophase of the first division of meiosis is divided into five stages: the leptotene, during which chromosomes form long slender strands; the zygotene, during which homologous chromosomes begin to pair; the pachytene, during which homologues become completely paired; the diplotene, during which chromosomes contract by coiling; and diakinesis, during which contraction nears the maximum. The second meiotic division resembles that in mitosis, but without DNA replication.[121]

melanic leucism See *leucism.*

melanic schizochroism See *schizochroism.*

melanism The replacement (in birds) by melanins of the carotenoid pigments normally present in some or all parts of the plumage, or the deposition of melanins in abnormally increased amounts in areas where they are normally present.[112] See also *leucism* and *schizochroism.*

  industrial m., see *Biston betularia.*

melano- A combining form meaning black, or denoting relation to melanin.

melanoameloblastoma Ameloblastoma exhibiting bluish black discoloration because of the presence of melanin granules.

melanoblast A cell originating from the neural crest that differentiates into a melanophore.

melanoblastoma A tumor made up of melanoblasts.

melanoma A tumor made up of melanin-pigmented cells. The behavior of these tumors is extremely unpredictable: they may remain dormant for long periods of time and suddenly spread rapidly. Of particular interest to comparative pathologists is the extremely common occurrence of these tumors in gray horses.[142]

Cloudman m. S91 A tumor found in 1937 at the base of the tail of a female DBA mouse by Cloudman at the Jackson Memorial Laboratory. A firm black subcutaneous tumor, it was found to be transplantable to other DBA mice. Subcutaneous transplants reach a diameter of 2.5 cm. eight weeks after inoculation and kill the host within nine to twelve weeks. The optimum transplantation interval is one month. Melanoma S91 grows in 80 to 100 per cent of DBA and BALB/c mice inoculated, and is invariably metastatic. However, it grows poorly in mice of other strains. In albino BALB/c mice, an amelanotic variant (amelanotic melanoma S91-A or C91AA) was selected and propagated by Algire. For comparison, see *Harding-Passey melanoma* of mice, a nonmetastatic melanoma histologically distinguishable from the Cloudman melanoma.[150]

Harding-Passey m., a melanoma found originally on the left ear of a brown non-inbred mouse in the laboratory of R. A. Passey at Leeds University, England, in 1925. It was subsequently subjected to passage by subcutaneous transplants by Harding and Passey and brought to the United States by J. B. Murphy of The Rockefeller Institute in 1928. Since then it has been propagated successfully as a nonmetastasizing melanoma by subcutaneous transplantation in a variety of inbred and non-inbred mouse strains. An amelanotic variant was developed by selection by Harding and Passey and by Sugiura.[150]

malignant m., a malignant tumor, usually developing from a nevus and consisting of black masses of cells with a marked tendency to metastasis.

melanophore A pigment cell containing melanin, especially such a cell in fishes, amphibians, and reptiles.

melanoschizochroism See *schizochroism.*

melanosis 1. A condition characterized by abnormal pigmentary deposits. 2. In insect pathology, a disease of queen honeybees, characterized by discoloration of the egg cells and trophocytes, which turn from yellow-brown to black. Affected queens become sterile. There are two types of melanosis in the queen honeybee: H-melanosis (also called *Arnhart's black-egg disease)* is caused by yeastlike microorganisms, whereas B-melanosis is caused by a bacterium, probably *Aerobacter cloacae.*

melting brood See *European foulbrood,* under *foulbrood.*

melting-out temperature (Tm) The temperature required to denature a nucleic acid, at which point the complementary bonds between strands are broken, and there is a loss of biological activity and an increase in absorption of ultraviolet light. This can be reversed by slow cooling (annealing).[90]

Mengo virus Reovirus-3.

meningioma A hard, slow-growing vascular tumor that occurs mainly along the meningeal vessels and superior longitudinal sinus, invading the dura and skull and leading to erosion and thinning of the skull.

menstruation Cyclic vaginal bleeding exhibited by sexually mature female members of the order Primates. In many subhuman primate genera, it is temporally similar to the cycle in women. In reproductive physiological experiments utilizing subhuman primates, the menstrual cycle is carefully calculated in individual females (by daily vaginal swabs) in order to estimate the ovulation time, which in *Macaca mulatta* follows by twelve to thirteen days the onset of menstruation. The normal cycle in *M. mulatta* ranges from 26 to 32 days, with a mode of 28 days. Menses (blood flow) lasts two to five days on the average. When impregnation occurs the menstrual cycle is abated.

6-mercaptopurine A purine analog used as a metabolic inhibitor (antimetabolite) in the treatment of certain types of cancer and as an immunosuppressant.

mercy killing See *euthanasia.*

mericlinal chimera See under *chimera.*

mero- A combining form meaning part.

merostome Any member of the phylum Arthropoda, subphylum Chelicerata, class Merostomata. One form, the king or horseshoe crab *Limulus polyphemus* (q.v.), is of great biological interest and is extensively used in research.

mescaline A poisonous alkaloid, 3,4,5-trimethoxyphenyl ethylamine, $(CH_3 \cdot O)_3 C_6 H_2 \cdot CH_2 \cdot CH_2 \cdot NH_2$, in the form of a colorless alkaline oil from *Lophophora williamsii.* It produces an intoxication with delusions of color and music.

meso- A prefix denoting middle, or intermediate.

mesoglea A layer of jelly-like material between the endoderm and ectoderm of a coelenterate, and thought to be the homologue of mesoderm in higher animals.

mesomorphy A type of body build in which tissues derived from the mesoderm predominate. There is relative preponderance of muscle, bone, and connective tissue, usually with heavy, hard physique of rectangular outline.

mesophilic Fond of moderate temperature; said of bacteria that develop at temperatures between 20 and 50° C. Cf. *psychrophilic* and *thermophilic.*

mesosome (plasmalemmosome; chondrioid; peripheral body) Intracytoplasmic membranous bacterial organelles that are formed by invagination of the cytoplasmic membrane. They are intermediate between nucleoid and membrane and play a role in the synthesis of the cell wall and the oxidation-reduction processes of the cell. They may be vesicular or lamellar whorls. The latter type disappears when protoplasts are formed.[32]

mesothelioma   A tumor developed from mesothelial tissue.

Mesozoic   Denoting the era extending from 250 to 63 million years ago; the age of reptiles. See *geologic time divisions.*

messenger RNA   That type of RNA which transmits information from chromosomal DNA to the site of protein synthesis in the cytoplasm.[90]

meta-   A prefix indicating (1) change, transformation, or exchange; (2) after or next; (3) the 1,3 position in derivatives of benzene.

metabolism   The sum of all the physical and chemical processes by which living organized tissue is formed and maintained, and also the transformation by which energy is made available for use by the organism.

    inborn error of m., any disease characterized by the absence or deficiency of an enzyme that catalyzes a biologically important process. Such defects may result in the accumulation of excessive substrate, as in storage diseases such as Gaucher's disease, or may result in excessive quantities of materials being excreted, as in phenylketonuria and galactosemia. In addition, there are many well defined hereditary errors of metabolism for which an enzyme defect has not yet been identified. Inborn errors are listed by group in the accompanying table, and animal models are listed when known. These genopathies are the problem diseases which lend themselves especially well to studies in comparative pathology and to possible future correction by genetic engineering.[12, 76, 147] See also *animal model* and *genetic disease.*

GENETICALLY DETERMINED METABOLIC DISEASES
INVOLVING ENZYME DEFECTS[12, 70, 90, 147]

DISEASES	ENZYME DEFECT (If known)	EFFECT AND MODE OF TRANSMISSION	ANIMAL MODEL (If known)*
CARBOHYDRATE METABOLISM			
Diabetes mellitus	– – –	Inadequate glucose oxidation, acidosis, atherosclerosis, hyperglycemia	Horse, hamster, sand rat, mouse, dog, cat, rat
Galactosemia	Galactose-1-phosphate uridyl transferase	Retarded growth, mental deficiency, cataracts; autosomal recessive	– – –
Pentosuria	– – –	Blocked glucuronic acid metabolism; sugars in urine; harmless	– – –
Fructosuria	Lack of hepatic fructokinase	Harmless	– – –
Hereditary fructose intolerance	1-Phosphofructoaldolase	Hypoglycemia	– – –
Hyperoxaluria	Probably glyoxalic acid– glycine transaminase	Calcium oxalate urolithiasis; autosomal recessive	– – –
GLYCOGEN STORAGE DISEASES (Glycogenoses)			
von Gierke's disease	Glucose-6-phosphatase	Hepatorenal glycogenosis	Dog, duck
Pompe's disease	α-1-4 glucosidase (acid maltase)	Generalized glycogenosis	– – –
Forbes' disease	Amylo-1,6-glucosidase	Debrancher deficiency of liver, heart muscle, leukocytes	– – –
Anderson's disease	Amylo-1,4-1,6-trans- glucosidase	Brancher deficiency of liver, etc.	– – –
McArdle-Schmid-Pearson disease	Muscle glycogen phosphorylase	Glycogenosis of skeletal muscle	– – –
Hers' disease	Liver glycogen phosphorylase	Glycogenosis of liver, leukocytes	– – –
AMINO ACID METABOLISM			
Familial goiter	Several types: iodine organification, etc.	Goiter, cretinism, etc.; autosomal recessive	Cow
Albinism	Tyrosinase or tyrosine deficiency	Inability to form melanin; may be recessive or dominant	Mouse, rabbit, horse, etc.
Hyperglycinuria	(?)	May be renal or overflow; may be associated with hypophosphatemic rickets; genetics not clear	– – –
Histidinemia	Histidase	Mental retardation; autosomal recessive	– – –
Hyperammonemia	Ornithine trans- carbamylase	Mental retardation; autosomal recessive	

*See Addendum, Table of Animal Models for references and additional examples.

DISEASES	ENZYME DEFECT (If known)	EFFECT AND MODE OF TRANSMISSION	ANIMAL MODEL (If known)*
AMINO ACID METABOLISM (Continued)			
Citrullinemia	(?)	Mental retardation; autosomal recessive	– – –
Argininosuccinicaciduria	Argininosuccinase	Mental retardation; autosomal recessive	– – –
Phenylketonuria	Phenylalanine hydroxylase	Central nervous system damage, mental deficiency; autosomal recessive	– – –
Alcaptonuria	Homogentisic acid oxidase	Failure to form tyrosine, homogentisic aciduria; autosomal recessive	– – –
Maple syrup urine disease	Amino acid decarboxylase	Mental deficiency; genetics not clear	Mouse(?)
Homocystinuria	Cystathione synthetase	Blockage of methionine metabolism, mental retardation, etc.; familial	– – –
LIPID METABOLISM			
Niemann-Pick disease	– – –	Sphingomyelin lipidosis, foam cells, hepatosplenomegaly	Mouse
Gaucher's disease	– – –	Cerebroside accumulation, hepatosplenomegaly	– – –
Tay-Sachs disease	– – –	Ganglioside lipidosis, dementia, death; autosomal recessive	Dog
Amaurotic familial idiocy	– – –	Cerebroside accumulation in CNS; blindness, mental deficiency, etc.	Dog
Globoid leukodystrophy (Krabbe's disease)	(?)	Perivascular demyelination and accumulation of "globoid" cells. Probably autosomal recessive.	Dog, cat.
Metachromatic leukodystrophy	(?)	Sulfatide accumulation, degeneration of myelin, dementia, death	Dog, mink, pig
Fabry's disease	(?)	Glycolipid accumulation in tissues; sex-linked recessive	– – –
Hyperlipoproteinemia	(?)	Elevated cholesterol and/or glycerides, xanthomatosis	– – –
High density lipoprotein deficiency (Tangier disease)	(?)	Cholesterol storage in foam cells	– – –
Abetalipoproteinemia	(?)	Absence of low-density lipoproteins, neuromuscular disorders; autosomal recessive	– – –
STEROID METABOLISM			
Virilizing adrenal hyperplasia (adrenogenital syndrome)	21-Hydroxylase	Failure of adrenocorticosteroid synthesis; progressive virilism; autosomal recessive	– – –
PURINE-PYRIMIDINE METABOLISM			
Gout	(?)	Excess uric acid, arthritis, renal lithiasis	Chicken
Xanthinuria	Xanthine oxidase	Xanthine replaces uric acid	– – –
Hereditary orotic aciduria	Orolidylic phosphorylase, carboxylase	Poor growth, anemia; autosomal	– – –
METAL METABOLISM			
Hepatolenticular degeneration (Wilson's disease)	Multiple	Defect in ceruloplasmin, copper deposition in liver and CNS	– – –
Hemochromatosis	(?)	Defective control of iron absorption, cirrhosis, pancreatic fibrosis	– – –

DISEASES	ENZYME DEFECT (If known)	EFFECT AND MODE OF TRANSMISSION	ANIMAL MODEL (If known)*
PORPHYRIN AND HEME METABOLISM			
Porphyria	Multiple	Overproduction of porphyrins, anemia, photosensitivity; autosomal recessive in some, dominant in others	Cow, swine, fox, cat, squirrel
Hyperbilirubinemia nonhemolytic Jaundice (Crigler-Najjar syndrome)	Glucurone transferase	Unconjugated bilirubin, kernicterus	Gunn rat
Hepatic dysfunction (Gilbert's disease)	– – –	Mild intermittent icterus, lassitude	Sheep
Chronic idiopathic jaundice (Dubin-Johnson syndrome)	– – –	Hepatic excretory, raised conjugated bilirubin	Sheep
MUSCLE, BONE, AND CONNECTIVE TISSUE			
Periodic paralysis	(?)	Episodic muscular weakness, abnormal potassium metabolism; autosomal dominant	– – –
Muscular dystrophies	Multiple	Random destruction of muscle fibers, creatinuria	Mouse, chicken, hamster, sheep
Central core disease	Phosphorylase(?)	Decrease of cell organelles; autosomal dominant	– – –
Nemaline myopathy	(?)	Abnormal fibrous protein constituents of muscle cell; autosomal recessive	– – –
Hurler syndrome (gargoylism)	(?)	Short stature, mental retardation, excessive chondroitin sulfate B, and heparin monosulfuric acid; autosomal recessive and X-linked	– – –
Hereditary amyloidosis	(?)	Accumulation of abnormal fibrous protein	Mouse
Pseudohypoparathyroidism	(?)	Metastatic ossification, mental retardation; X-linked	– – –
Hypophosphatasia	Alkaline phosphatase	Severe skeletal defects, inadequate calcification; autosomal recessive	– – –
BLOOD AND THE BLOOD-FORMING TISSUES			
Hereditary spherocytosis	(?)	Congenital hemolytic anemia; autosomal dominant	Deer mouse
Hereditary hemolytic anemia	Pyruvate kinase deficiency	Hemolytic anemia; autosomal recessive	– – –
Clotting defects (hemophilia)	– – –	Deep hemorrhages; X-linked	Dog, horse, swine (see *hemophilia*)
Idiopathic paroxysmal myoglobulinemia	Muscle phosphorylase	Deficient glycogen-to-glucose transformation under anaerobic conditions	– – –
Hemoglobinopathy (q.v.)	– – –	Abnormal electrophoresis; symptoms vary according to the type of defects	Deer
Methemoglobinemia	Methemoglobin reductase	Inability to reduce methemoglobin, cyanosis; dominant or recessive	– – –
Hereditary sensitivity to drugs	Glucose-6-phosphate dehydrogenase	Decreased G-6-phosphatase; X-linked	Sheep
EPITHELIAL TRANSPORT			
Familial vitamin D-resistant rickets	– – –	Rickets or osteomalacia, hypophosphatemia; X-linked dominant	Dog

123

Genetically Determined Metabolic Diseases Involving Enzyme Defects (Continued)

Diseases	Enzyme Defect (If known)	Effect and Mode of Transmission	Animal Model (If known)*
EPITHELIAL TRANSPORT (Continued)			
Fanconi syndrome	– – –	Osteomalacia, glycosuria, aminoaciduria, increased phosphorus clearance	– – –
Renal glycosuria	– – –	Urine contains glucose when blood level is normal; dominant	– – –
Renal tubular acidosis	– – –	Elevated blood chloride, hypokaluria, renal calcinosis; dominant	– – –
Cystinuria	– – –	Excessive ornithine, lysine, arginine, and ornithine in urine, urolithiasis; may be recessive or incomplete dominant	Dog
Hartnup disease	Tryptophan metabolism	Pellagra-like rash, cerebellar ataxia, amino-aciduria; autosomal recessive	– – –
Mucoviscidosis (cystic fibrosis)	(?)	Defect of eccrine, sweat glands, abnormal saliva salt concentration, chronic respiratory and enteric disorders; autosomal recessive	– – –

metacentric   Denoting a chromosome with a centrally located centromere. See *acrocentric*, *submetacentric*, and *telocentric*.

metachromasia   A color change exhibited when pure aniline dyes or their fractions become bound to chromotropes either in tissue sections or in aqueous solutions.[57]

metachromatic dye   A substance that stains tissues more than one color, as toluidine blue, alcian blue, azure B, etc.

metamerism   Repetition of segments (somites) along the long axis of an animal's body, a trait exhibited by many invertebrates, including annelids and arthropods, and by some vertebrates.

metaphase   The middle stage of mitosis during which occurs the lengthwise separation of the chromosomes in the equatorial plate. See *mitosis*.

metaplasia   The change in the type of adult cells in a tissue to a form which is not normal for that tissue.

metastasis   The transfer of disease from one organ or part to another not directly connected with it. It may be due either to the transfer of pathogenic microorganisms (e.g., tubercle bacilli) or to the transfer of cells, as in malignant tumors.

Metastrongylus elongatus   A member of the superfamily Metastrongyloidea found in the lungs of pigs and known as porcine lungworm.

-meter   A word termination designating relationship to measurement, or denoting especially an instrument used in measuring.

methenamine silver nitrate   A stain used in the Gomori technic to demonstrate argyrophilic tissue components; also used to stain glycogen and mucin and for certain fungi.[153]

methotrexate   An antimetabolite that is a folic acid antagonist; used as an oncolytic drug and immunosuppressant.

methyl blue   An acid triphenylmethane dye. Solubility at 15° C.: water 50 per cent, absolute alcohol nil, and glycerol 25 per cent.

methylcholanthrene   A carcinogenic hydrocarbon.

methylene blue   A basic dye of the thiazine group. Solubility at 15° C.: water 9.5 per cent, absolute alcohol 6 per cent, and glycerol 15 per cent. It is used with basic fuchsin as a differential stain for nucleic acids, with carbol fuchsin for bacterial flagella and capsules, and with basic fuchsin and eosin for blood, bacteria, and spirochetes.[57]

methylglyoxalase   An enzyme that catalyzes the change of methylglyoxal to lactic acid.

methyl green   A basic triphenyl dye. Solubility at 15° C.: water 8 per cent, absolute alcohol 3 per cent, and glycerol 12.5 per cent. It is used with acid fuchsin for staining lignified tissues and chromosomes, and with erythrosin in plant cytology. It selectively stains DNA and is frequently used in combination with pyronin to stain nucleic acids.[57]

methymycin   See *macrolide*.

metonymy   Disorder of thinking in which the patient uses, instead of the correct term, a poor approximation to it.

metric system   See table for prefixes used in the metric system.

METRIC PREFIXES

Prefix	Symbol	Multiple
deka-	da	10
hecto-	h	10^2
kilo-	k	10^3
mega-	M	10^6
giga-	G	10^9
tera-	T	10^{12}
deci-	d	10^{-1}
centi-	c	10^{-2}
milli-	m	10^{-3}
micro-	μ	10^{-6}
nano-	n	10^{-9}
pico-	p	10^{-12}
femto-	f	10^{-15}
atto-	a	10^{-18}

metro-   A combining form denoting relationship to the uterus; also used as a prefix meaning to measure.

metrology   The science that deals with measurement.

-metry   A word termination meaning the act of measuring or the measurement of, the object measured being indicated by the word stem to which it is affixed, as hemoglobulinometry.

mice   See *mouse.*

Michigan Academy of Sciences, Arts, and Letters   Ann Arbor, Mich.

micro-   A combining form designating small size; used in naming units of measurement to indicate one-millionth (10^{-6}) of the unit designated by the root with which it is combined.

microautoradiography   See *autoradiography.*

microbial control   That part of biological control (q.v.) concerned with the use of microorganisms (including viruses) to control undesirable animals or plants. Pathogens may exert their controlling effect by means of their invasive properties, toxins, enzymes, or other substances.

microbial insecticide   A pathogenic microorganism or its products (toxins, etc.) used to suppress an insect population. The terms "microbial pesticide," "biotic insecticide," and "microbial control product" are also used. See also *biotic insecticide.*

microcinematography   The photographing of living cells under the phase-contrast microscope, usually employing motion-picture film with one frame being exposed at selected intervals and then projecting the film at ordinary speed (usually 24 frames per second). Thus if one frame per second is exposed there is a speed-up factor at projection of 24; if one per minute, a factor of 60×24, or 1440. Cell movements, phagocytosis, mitosis, etc., then can be viewed as dynamic processes.

The Microcirculatory Society, Inc.   Department of Physiology, School of Medicine, University of Arizona, Tucson, Ariz. 85721.

microevolution   An evolutionary pattern occurring over a short span of time. Cf. *macroevolution.*

microfauna   The animal life, visible only under the microscope, that is present in or characteristic of a special location, as the protozoan population of the ruminant stomach.

microfeeding   Forced feeding of small volumes of solutions or suspensions to insects and other small animals, usually by peroral inoculation by means of a microcatheter.

microflora   The plant life, visible only under the microscope, which is present in or characteristic of a special location, e.g., the bacterial population of the mouth of normal animals.

microfluorometry   A technic to measure fluorescent emissions from cells as they flow across a light beam.

microides   Sabouraud's term for small ectothrix chains in dermatophyte-infected hair, *e.g., Trichophyton mentagrophytes.*

microinjector   A device for injecting measured, minute amounts of fluids. It usually consists of a fine metal or glass needle adapted to a syringe, and of a mechanism for the advancement of the piston (micrometer or ratchet).

micromania   A delusional belief that one's own body has become reduced in size or one's personality reduced in importance.

micromelia   A developmental anomaly characterized by abnormal smallness or shortness of the limbs.

micrometer   An instrument for measuring objects seen through the microscope.

   eyepiece m. (ocular m.), a micrometer used in connection with the eyepiece of a microscope.

   ocular m., eyepiece m.

   stage m., a micrometer fastened to the stage of a microscope.

microorganism   A minute living organism of microscopic or ultramicroscopic size. For a comparison of various forms, see table on page 126.

microphobia   Morbid dread of small objects.

microscope   An instrument that is used to obtain an enlarged image of small objects and to reveal details of structure not otherwise distinguishable.[153]

   binocular m., a microscope that has two eyepieces, making possible simultaneous viewing with both eyes.

   centrifuge m., a microscope built into a high-speed centrifuge, by which a magnified image of a specimen undergoing centrifugal force may be produced.

   comparison m., an instrument that permits simultaneous viewing of parts of images of two separate specimens, involving two microscopes bridged together with a comparison eyepiece, or one microscope with two body tubes and lens systems.

   compound m., one that consists of two lens systems, one above the other, in which the image formed by the system nearer the object (objective) is further magnified by the system nearer the eye (eyepiece).

   darkfield m., one with a central stop in the condenser, permitting diversion of the light rays and illumination of the object from the

BIOLOGICAL AND CHEMICAL COMPARISON OF MICROORGANISMS AND VIRUSES*

	GROW ON ARTIFICIAL MEDIA	DIVIDE BY BINARY FISSION	CONTAIN BOTH DNA AND RNA	CONTAIN RIBO-SOMES	COAT CONTAINS MURAMIC ACID	RESPOND TO SOME ANTIBIOTICS EFFECTIVE AGAINST BACTERIA	SENSITIVE TO INTER-FERON
Bacteria	+	+	l	l	Sometimes	+	−
Mycoplasmata	+	+	+	+	−	+	−
Rickettsiae	−	+	+	+	+	+	−
Chlamydiae	−	+	+	+	+	+	+
Viruses	−	−	−	−	−	−	+

*From F. Fenner: The Biology of Animal Viruses. Academic Press, New York, 1968.

side, so that the details appear light against a dark background.[153]

electron m., one in which an electron beam, instead of light, forms an image for viewing on a fluorescent screen, or for photography.

fluorescence m., one in which light of one wavelength is used to illuminate the specimen, and the image seen is due to light of longer wavelength, re-emitted by the specimen.[153]

infrared m., one in which radiation of 800 mμ or longer wavelength is used as the image-forming energy.

interference m., a microscope for observing the same kind of refractile detail as that observed with the phase microscope, but utilizing two separate beams of light which are sent through the specimen and combined with each other in the image plane.

phase-contrast m., a microscope which alters the phase relationship of the light passing through and that passing around the object, the contrast permitting visualization of the object without the necessity for staining or other special preparation.

polarizing m., one equipped with a polarizer, analyzer, and means for measurement of the alteration of the polarized light by the specimen.

Schlieren m., one in which light is deviated by the insertion of one or two diaphragms in the optical system, to reveal differences in refractive index in a specimen.

stereoscopic m., a binocular biobjective microscope, or a binocular monobjective microscope modified to give a three-dimensional view of the specimen.

stroboscopic m., one that utilizes flashing illumination, permitting analysis of motion in the specimen.

ultraviolet m., a microscope which utilizes reflecting optics or quartz and other ultraviolet-transmitting lenses, with radiation of less than 400 mμ wavelength as the image-forming energy.

Microsporidia An order of protozoan parasite common in arthropods.[109]

microsporidiosis Infection with Microsporidia; seen in mosquito larvae, honeybees, and silkworms. See *nosema disease.*[109]

Microsporum A genus of imperfect keratinophilic fungi that exhibit a slow-growing or a fast-growing (cottony) colony and are most commonly the etiologic agent of ringworm.[36, 142] *M. audouini* causes ringworm in the dog, monkey, guinea pig, and man; *M. canis* in the dog, cat, horse, monkey, chinchilla, and man; *M. distortsem* in the monkey and man; *M. gypseum* in the dog, cat, horse, fowl, guinea pig, rat, and mouse; and *M. nanum* in swine.

microsymbiont This term is sometimes used to designate the smaller organism, or microorganism, of a symbiotic association. See also *symbiont.*

microtome An instrument for cutting tissues to be examined under the microscope. There are several types, including the rotary microtome, the sliding microtome, the freezing microtome for cutting frozen sections, and the cryostat microtome, which has a controlled temperature chamber.[153] See also *ultramicrotome.*

microtubule A filamentous tubular structure seen by electron microscopy in the cytoplasm of many types of cells. It is about 250 Å in diameter and probably functions in cell motility and as a component of the mitotic spindle.[38]

mikamycin See *streptogramin.*

milk See *pigeon milk.*

milk agent Bittner mammary tumor virus.

milk factor Bittner mammary tumor virus.

milk fever A colloquial name for a frequently occurring, sudden, acute hypocalcemia of dairy cattle which occurs immediately after parturition.

milk influence Bittner mammary tumor virus.

milky disease Any of a group of maladies of scarabaeid larvae, caused by species of the genus *Bacillus.* Type A milky disease of the white grub of the Japanese beetle (*Popillia japonica*) is caused by *Bacillus popilliae,* whereas type B milky disease (marked by extensive formation of blood clots, impairment of circulation, and gangrene of the appendages) is caused by *B. lentimorbus.* Milky disease of both types occurs in numerous other species of scarabs. As the disease progresses, the bacteria multiply and sporulate in the insect's blood to produce marked turbidity of the normally clear fluid. The appearance of the blood at this stage is the basis for the name "milky" disease.

milli- A prefix used in naming units of measurement to indicate one one-thousandth (10^{-3}) of the unit designated by the root with which it is combined.

millipede (thousand-legged worm) Any member of the phylum Arthropoda, subphylum Mandibuluta, class Myriapoda, subclass Diplopoda. The millipedes have a head with simple eyes, a thorax of four single somites, and an abdomen of 20 to 100 double somites, depending on the species, each with two pairs of seven-jointed walking legs. Their food consists of dead plant or animal matter. They do not bite and are not poisonous. Examples are *Spirobolus* and *Julus virgatus*. See also *arthropod*.

mimesis Mimetic behavior; see under *behavior*.

miniature swine Swine which as adults reach a weight of 79 to 90 kg., as compared to 225 kg. for normal swine. Their relatively small size, omnivorous diet preference, and several anatomic and physiologic characteristics shared with man provide advantages for several areas of research, including nutrition, immunology, dentition studies, radiobiology, and cardiovascular studies.[19]

mink A small semiaquatic carnivore, *Mustela vison*, of the family Mustilidae, which occurs in the wild state in the United States and Canada and is raised commercially for its fur, which makes coats of great beauty and durability. There are about 30 phenotypes or "color phases" of mink. Of considerable biomedical importance is the mutant animal known as the Aleutian mink, which in the homozygous recessive state exhibits an inherited defect of lysosomes called the Chediak-Higashi syndrome (q.v.). Also of interest to experimental biologists is an immunoproliferative disease caused by a filterable agent (see Aleutian disease). Several other infectious diseases and inherited defects are of experimental significance.

mink encephalopathy See under *encephalopathy*.

minomycin An antibiotic produced by a species of *Streptomyces* that is active against gram-positive bacteria. Its mechanism of action is poorly understood but probably involves interference with protein or nucleic acid metabolism.[49]

Miocene Denoting the epoch in the Tertiary period extending from 25 to 13 million years ago. See *geologic time divisions*.

miscegenation The intermarriage or union of persons of different races, or the procreation of persons of mixed race.

miso- A combining form meaning hatred of.

misogamy Morbid aversion to marriage.

misogyny Aversion to women.

misopedia Morbid dislike of children.

Mississippi Academy of Sciences Drawer CQ, State College, Miss. 39762.

Mississippian Denoting an epoch in the

Carboniferous period. See *geologic time divisions*.

Missouri Academy of Science 9715 Mercier, Kansas City, Mo. 64114.

mithramycin See *chromomycin*.

mito- A combining form meaning threadlike, or denoting relationship to a thread.

mitochondrion (pl. *mitochondria*) An organelle which occurs in the cytoplasm of most cells except bacteria and blue-green algae. Mitochondria are composed of double unit-membrane structures, the inner of which is convoluted into ridges called cristae. They are the site of oxidative metabolism.[38]

mitogen A compound capable of stimulating mitosis. Some of the common mitogens used in experimental biology are phytohemagglutinin (q.v.), pokeweed mitogen, and antigens to which an animal has been sensitized. These materials act primarily on the lymphoid system, both in vivo and in vitro.

mitomycin Any of a group of antibiotics produced by a species of *Streptomyces* and closely related to another group, the porfiromycins, which exhibit inhibitory effects on the transforming capacity of pneumococci, inhibit cell division of several species of bacteria, and in higher concentrations are bactericidal. The mitomycins interfere with DNA metabolism probably by the formation of mitomycin cross-links between the complementary DNA strands.[36, 49]

mitosis A method of indirect division of a cell, consisting of a complex of various processes, by means of which the two daughter nuclei normally receive identical complements of the number of chromosomes characteristic of the somatic cells of the species. Mitosis is divided into four phases. 1. Prophase: formation of a duplicate spireme; disappearance of the nuclear membrane; breaking up of the spireme into chromosomes; appearance of the achromatic spindle; formation of polar bodies. 2. Metaphase: arrangement of chromosomes in the equatorial plane of the central spindle to form the monaster; chromosomes separate into exactly similar halves. 3. Anaphase: the two groups of daughter chromosomes separate and move along the fibers of the central spindle, each toward one of the asters, forming the diaster. 4. Telophase: the daughter chromosomes resolve themselves into a reticulum and the daughter nuclei are formed; the cytoplasm divides, forming two complete daughter cells.

heterotypic m., mitosis in which the halves of bivalent chromosomes move away from each other toward the poles, as occurs in the first, or reductional, division of meiosis.

homeotypic m., the ordinary type of cell division in mitosis, as occurs also in the second, or equational, division of meiosis.

multicentric m., pluripolar m.

pathologic m., atypical, asymmetrical mitosis indicative of malignancy.

pluripolar m., cell division that results in

the formation of more than two daughter cells.

model   See *animal model.*

modifier   A gene that alters the phenotypic expression of another gene of which it is not an allele.

molecular anatomy   The biochemical and biophysical dissection of cell organelles and macromolecules to determine their function in relation to the total cell function.

molecular biology   The study of biological phenomena at the molecular level by the use of biochemical and biophysical technics.

molluscum   A group of skin diseases characterized by the formation of soft, rounded cutaneous tumors.

   m. contagiosum (m. epitheliale), a skin disease of anthropoid apes and man caused by a poxvirus and marked by the formation of firm, rounded skin tubercles containing a semifluid caseous matter or solid masses made up of fat, epidermis, and peculiar capsulated bodies (molluscum corpuscles). The tubercles usually appear upon the face, especially below the eyes and on the bridge of the nose. There are intracytoplasmic accumulations of virions (molluscum bodies). The infection in the chimpanzee is an excellent model for comparison to the human disease.[3, 114]

   m. fibrosum, m. pendulum, m. simplex, diseases marked by the development of multiple fibromas of the skin, which often form pendulous growths. They arise from the corium or the subcutaneous tissue.

   m. verrucosum, a late stage of molluscum contagiosum in which the growths have become wartlike masses.

mollusk   Any member of the phylum Mollusca. The group has many divergent morphological types, but they are all characterized by bilateral symmetry, no segmentation, a calcareous exoskeleton or shell secreted by a mantle, an anterior head, a ventral foot for locomotion, a complete digestive tract, a two- or three-chambered heart, blood vessels, respiratory gills, a reduced coelom, and a nervous system of paired ganglia. Sexes are usually separate, although some forms are bisexual. Most forms are marine, some inhabit fresh water, and a few forms are terrestrial.

Five classes are recognized: Amphineura, including the chitons; Scaphapoda, the tooth shells (e.g., *Dentalium*); Gastropoda, the univalve mollusks (spiral shells usually), including the snails, slugs, and abalone; Pelecypoda, bivalve mollusks (hinged shells), including oysters, clams, mussels, and scallops; and Cephalopoda, including the squids and octopuses.

Moloney leukemia virus   The Moloney virus originated from a cell-free extract of a sarcoma 37 implant in a BALB/c mouse. The original preparation induced lymphoid leukemia in 100 per cent of BALB/c mice inoculated, after a latent period of about seven months. After several mouse passages, the virus recovered from the spleen or lymph nodes was capable of inducing lymphoid leukemia in BALB/c, C3H, DBA/2, R111, and C57B mice or their hybrids, in Sprague-Dawley and Osborne-Mendel rats, and in hamsters. When the virus was inoculated into thymectomized mice, a reticulum cell sarcoma developed. The virus may be maintained without cytopathologic effect in a variety of cell culture lines, and can be neutralized in vitro or in vivo by immune rabbit serum. Its chemical and ultrastructural properties have been described in detail.[53, 114]

monactin   See *nonactin.*

Monckeberg's arteriosclerosis   See *arteriosclerosis.*

Moniezia   A genus of anoplocephalid tapeworms which parasitize lambs and New World monkeys. The intermediate host of this parasite is the oribatid mite.[21]

Monilia   Former name for *Candida.*

Moniliformis moniliformis   See *helminth parasites,* under *rat.*

monkey   See *primate.*

mono-   A combining form denoting one or single; limited to one part; in chemistry, combined with one atom.

monoamine oxidase   An enzyme that catalyzes the oxidation of amines to aldehydes, ammonia, and hydrogen peroxide. It is used as a histochemical indicator for the presence of catecholamines in anaphylactic reactions.[160]

monoblastoma   A neoplasm containing monoblasts and monocytes.

monocentric   Denoting a chromosome that has a single centromere.

monocin   See *bacteriocin.*

monodactyly   A developmental anomaly characterized by the presence of only one digit on a hand or foot.

monogenic   Denoting a character determined by a single gene.

monolayer   A single layer, such as a monolayer of cells in cultures used in studies of viruses.

monolepsis   The transmission to the offspring of the characters of one parent, to the exclusion of those of the other.

monophasia   Aphasia with ability to utter but one word or phrase.

monophobia   Morbid dread of being left alone.

monophyletic   Arising or descending from a single cell type.

monotreme   Any of a group of oviparous mammals which include the platypus and echidna.

monoxenic   Associated with a single species of microorganisms; said of otherwise germ-free animals contaminated by a single type of organism.

monoxenous   Requiring only one host in order to complete the life cycle. Cf. *heteroxenous.*

monozygotic   Denoting twins formed from one fertilized egg. Cf. *dizygotic.*

Montana Academy of Sciences University of Montana, Missoula, Mont. 59801.

morbid drone-laying (drone broodiness) A disease of queen honeybees of unknown etiology, in which the epithelial cells of the spermathecae of affected queen bees contain intranuclear acidophilic inclusion bodies. The spermatozoa within such spermathecae curl into ringlets and degenerate. Each ringlet consists of only one spermatozoon (Arnhart's "Ringelsamen").[148]

Morgan unit A measurement of relative distance between genes on a chromosome.

Morison's cell inclusion Any of the strongly basophilic cytoplasmic inclusions appearing in the hindgut epithelium of bees showing symptoms of chronic paralysis. The inclusions are largest in the cells immediately posterior to the opening of the malpighian tubules.[148]

-morph A word termination denoting relationship to form or shape; such as an individual possessing a certain form, indicated by the preceding root, as mesomorph.

morula An early stage of embryonic development, when cleavage has resulted in a solid ball (mulberry-like) of cells.

mosaicism The state of being composed of cells of different chromosome number, genotype, or phenotype, all of which have been derived from a single zygote. Numerical aberrations are believed to result from a failure of proper pairing and separation of homologous chromosomes during mitosis, e.g., loss of a Y chromosome from some XY cells, leading to an XO/XY mosaic. Exposure to ionizing radiation or carcinogens may produce a change in genotype of a portion of the body, as in tumor formation. According to the Lyon hypothesis, normal female mammals are mosaics for phenotypic expression of genes located on the X chromosome, because one of the X chromosomes in each cell has been randomly inactivated. Cf. *chimerism* and see *late-replicating X chromosome*, under *chromosome*.

mosquito 1. A popular name for gnatlike, blood-sucking, and venomous insects of the family Culicidae and of various genera, chiefly *Culex, Aedes, Anopheles, Mansonia, Haemagogus, Psorophora, Theobaldia,* and *Chagasia*. Mosquitoes are important disease vectors. 2. An apparatus for drawing blood from a vessel in sterile condition.

motile Having spontaneous but not conscious or volitional movement.

motivation In behavioral science, a term referring to the broad class of variables controlling behavior. The concept is broader than that of drive (q.v.) and includes such notions as preferences, appetites, etc.

mouse A small rodent of the family Muridae found throughout the world. Specific kinds of mice are designated by compound terms such as harvest mouse (*Mycromys* of Eurasia), wood mouse (*Apodemus* of Eurasia), white-footed mouse (*Peromyscus* of America), and pocket mouse (*Perognathus* of North America). The house mouse (*Mus musculus*), the genus type, measures from 65 to 95 mm. in length and weighs 18 to 30 gm. The white laboratory mouse is a domesticated variant of the house mouse.[51, 88, 138]

    arthropod parasites of m., see *arthropod parasites*, under *rat*.

    helminth parasites of m., see *helminth parasites*, under *rat*.

    inbred m., see *inbred strain*. Many families of mice which meet the criteria of inbred strain have been developed over the past 50 years and have aided immensely in carrying out experiments with drugs, oncogenic viruses, transplantation, and many other studies.[51, 53, 138] See table for a selected list of strains, and see Staats[146] in Bibliography for a complete list.

    multimammate m., a small African rodent, *Praomys natalensis (Rattus natalensis; Mastomys coucha)*. The males may weigh up to 100 gm. In the wild, it often prefers cohabitation in human dwellings. Anatomically it resembles the rat more than the mouse, as in the absence of a gallbladder. The animal was introduced as a laboratory species in 1939 and is used especially in cancer research. It is called the multimammate mouse because of the presence of eight to ten pairs of teats and, although the average litter size is eight, numbers as high as 16 are not unusual.[80]

    New Zealand black m. (NZB m.), see *NZB mouse disease*.

    protozoan parasites of m., see *protozoan parasites*, under *rat*.

    Swiss m., a strain of albino mice brought to the United States in 1926 by Lynch and used widely in laboratory experiments.[88] See diagram on page 130.

mouse adenovirus A virus found in certain laboratory mouse colonies in the absence of any detectable clinical illness. In suckling mice, fatal infection may be induced by in-

SOME STRAINS OF INBRED MICE*

SYMBOL	COLOR	DEVELOPER OF STRAIN
A	Albino	Strong
Ak	Albino	Furth
BALB	Albino	Bagg
CBA	Black agouti	Strong
C3H	Black agouti	Strong
C57 Brown	Non-agouti brown	Little
C57 Black	Black	Little
C58	Black	MacDowell
DBA/2	Non-agouti dilute-brown	Little
I	Dilute-brown, piebald pink-eyed	Strong
R III	Albino	Dobrovolskaia-Zavadskaia
Swiss†	Albino	Lynch

*From L. Gross: Oncogenic Viruses. Pergamon Press, New York, 1961.

†Only some of the substrains employed are inbred, or partially inbred. For that reason, the characteristics may vary among the different sublines.

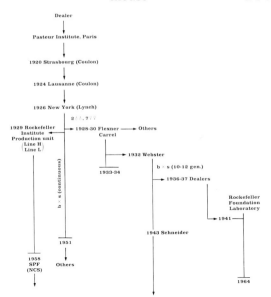

Figure 4. Brief outline of the history of the Swiss mouse. (From C. J. Lynch: The so-called Swiss mouse. Lab. Animal Care, 19(No. 2):214–220, 1969.)

tranasal, intracerebral, or intraperitoneal inoculation of the virus, with production of a generalized disease characterized by intranuclear inclusion bodies in brown fat, myocardium, adrenal cortex, kidney, and salivary gland. In weaned mice, the agent produces a clinically silent infection, occasionally with mild myocarditis and adrenal focal necrosis.[63, 114]

mouse hepatitis   See under *hepatitis.*

mouse opossum   A small marsupial, genus *Marmosa,* native to South America. The young, born after 14 to 15 days of gestation, are not carried in a pouch but are attached to mammae and easily accessible to investigators.

mouse papular virus   An agent causing papular dermatitis in laboratory mice. The lesion is often inapparent, being merely a small swelling concealed beneath the body hair. On the feet and tail, it is more visible and may superficially resemble chronic ectromelia. Eosinophilic intracytoplasmic inclusion bodies are seen in epidermal cells at the periphery of the lesion. Serologically it is not related to vaccinia or ectromelia viruses. Although it has not been observed since the original description by Kraft, it is important in the differential diagnosis of ectromelia.[77]

mouse pneumonitis   See under *pneumonitis.*

mouse poliomyelitis   See *Theiler's mouse encephalomyelitis,* under *encephalomyelitis.*

mousepox   *Ectromelia,* def. 1.

mouse unit   The least amount of estrus-producing hormone which will cause in a spayed mouse a characteristic change in the vaginal epithelium.

moustached monkey   Any member of the species *Cercopithecus cephus.* See *primate.*

MSX disease   A code name meaning "multinucleated sphere of unknown affinities." Found in the American oyster, *Crassostrea virginica,* along the middle Atlantic coast of the United States, the disease is caused by the haplosporidian *Minchinia nelsoni,* which lives in the connective tissues surrounding the gut. It causes serious mortality rates in high salinity areas during late summer and early fall.

mucoid enteritis   See under *enteritis.*

mucormycosis   An infection caused by any of several species of coenocytic (nonseptate) fungi which may occur in dogs, cattle, and occasionally swine. The lesions are most commonly granulomatous and frequently involve the lymph nodes. There have been occasional reports of these organisms as the cause of gastric erosions. They may also be the cause of abortions in cattle.[142]

multi-   A combining form signifying many or much.

Multiceps multiceps   A cyclophyllidean cestode known as the dog tapeworm, which also may parasitize the fox, coyote, and man. Its larval stage is called *Coenurus cerebralis* owing to the appearance of its cysts in the nervous system.[21] See table of *Common Cestode Parasites,* and *cestodiasis.*

multimammate mouse   See under *mouse.*

multiple schedule   See *schedule of reinforcement,* under *reinforcement.*

multiple T-maze   See under T-*maze.*

murine chronic respiratory disease   See under *respiratory disease.*

murine encephalomyelitis virus   A group of neurotropic viruses capable of producing flaccid paralysis due to destruction of the gray matter of the spinal cord (Theiler's mouse poliomyelitis). FA and GD VII viruses are included in this group. Other neurotropic viruses which do not cause demyelination are SKC Columbia strain of Jungleblut, EK virus, herpes simplex virus, and eastern encephalitis virus.[63, 114]

murine pseudotuberculosis　　See under *pseudotuberculosis.*

Murphy-Sturm lymphosarcoma　　See under *lymphosarcoma.*

muscardine　Mycoses of insects in which the fruiting bodies of the pathogenic fungi ("muscardine fungi") arise on the exterior of the insect, producing a thick covering about the animal. Originally, the term muscardine was used in reference to muscardine of the silkworm. But today it is used, accompanied by a modifier, to denote specific mycoses of a number of insects, such as white muscardine of the chinch bug, and green muscardine of the European corn borer.

　green m., a mycosis of various larval, pupal, and adult insects, caused by the hyphomycetous fungus *Metarrhizium anisopliae.* Infection occurs principally by mycelial penetration through the insect's integument. After death of the host, if external conditions are suitable, the hyphae emerge through the integument and produce spores, which become olive green in color as they mature. See also *muscardine.*

　m. of the silkworm, a mycosis of silkworm larvae, caused by the hyphomycetous fungus *Beauveria bassiana.* Infection occurs by mycelial penetration through the larval integument. In serocultural practice, the disease is transmitted from one generation of silkworms to the next by the conidia which have accumulated in neglected rearing rooms. Particularly severe epizootic appearances of the disease were described in the eighteenth and nineteenth centuries. Agostine Bassi, the "founder of parasitology," was the first to prove, in 1834, that muscardine of the silkworm is contagious and that the fungus is the causative agent of the disease. *Beauveria bassiana* infects numerous additional species of insects.

　white m., a mycosis of various larval, pupal, and adult insects, caused by the hyphomycetous fungus *Beauveria bassiana,* also known as "white fungus." Infection occurs by mycelial penetration through the insect's integument. After death of the host, hyphae fill the body cavity, finally emerging through the integument. Under suitable external conditions, the typical white mycelial growth and white conidia cover the insect's body. The disease occurs (frequently in epizootic proportions) in populations of the chinch bug, *Blissus leucopterus,* of the silkworm (see *muscardine of the silkworm*), of the European corn borer, *Ostrynia nubilalis,* and of other species.

mutable site　The location on a chromosome at which mutation is most likely to occur.

mutagenic　Denoting an environmental factor capable of causing mutation.

mutase　An enzyme that hastens oxidation-reduction reactions.

mutation　A change in form, quality, or some other characteristic. In biology, a permanent transmissible change in the characters of an offspring from those of its parents; also, an individual showing such a change; a sport.[121]

　induced m., a genetic mutation caused by external factors which are experimentally or accidentally produced.

　natural m., a genetic mutation occurring without the intervention of any known external factors.

　somatic m., a genetic mutation occurring in a somatic cell, providing the basis for a mosaic condition.

mutualism　A symbiotic relationship between a host and its parasite in which the symbionts are mutually dependent upon and beneficial to each other. Some examples are termites and the intestinal protozoa, which hydrolyze cellulose for the termites, and the bacteria and protozoa which perform similar functions in ruminants and other herbivores.[159]

mycelium　Filamentous mat or vegetative whole of a fungal plant.

mycetismus　Poisoning caused by a fungus, as that resulting from ingestion of poisonous mushrooms.

mycetocyte　A cell containing intracellular mutualistic and commensalistic microsymbionts. One of many cells making up the mycetome.

mycetome　In various invertebrate animals, the structure or organ which houses symbionts. The cells making up the mycetome and containing the symbionts are known as mycetocytes.

myco-, myc-, mycet-　A combining form denoting relationship to fungus.

Mycobacterium　See *tuberculosis.*

Mycological Society of America　U.S. Army Natick Laboratories, Natick, Mass. 01762.

Mycoplasma　See *mycoplasmosis.*

mycoplasmosis　A disease caused by or associated with microorganisms of the order Mycoplasmatales, single genus *Mycoplasma,* currently classified within the bacteria (Schizomycetes). Known previously as the pleuropneumonia-like organisms (PPLO), *Mycoplasma* can be grown, like bacteria, on artificial media enriched with serum, yeast extract, and other necessary components. But unlike bacteria, most require cholesterol as a necessary nutrient (for a comparison of mycoplasmata and other microscopic forms, see *microorganism*). Under the microscope, colonies on agar have a characteristic "fried-egg" appearance due to the yellowish raised central part that grows down into the media and is surrounded by a lighter and more flat peripheral zone.

　The basic reproductive unit varies in size from 125 to 300 mμ, which is of the same order as that of large viruses, e.g., poxvirus; consequently they are just visible with the light microscope, but will pass ordinary bacterial filters. From these units one or more filaments grow out and by continuous dichotomous branching produce a regular mycelium. The filaments constrict, undergo fragmentation, and form new cells. Electron micrography has shown the structure of the *Mycoplasma* cell membrane to be that of a unit membrane (q.v.), rather than the cell wall common to bacteria. Associated with the lack of a true cell wall is the absolute insusceptibility to penicillin (with the sole exception of *M. neurolyticum*) that is a general property of the order. The mycoplasmas are extremely widespread in nature, occurring as free-living commensals, as well as pathogens (see table).[16, 62]

In the older literature, these organisms are referred to as coccobacilliform bodies (of Nelson). In addition, various generic names have been proposed in previous classifications, including *Coccobacillus, Micromyces, Asteromyces, Borrelomyces, Borimyces,* and *Asterococcus.* The first organism of the group to be discovered was *M. mycoides* (the type species), the cause of bovine pleuropneumonia.

myelin figure Any of a number of types of multilayered membranous structures found within the cytoplasm of many cell types, both normal and abnormal. Their significance is not understood.[38]

myelo-, myel- Combining form denoting relationship to marrow, often used in specific reference to the spinal cord.

myeloblastoma A focal malignant tumor observed in chronic or acute myelogenous leukemia, composed of myeloblasts and lacking green coloration.

myelocytoma Chronic myelocytic leukemia; myeloma.

   canine cutaneous m., a tumor of the subcutaneous tissue of the dog, which resembles myeloma but is benign. The cells

are of heterogeneous type, including neutrophilic and eosinophilic leukocytes.[142]

myiasis Invasion of tissue by larval forms of flies. The principal parasites of this group include the horse botflies, genus *Gasterophilus,* which parasitize members of the family Equidae. Important species are *G. intestinalis,* larvae of which attach to the mucosal layer of the stomach of horses; *G. hemorrhoidalis,* which also parasitizes the stomach; *G. nasalis,* the larvae of which attach to the mucosa of the pylorus and duodenum; and *G. pecorum,* which occurs in Europe, but not in the United States, attaches to the stomach mucosa. *Oestrus ovis,* the blowfly of sheep, deposits its larvae in the nose, from where they migrate into the nasal cavity and nasal sinuses. *Callitroga hominivorax* (q.v.), the screwworm, is the most prominent American species.

Heelflies of the genus *Hypoderma,* principally two species, *H. bovis* and *H. lineatum,* attack cattle. The larvae are laid in the hairs of the legs, flanks, or dewlap of cattle, penetrate the skin, and migrate until they eventually reach the subcutaneous tissues of the back. There the larvae remain until the next stage of the life cycle, in which the larvae emerge through the skin to form pupae on the ground. The holes formed in the skin during this process result in heavy economic losses to farmers.

Myleran Trademark for busulfan.

myo-, my- Combining form denoting relationship to muscle.

Diseases Caused by *Mycoplasma*

Host	Species	Disease
Man	*M. pneumoniae* (Eaton agent)	Atypical pneumonia
Sheep, goats	*M. mycoides* var. *capri* *M. agalactiae*	Contagious pleuropneumonia Mastitis, metritis
Cow	*M. mycoides* *M. l ovigenitalium*	Contagious pleuropneumonia Mastitis, metritis
Swine	*M. hyorhinis* *M. granularum* *M. hypopneumoniae*	Polyserositis, arthritis Arthritis Enzootic pneumonia
Dog	*M. spumans* *M. canis* *M. maculosum*	None known None known (pneumonia?) None known
Mouse	*M. neurolyticum*	Rolling syndrome
Rat	*M. arthritidis*	Polyarthritis
Mouse, rat	*M. pulmonis*	Chronic respiratory disease complex
Chicken, turkey	*M. gallisepticum*	Chronic respiratory disease complex
Chicken	*M. gallinarum* *M. synoviae* *M. iners*	None known Infectious synovitis None known
Turkey	*M. meleagridis*	Air sacculitis
Duck	*M. anatis*	Sinusitis

Myobia musculi See *arthropod parasites,* under *rat.*

myoblastoma A tumor of striated muscle made up of groups of cells which resemble primitive myoblasts. See *rhabdomyosarcoma* and *leiomyosarcoma.*

Myocoptes musculinus See *arthropod parasites,* under *rat.*

Myocoptes romboutsi See *arthropod parasites,* under *rat.*

myoepithelioma HD A spontaneously arising myoepithelioma of the salivary gland found in an A/HeN female mouse in the laboratory of Heston at the National Cancer Institute in 1953. Subcutaneous transplants grow progressively in 90 per cent of A/HeN hosts, with occasional pulmonary and lymph node metastases. Most animals exhibit a marked concurrent leukemoid reaction. Similar spontaneously occurring tumors have been observed in BALB/c mice.[150]

myofibrosarcoma HS-6 (sarcoma HS-6) A sarcoma induced by multiple injections of a 9,10-dimethyl-1,2-benzanthracene solution into the subpanniculus over the lumbar area of a female Syrian hamster in 1944 in the laboratory of E. D. Crabb at the University of Colorado. A local tumor arising at the injection site in one hamster was propagated in others, and a metastatic subline (HS-6) selected for serial transplantation. The tumor generally kills the host within 28 days.[150]

myokinase A heat-stable protein constituent of skeletal muscle, which activates the yeast hexokinase system, thus making possible the transfer of phosphate from adenosine diphosphate to fructose or glucose.

myositis Inflammation of a voluntary muscle.

eosinophilic m., a rare disease involving the masseter, temporalis, and pterygoid muscles of the dog. Lesions are characterized by prominent swelling and pain. There is usually a marked increase in peripheral blood eosinophil leukocytes. The cause of the disease is unknown. Although parasites have been suspected, no proof for their causative relationship has been obtained. A similar myositis has been described in cattle, but this disorder is more likely to be chronic, is characterized by the formation of granulomata and giant cells, and is seen in skeletal muscle and also in cardiac muscle. Parasites such as *Sarcocystis* or *Trichina* have been accused of being the cause in cattle.

m. of guinea pig (Saunder's myositis), a disease characterized by inflammation of the skeletal muscles. In the original (and only) description of this form of myositis, the clinical symptoms included swelling and pain in the large muscle groups of the hind legs, with involvement of the forelegs several days later, followed by prostration and death, presumably of starvation. The only gross lesions were petechiae of the affected muscle masses and lymphadenopathy of the nodes draining these areas. The key histologic lesions were hemorrhage and inflammatory cellular infiltrates in affected muscles. Although no infectious agent could be isolated the disease was transmitted to other guinea pigs by inoculations of the original clinical material only.[131]

mysophilia A form of paraphilia in which there is a lustful attitude toward excretions.

mysophobia Morbid dread of filth or contamination.

mytilotoxism (mussel poisoning) Severe and sometimes fatal poisoning that occasionally follows the eating of mussels.

myxadenoma An epithelial tumor with the structure of a mucous gland.

myxofibroma A fibroma containing myxomatous tissue.

myxoma A tumor composed of mucous tissue.

myxomatosis (big head; mosquito disease) A highly infectious and fatal disease of the domestic laboratory rabbit (*Oryctolagus cuniculus*), caused by a poxvirus and first described in epizootic form by Sararelli in South America in 1898. The natural host is the wild rabbit (*Syvilagus*) of the Americas, in which the disease is much less virulent or even asymptomatic. In the United States there are no wild members of the genus *Oryctolagus*, hence maintenance of a natural reservoir in this country has an uncertain status at present, although California is classified as an endemic area. Natural transmission of the disease requires an arthropod vector, generally the *Aedes* or *Culex* mosquito, or the rabbit flea *Spilopsyllus*.

The disease was first introduced into Europe and Australia for the express purpose of limiting the population of feral *Oryctolagus* rabbit. It was shown that the virus, regularly lethal in ten days at first, could be modified by passage in successively more resistant rabbits to produce strains of progressively diminishing virulence. From the Australian studies, a group of agents of graded virulence were isolated. On the basis of this evidence, and also that of the Berry-Dedrick phenomenon, it has been recognized that a Shope fibroma-myxoma spectrum of virulence exists. Shope realized that *Oryctolagus* rabbits which recovered from Shope fibroma infections were solidly immune to myxomatosis, but only later could the following graded spectrum be constructed: the least virulent is the 1A strain, followed by the OA and Boerlage strains of fibroma virus, and then the strains (from Australia) of myxoma virus of increasing virulence. Heat-inactivated viruses of each strain in this classification are capable of yielding an enhancing factor for those lower in the classification.

The incubation period of myxomatosis is variable, but experimental infections usually first manifest themselves in seven to ten days with a soft gelatinous, hemorrhagic swelling at the site of injection. This is followed by a discharge from the eyes, subcutaneous edema with a predilection for the head, anorexia, and fever. The ears may droop as a result of fluid accumulations. Irregular subcutaneous swellings develop, especially at mucocutaneous borders, that are elevated, round or oval, often vesiculated, and occasionally attached to the underlying muscle. Lymph nodes draining these areas become enlarged and hemorrhagic. The "tumors" are mucoid, gelatinous, and reddish in gross cross-section. The spleen is enlarged and most serous surfaces show petechiae.

Microscopic lesions include hypertrophy and hyperplasia of epithelial cells, hydropic degeneration, and vacuolation of the cytoplasm with eosinophilic clumps simulating inclusion bodies. The dermis is myxomatous, like Wharton's jelly, with large stellate and spindle-shaped (myxoma) cells which represent hypertrophied fibroblasts and are the key microscopic finding. There is accompanying hyperplasia and hypertrophy of endothelial cells within the myxomatous mass.

Recovery from spontaneous infection (rare) confers lasting immunity, but no killed-virus preparation has been shown to be useful for vaccination. Nor does any treatment exist. Prevention involves steps designed to exclude access to susceptible rabbits by the arthropod vectors.[30, 39, 40] See also *Berry-Dedrick phenomenon,* and see *Shope fibroma,* under *fibroma.*

myxosarcoma   A sarcoma containing myxomatous tissue.

myxovirus   A large ribovirus which received its name because of its affinity for mucoproteins. See *classification,* under *virus.*

N

NAD   Nicotinamide adenine dinucleotide. Formerly called diphosphopyridine nucleotide (DPN).

NADP   Nictonamide adenine dinucleotide phosphate. Formerly called triphosphopyridine nucleotide (TPN).[90]

nagana   A disease of horses and cattle of Central Africa, due to the presence of the parasite *Trypansoma brucei* in the blood. The parasite is transmitted by the bite of the tsetse fly and other species of Glossina. Several wild animals, including the hyena, serve as the reservoir of the disease.

Nairobi disease of sheep   A viral disease characterized by acute hemorrhagic gastroenteritis. The etiologic agent is an arbovirus, transmitted by the adult form of a tick, *Rhipicephalus appendiculatus.*[16, 66]

nanivirus   A name suggested, and then discarded, for the very small RNA viruses. See *picornavirus* in the *classification of viruses,* under *virus.*

nano-   A combining form designating small size; used in naming units of measurement to indicate one-billionth (10^{-9}) of the unit designated by the root with which it is combined.

nanomelia   A developmental anomaly characterized by abnormal smallness of the limbs. See also *phocomelia.*

Nanophyetus   A genus of trematodes, formerly known as *Troglotrema.*

   N. salmincola, a trematode that serves as the vector for the organism *Neorickettsia helminthoeca,* the cause of salmon disease in the dog. The metacercariae excyst and develop into adults in the small intestine of the dog. See *salmon disease.*

   N. schikhobalowi, a species reported in man in eastern Siberia.

nanoplankton   Microscopic forms of plankton.

naphthochrome green   An acid dye of the hydroxy-trianyl-methane group. Solubility at 15° C.: water 3 per cent, absolute alcohol 1.5 per cent, and glycerol 15 per cent.

naphthol yellow   An acid dye of the nitro group. Solubility at 15° C.: water 12.5 per cent, absolute alcohol 0.65 per cent, and glycerol 11 per cent. It is used with trypan blue as a nuclear stain for plant material.[57]

narco-   A combining form denoting relationship to stupor or to a stuporous state.

narcolepsy   A condition marked by an uncontrollable desire for sleep or by sudden episodes of sleep occurring at intervals. Called also *paroxysmal sleep* and *sleep epilepsy.*

narcomania   1. An insane desire for narcotics. 2. Alcoholic insanity.

National Academy of Sciences   National Academy of Engineering, National Research Council, 2101 Constitution Avenue, N.W., Washington, D.C. 20418.

National Association for Research in Science Teaching   Michigan State University, East Lansing, Mich. 48823.

National Science Teachers Association   1201 16th Street, N.W., Washington, D.C. 20036.

National Society for Medical Research   1330 Massachusetts Avenue, N.W., Suite 103, Washington, D.C. 20005.

nauplius   The free-swimming larva of a crustacean.

navel-ill   Omphalitis.

NCI   Abbreviation for National Cancer Institute.

Neanderthal man   A subspecies of primitive man who inhabited Europe, North Africa, and the Near East during the upper Pleistocene epoch.

Nebraska Academy of Sciences, Inc.   209 Morrill Hall, 14th and U Streets, Lincoln, Nebr. 68508.

Necator americanus   A hookworm of man

found in southern United States, Central South America, and the Caribbean area.[21]

necro- A combining form denoting relationship to death or to a dead body.

necrobacillosis Schmorl's disease.

necrophilism Morbid attraction to corpses; sexual intercourse with a dead body.

necrophobia 1. Morbid fear of death. 2. Morbid dread of dead bodies.

necropsy Examination of a body after death.

need 1. In behavioral science, a state in an animal considered to be of such disadvantage that its continuance may lead to death of the animal. 2. A state of homeostatic imbalance.

negative staining A technic used to prepare specimens for electron microscopy in which the material is embedded in electron-dense material and is seen as a negative image. It is especially useful for studies of virus structure.

Negri body An oval or round inclusion seen in the cytoplasm of nerve cells of animals infected with rabies virus. Previously, this identification was the definitive diagnostic method for rabies infection, but it has been replaced by fluorescent-antibody technics.

nemato- A combining form denoting relationship to a nematode, or to a threadlike structure.

nematocyst A minute stinging structure, found in the cnidoblasts of coelenterates and in certain other species, used for anchorage, for defense, and for the capture of prey.

Nematoda A class of worms, the roundworms or threadworms. Parasitic forms invade the host's eyes, mouth, tongue, stomach, intestine, lungs, liver, and the body cavities. Although some are harmless, others cause severe diseases in man and anomen.

nematode (roundworm) An endoparasite belonging to the class Nematoda.

nematodiasis Infestation by a nematode parasite.[21]

cerebrospinal n., invasion of the central nervous system by the larvae of certain nematodes that occasionally wander into the brain or spinal cord and cause inflammation and degeneration which result in central nervous system abnormalities. The parasites usually involved are *Setaria digitata* and *Neurofilaria cornellensis.*

pulmonary n., an infection with lungworms that have a wide species spectrum, including the cat, dog, mouse, deer, swine, fox, horse, cow, and rabbit. The parasites are roundworms, mostly of the superfamilies Metastrongyloidea and Filaroidea. Some of them may be important vectors of disease.[142] See *porcine influenza,* under *influenza.*

Nematomorpha A class of the phylum Aschelminthes, the principal member being the fordian (horsehair) worm. The hair snake or horsehair worm resembles a nematode in that the body is smooth and threadlike, 30 to 90 cm. in length, with an opaque cuticle. The larvae are parasitic in insects; the adults are free-living in fresh water. They differ from nematodes in having a lined body cavity filled with parenchyma, a single nerve cord, and separate gonads and reproductive ducts. The class includes two orders, Gordioidea and Nectonematoidea.

neo- A combining form meaning new or strange.

Neoascaris vitulorum A nematode of the family Ascaridae found in the small intestine of cattle, primarily calves.[21]

Neolithic Age (New Stone Age) The time commencing about 10,000 years ago, during which agriculture and animal husbandry became part of human culture. See *geologic time divisions.*

neophobia Abnormal dread of new things.

neoplasm A new and abnormal growth, a tumor. See accompanying table for the common types of neoplasms affecting domestic animals.

(*Text continued on page 140.*)

INCIDENCE OF VARIOUS NEOPLASMS OF DOMESTIC ANIMALS *

LOCATION AND KIND OF NEOPLASM	CANINE	EQUINE	BOVINE	OVINE	PORCINE	FELINE	TOTAL
Skin, Adnexa, Subcutis, and Adjoining Tissues							
Carcinoma, squamous, epidermoid	212	12	18	6	0	21	269
Basal cell carcinoma, includes sweat gland and sebaceous gland carcinomas and adenomas	428	4	24	3	2	19	480
Perianal adenoma	321	0	0	0	0	0	321
Papilloma	71	3	26	1	0	9	110
Fibro(sarco)ma, chondro(sarco)ma, myxo(sarco)ma, neurofibro-(sarco)ma	478	53	34	3	1	23	592
Lipoma	94	4	2	1	1	0	102
Hemangio(sarco)ma	112	10	8	0	0	0	130
Lymphangioma	4	2	1	0	0	0	7
Melanoma, benign and malignant	257	36	17	1	20	7	338
Mast cell tumor	388	0	3	0	0	2	393
"Cutaneous myelocytoma"	50	0	0	0	0	0	50
Equine "sarcoid"	0	93	0	0	0	0	93
Canine transmissible tumor, nongenital locations	205	0	0	0	0	0	205
Hemangiopericytoma	39	0	1	0	0	2	42

(*Table continues*)

*Adapted from H. A. Smith and T. C. Jones: Veterinary Pathology. 3rd ed. Lea & Febiger, Philadelphia, 1966.

Incidence of Various Neoplasms of Domestic Animals (Continued)

Location and Kind of Neoplasm	Canine	Equine	Bovine	Ovine	Porcine	Feline	Total
Region of Mouth, Including Lips, Gums, Pharynx, Salivary Glands							
Carcinoma	44	8	2	0	0	7	61
Papilloma	16	0	3	0	2	1	22
Adamantinoma	6	1	1	0	0	0	8
Odontoma	1	0	0	0	0	0	1
Epulis	44	0	0	0	0	0	44
Fibro(sarco)ma	104	4	0	0	0	0	108
Hemangio(endothelio)ma	1	0	2	0	0	0	3
Lymphangioma	0	0	1	0	0	0	1
Neurofibro(sarco)ma	1	3	0	0	0	0	4
Melanoma, benign and malignant	64	0	0	0	0	0	64
Parotid adenocarcinoma	2	2	0	0	0	0	4
Tongue							
Carcinoma, squamous cell	4	0	0	0	0	0	4
Papilloma	0	0	1	0	0	0	1
Sarcoma	8	0	0	0	0	0	8
Myxoma	0	1	0	0	0	0	1
Melanoma	3	0	0	0	0	0	3
Canine transmissible tumor	1	0	0	0	0	0	1
Esophagus							
Carcinoma, squamous cell	2	1	1	0	0	10	14
Papilloma	0	0	2	0	0	0	2
Myxofibroma, neurofibroma	0	0	5	0	0	0	5
Sarcoma	6	0	0	0	0	1	7
Bone-forming sarcoma	11	0	0	0	0	0	11
Stomach							
Adenocarcinoma	10	0	0	0	0	0	10
Adenoma	1	0	0	0	0	0	1
Sarcoma	2	0	1	0	0	0	3
Leiomyo(sarco)ma	7	0	0	1	0	0	8
Rumen							
Carcinoma, squamous cell	–	–	1	0	–	–	1
Papilloma	–	–	6	0	–	–	6
Fibromyxoma	–	–	2	0	–	–	2
Omasum							
Papilloma	–	–	2	0	–	–	2
Intestines, Including Rectum							
Adenocarcinoma	41	1	3	2	1	3	51
Papilloma	1	0	0	0	0	0	1
Sarcoma	17	0	0	0	0	3	20
Myxofibroma	0	0	1	0	0	0	1
Neurofibroma	0	0	1	0	0	0	1
Leiomyo(sarco)ma	21	4	3	0	0	0	28
Lymphangioma	0	0	1	0	0	0	1
Liver							
Hepatoma, liver cell carcinoma	39	2	26	9	6	0	82
Bile duct tumor	21	0	26	8	0	0	55
Fibroma	1	0	0	0	0	0	1
Neurofibroma	1	0	1	0	0	0	2
Sarcoma	1	0	1	0	0	0	2
Hemangio(endothelio)ma	4	3	7	1	0	1	16
Paraganglioma	0	1	2	0	0	0	3
Gallbladder							
Adenocarcinoma	11	0	2	0	0	0	13
Adenoma	1	0	11	0	0	0	12
Leiomyoma	0	0	1	0	0	0	1
Pancreas							
Adeno(carcino)ma	27	0	4	1	0	5	37
Islet cell tumor	3	0	0	0	0	0	3
Fibrosarcoma	0	0	1	0	0	0	1
Leiomyoma	1	0	0	0	0	0	1

LOCATION AND KIND OF NEOPLASM	CANINE	EQUINE	BOVINE	OVINE	PORCINE	FELINE	TOTAL
Peritoneal Cavity							
Mesothelioma	0	3	24	0	0	0	27
Lipoma	3	6	8	0	1	1	19
Fibrosarcoma	1	0	0	0	0	0	1
Neurofibrosarcoma	0	0	1	0	0	0	1
Hemangioendothelioma	3	2	0	0	0	0	5
Lymphangioendothelioma	0	1	0	0	0	0	1
Neuroblastoma	0	1	1	0	0	0	2
Nasal Passages and Sinuses							
Carcinoma, squamous-cell or medullary	20	7	0	2	0	0	29
Adenocarcinoma	5	0	0	0	0	1	6
Papilloma	1	0	0	0	0	0	1
Fibro(sarco)ma	11	1	3	0	0	0	15
Chondrosarcoma	2	0	0	0	0	0	2
Osteo(sarco)ma	3	0	0	0	0	0	3
Rhabdomyoma	1	0	0	0	0	0	1
Hemangioendothelioma	2	1	0	0	0	0	3
Larynx							
Carcinoma, squamous-cell	1	0	0	0	0	0	1
Trachea							
Carcinoma, squamous cell	2	0	0	0	0	0	2
Sarcoma	1	0	0	0	0	0	1
Lungs							
Carcinoma, squamous cell, small round cell, "oat seed" cell	29	1	36	3	1	0	78
Adenocarcinoma, bronchial	2	1	15	2	0	0	20
Sarcoma	3	0	0	0	2	0	5
Hemangio(endothelio)ma	1	0	3	1	0	0	5
Lymphangioma	0	0	1	0	0	0	1
Pleura							
Mesothelioma	3	0	19	0	1	0	23
Sarcoma	0	0	2	0	0	0	2
Neurofibrosarcoma	0	0	5	0	0	0	5
Myxoma	0	0	0	0	1	0	1
Hemangio(endothelio)ma	2	1	1	0	0	0	4
Lymphangioma	0	1	1	0	0	0	2
Heart							
Hamartoma	0	0	1	0	1	0	2
Leiomyo(sarco)ma	0	0	2	0	0	0	2
Rhabdomyo(sarco)ma	1	0	1	1	0	0	3
Hemangio(endothelio)ma	0	0	4	0	0	0	4
Fibro(sarco)ma	0	0	11	1	0	0	12
Neurofibroma	0	0	3	0	0	0	3
Pericardium							
Mesothelioma (endothelioma)	0	0	3	0	0	0	3
Kidney							
Nephroblastoma (embryonal nephroma)	2	2	12	2	50	1	69
Carcinoma and adenocarcinoma	15	7	8	2	0	1	33
Adenoma	1	2	0	0	0	0	3
Hypernephroma	0	2	11	2	1	0	16
Sarcoma	0	1	3	0	0	0	4
Hemangio(endothelio)ma	0	0	1	2	0	0	3
Hamartoma	0	1	0	0	0	0	1
Urinary Bladder							
Carcinoma	13	1	5	0	0	0	19
Papilloma	3	0	1	0	0	0	4
Fibroma	6	0	0	0	0	0	6
Leiomyoma	1	0	1	0	0	0	2
Hemangioendothelioma	1	0	1	0	0	0	2

137

LOCATION AND KIND OF NEOPLASM	CANINE	EQUINE	BOVINE	OVINE	PORCINE	FELINE	TOTAL
Urethra							
Adeno(carcino)ma	1	0	0	0	0	0	1
Adenoma	1	0	0	0	0	0	1
Mammary Gland							
Adenocarcinoma	520	4	0	0	0	10	534
Carcinoma, squamous cell	8	0	0	0	0	0	8
Adenoma	167	0	1	0	0	1	169
Mixed mammary tumor	213	0	0	0	0	0	213
Fibro(sarco)ma	19	1	0	1	0	1	22
Lipoma	1	0	0	0	0	1	2
Leiomyosarcoma	4	0	0	0	0	0	4
Hemangioma	2	0	0	0	0	0	2
Vagina, Vulva							
Carcinoma, squamous cell	1	7	10	0	0	0	18
Fibroma	82	0	10	0	0	0	92
Lipoma	5	0	4	0	0	0	9
Leiomyo(sarco)ma	31	0	1	0	0	0	32
Melanoma	1	0	0	0	0	0	1
Canine transmissible tumor	33	0	0	0	0	0	33
Uterus							
Adenocarcinoma	3	0	8	0	0	0	11
Papilloma	0	0	0	0	1	0	1
Fibroadenoma	4	0	0	0	0	1	5
Sarcoma	0	0	1	0	0	0	1
Leiomyo(fibro)(sarco)ma	12	0	16	2	0	0	30
Cervix							
Carcinoma, squamous cell	0	0	1	0	0	0	1
Adenocarcinoma	0	0	1	0	0	0	1
Fibroma	5	0	0	0	0	0	5
Leiomyoma	0	0	1	0	0	0	1
Ovary							
Adenocarcinoma, cystadenocarcinoma or cystadenoma	40	1	8	0	1	2	52
Granulosa cell tumor	28	2	44	5	0	0	79
Dysgerminoma	6	0	0	0	0	0	6
Fibro(myxo)(chondro)sarcoma	2	0	0	0	0	0	2
Hemangio(endothelio)ma	1	0	0	0	0	0	1
Lymphangioma	0	1	0	0	0	0	1
Teratoma, dermoid cyst	2	4	0	0	0	0	6
Testis							
Seminoma	175	3	0	0	0	0	178
Sertoli cell (sustentacular cell) tumor	163	0	2	0	0	0	165
Interstitial cell tumor	69	2	0	0	0	0	71
Carcinoma (teratoma)	1	0	3	0	0	0	4
Hemangioma	3	1	0	1	0	0	5
Prostate							
Adenocarcinoma	10	0	0	0	0	0	10
Cystadenoma	8	0	0	0	0	0	8
Leiomyo(sarco)ma	4	0	0	0	0	0	4
Spermatic Cord							
Sarcoma	1	0	0	0	0	0	1
Rhabdomyoma	1	0	0	0	0	0	1
Penis, Prepuce							
Carcinoma, squamous cell	8	40	1	0	0	0	49
Papilloma, fibropapilloma	4	3	0	0	0	0	7
Fibro(sarco)ma	1	0	40	0	0	0	41
Canine transmissible tumor	55	0	0	0	0	0	55
Conjunctiva and Membrana Nictitans							
Carcinoma, squamous cell	14	45	138	7	0	1	205
Papilloma	6	0	2	0	0	0	8

LOCATION AND KIND OF NEOPLASM	CANINE	EQUINE	BOVINE	OVINE	PORCINE	FELINE	TOTAL
Fibro(sarco)ma	4	2	0	0	0	0	6
Hemangio(endothelio)ma	1	0	0	0	0	0	1
Melanoma	5	1	0	0	0	0	6
Teratoma	1	0	1	0	0	0	2
Lacrimal Glands							
Adenocarcinoma	3	0	2	1	0	0	6
Adenoma	4	0	0	0	0	0	4
Eyeball							
Carcinoma, squamous cell	1	7	94	1	0	0	103
Adenoma	1	0	0	0	0	0	1
Papilloma	2	2	1	0	0	0	5
Fibro(sarco)ma	2	1	0	0	0	0	3
Leiomyosarcoma	1	0	0	0	0	0	1
Rhabdomyosarcoma	1	0	0	0	0	0	1
Hemangioma	2	0	0	0	0	0	2
Melanoma	11	0	0	0	0	0	11
Retinoblastoma	1	0	0	0	0	0	1
Ear							
Papilloma	2	0	0	0	0	0	2
Ceruminous gland tumor	6	0	0	0	0	5	11
Chondroma	0	1	0	0	0	1	2
Musculoskeletal Tissues							
Osteogenic sarcoma	136	0	2	1	1	11	151
Osteoma	7	2	1	1	1	1	13
Giant cell tumor, "osteoclastoma"	2	1	2	0	1	0	6
Chondro(sarco)ma	11	1	7	1	0	0	20
Fibrosarcoma	12	4	0	1	0	0	17
Leiomyosarcoma	1	0	0	0	0	0	1
Rhabdomyosarcoma	5	1	2	1	0	2	11
Lipoma	5	1	0	0	0	0	6
Hemangioma	5	0	1	0	0	0	6
Synovioma	13	0	0	0	0	0	13
Thyroid							
(Adeno)carcinoma	33	0	3	1	1	0	38
Adenoma	11	1	18	8	0	0	38
Mixed tumor	1	0	1	0	0	0	2
Adrenal Cortex							
Carcinoma	5	0	19	8	0	0	32
Adenoma	12	2	15	9	0	0	38
Adrenal Medulla and Chromaffine Tissues							
Neuroblastoma	0	0	8	0	0	0	8
Pheochromocytoma, medullary adenoma	1	1	16	0	0	0	18
Aortic body tumor	28	0	0	0	0	0	28
Carotid body tumor	1	0	0	0	0	0	1
Pituitary							
Chromophobe adenoma	0	0	0	0	0	1	1
Parathyroid							
Carcinoma	1	0	0	0	0	0	1
Adenoma	2	0	0	0	0	0	2
Hemic and Lymphoid Tissues							
Malignant lymphoma	247	2	369	14	58	17	707
Malignant myeloma and myeloid leukemia, including "chloromas"	9	12	15	0	0	0	36
Plasmacytoma	0	1	0	0	0	0	1
Hodgkin's-like growths	0	0	0	0	9	0	9
Thymoma	6	1	18	6	3	0	34
Lymphoepithelioma of thymus	0	0	6	3	0	0	9

139

INCIDENCE OF VARIOUS NEOPLASMS OF DOMESTIC ANIMALS (Continued)

LOCATION AND KIND OF NEOPLASM	CANINE	EQUINE	BOVINE	OVINE	PORCINE	FELINE	TOTAL
Spleen							
Hamartoma	3	0	0	0	0	0	3
Fibrosarcoma	5	0	0	0	0	0	5
Leiomyosarcoma	6	0	2	0	0	0	8
Hemangio(endothelio)ma	25	4	1	0	0	0	30
Nervous tissues							
Glioma, unspecified	3	0	0	0	0	0	3
Astrocytoma	5	0	1	0	0	0	6
Spongioblastoma	2	0	0	0	0	0	2
Medulloblastoma	0	0	3	0	0	0	3
Oligodendroglioma	6	0	0	0	0	0	6
Ependymoma	5	0	0	0	0	0	5
Meningioma	2	1	3	0	0	0	6
Carcinoma of choroid plexus	1	0	0	0	0	0	1
Cholesteatoma of choroid plexus or lateral ventricle	0	8	0	0	0	0	8
Neurilemmoma ("Schwannoma")	1	2	2	1	0	0	6
Neurofibroma	46	1	13	0	0	0	60
Hemangioma	1	0	0	0	0	0	1
Sarcoma	0	0	2	0	0	0	2
Melanoma of meninges	0	0	1	0	0	0	1
Totals	5854	464	1371	129	167	174	8159

neoplasm (*continued*)

skin n., any tumor of the skin, such as squamous cell carcinoma, mast cell tumor, etc. Because of its accessibility, several tumors of viral origin have developed in the skin. See table.

testicular n., a tumor of the testes. Among anomen, the dog has by far the highest incidence of the three types of neoplasms of the testicle.[142] These types, which occur with about equal incidence in the dog, are as follows. *Seminoma* is a malignant tumor derived from germinal epithelium, which does not metastasize as frequently as it does in man, in whom it is also common. *Sertoli cell tumor* is a benign tumor (tubular adenoma) from Sertoli or sustentacular cells, which produces feminizing hormone. It occurs almost exclusively in the dog, the human counterpart being extremely rare. *Interstitial cell tumor* (Leydig cell) is a benign tumor which arises in the interstitial or androgen-secreting cells of the interstitial tissue.

VIRUSES MANIFESTED IN NATURAL INFECTIONS BY SKIN NEOPLASMS*

VIRUS	HOST	Local Lesion	Generalized Lesions	MECHANISM OF TRANSMISSION (OTHER THAN INOCULATION)
Poxvirus group				
Cowpox	Cow	+	–	Mechanical – trauma
Myxoma	*Sylvilagus brasiliensis*	+	–	Mechanical – arthropod vectors
	Oryctolagus cuniculus	+	+ (throughout organism)	Mechanical – arthropod vectors
Rabbit fibroma	*Sylvilagus floridanus*	+	–	Mechanical – arthropod vectors
	Oryctolagus cuniculus	+	Rarely (on skin only)	Not transmissible
Hare fibroma	*Lepus europaeus*	+	Sometimes (mainly on skin)	Probably mechanical – arthropod vectors
Squirrel fibroma	*Sciurus carolinensis*	+	Sometimes (mainly on skin)	Mechanical – arthropod vectors
Yaba monkey tumor poxvirus	*Macaca rhesus*	+	–	Not known
Molluscum contagiosum	Man	+	+ (on skin only)	Probably mechanical – trauma
Swinepox	Swine	+	+ (on skin only)	Mechanical – arthropod vectors
Birdpox	Birds	+	Sometimes (throughout organism)	Mechanical – arthropod vectors (also by respiratory route)
Papovavirus group				
Rabbit papilloma	*Sylvilagus floridanus*	+	–	Mechanical – arthropod vectors
Human wart	Man	+	–	Mechanical – trauma

*From F. Fenner: The Biology of Animal Viruses. Academic Press, New York, 1968.

Neorickettsia A genus of the tribe Ehrlichieae, family Rickettsiaceae, order Rickettsiales. It includes a single species, *N. helminthoeca*, which causes salmon disease in dogs, and is found in the intestinal trematode *Nanophyetus salmincola*, which is considered to be the vector of infection.

neoteny The tendency to retain larval characteristics even though sexual maturity is reached and reproduction can occur, as in the axolotl.

neotropical Having a distribution that includes parts of Central and South America.

nephritis Inflammation of the kidney; a diffuse progressive degenerative or proliferative lesion affecting in varying proportion the renal parenchyma, the interstitial tissue, and the renal vascular system. See also *glomerulonephritis*.

nephro-, nephr- Combining form denoting relationship to the kidney.

nephroma A tumor of the kidney tissue; a tumor of the kidney.

  ombryonal n., an embryonal malignant tumor consisting of two components, glandular tissue of the kidney and connective tissue, both apparently neoplastic. This tumor is quite common in young swine.

nesidioblastoma An islet cell tumor of the pancreas.

neurilemoma A neoplasm of peripheral nerve neurilemma cells. This tumor is very similar to and sometimes indistinguishable from neurofibroma, and is very common in animals, especially cattle.

neuro-, neur- Combining form denoting relationship to a nerve or nerves, or the nervous system.

neuroblastoma A malignant tumor of the nervous system composed chiefly of neuroblasts.

  n. C-1300 (tumor C-1300), an undifferentiated round cell tumor, possibly a neuroblastoma, arising spontaneously in the region of the spinal cord in a four-month-old A/Jax strain mouse from the Jackson Memorial Laboratory in 1940. The tumor grows progressively in a variety of inbred mouse strains, killing the host in 21 to 30 days.[150]

neurofibroma A connective tissue tumor of the nerve fiber fasciculus, formed by proliferation of the perineurium and endoneurium. Cf. *neurilemoma*.

neuroglioma Glioma containing nerve cells; a tumor made up of neuroglial tissue.

neuroma A tumor or new growth largely made up of nerve cells and nerve fibers; a tumor growing from a nerve.

  amputation n., a tumor-like reactive growth containing many nerve fibers which occurs at the site of healing of an amputation.

  traumatic n., an unorganized bulbous or nodular mass of nerve fibers and Schwann cells produced by hyperplasia of nerve fibers and their supporting tissues after accidental or purposeful sectioning of the nerve.

neurotransmitter A chemical present at a nerve synapse which is responsible for transmission of nerve impulses. Some of these substances are acetyl choline, norepinephrine, and perhaps serotonin and dopamine.

neutral red A basic dye of the azine group. Solubility at 15° C.: water 4 per cent, absolute alcohol 1.8 per cent, and glycerol 12.25 per cent. It is used with Janus green for supravital staining of blood and with tannins and pine-leaf for vacuoles.[57]

neutrophil A cell or structural element, particularly a leukocyte, stainable by neutral dyes; a polymorphonuclear neutrophilic leukocyte.

Newcastle disease (ND) An economically serious viral disease of galliform birds primarily, but also of psittacine and passerine species. It is known by at least 15 synonyms, including avian pest, avian distemper, and ranikhet. The disease affects birds of all ages, but is most lethal in juveniles. The agent of Newcastle disease is a paramyxovirus of a subgroup including mumps, Sendai, and parainfluenza viruses. A variety of tissues and organs are affected, but the symptoms are related primarily to respiratory infection and encephalitis. Economic effects in mature poultry include depressed egg production. Diagnosis is based on hemagglutinating properties of the virus and hemagglutination-inhibition properties of specifically immune serum. The ND agent is considered zoonotic, since occasional cases of ND conjunctivitis have been reported in man.[11, 112, 114]

New England Colloquy of Comparative Pathologists New England Regional Primate Center, Southborough, Mass. 01772.

New England Society of Pathologists Department of Pathology, Dartmouth Medical School, Hanover, N.H. 03755.

new fuchsin A basic tryphenyl-methane dye. Solubility at 15° C.: water 1 per cent, absolute alcohol 1 per cent, and glycerol 10 per cent. It is used with Congo red for bacterial cell walls, and to stain acid-fast bacteria.[37, 57]

New Jersey Academy of Science Box B, Rutgers, The State University, New Brunswick, N.J. 08903.

New York Academy of Medicine 2 E. 103rd Street, New York, N.Y. 10029.

New York Academy of Sciences 2 E. 63rd Street, New York, N.Y. 10021.

New York bee disease See *European foulbrood*.

New York Microscopical Society Central Park West at 79th Street, New York, N.Y. 10024.

New York Society of Electron Microscopists Department of Anatomy, Albert Einstein College of Medicine, The Bronx, N.Y. 10461.

New York Society for Comparative Pathology The Rockefeller University, New York, N.Y. 10021.

New York State Society for Medical Research, Inc. 50 E. 41st Street, New York, N.Y. 10017.

New York Zoological Society   630 5th Avenue, New York, N.Y. 10020.

NHI   Abbreviation for National Health Insurance and National Heart Institute.

NIAID   Abbreviation for National Institute of Allergy and Infectious Diseases.

NIAMD   Abbreviation for National Institute of Arthritis and Metabolic Diseases.

NICHD   Abbreviation for National Institute of Child Health and Human Development.

nicotinamide   The amide of nicotinic acid, a component of the vitamin B complex.

   n. adenine dinucleotide (NAD), a coenzyme widely found in nature and involved in numerous enzymatic reactions, the dinucleotide of nicotinamide and of adenine. The products of hydrolysis are one molecule of adenine, one molecule of nicotinamide, two molecules of *d*-ribose, and two molecules of phosphoric acid.[90, 118] Called also codehydrogenase I, coenzyme I (CoI), cozymase, dihydroco-enzyme I, and diphosphopyridine nucleotide (DPN).

   n. adenine dinucleotide phosphate (NADP), a coenzyme required for a limited number of reactions, and similar to NAD, except for the inclusion of three phosphate units.[90] Called also coenzyme II (CoII), codehydrogenase II, coferment, triphosphopyridine nucleotide (TPN), and Warburg's coenzyme.

nidicolous birds   Those that remain in the nest for some time after being hatched.

nidifugous birds   Those that leave the nest soon after being hatched.

NIDR   Abbreviation for National Institute of Dental Research.

nigericin   An antibiotic produced by a species of *Streptomyces*, which inhibits gram-positive bacteria, has weak activity against gram-negative bacteria and considerable activity against mycobacteria. Its activity is based on inhibition of oxidative metabolism in the Krebs cycle.[36, 49]

Nigg pneumonitis   See *mouse pneumonitis*, under *pneumonitis*.

night monkey   Any member of the species *Aotus trivergatus*. See *primate*.

NIGMS   Abbreviation for National Institute of General Medical Sciences.

NIH   Abbreviation for National Institutes of Health.

Nile blue   A basic dye of the oxazine group. Solubility at 15° C.: water 6 per cent, absolute alcohol 5 per cent, and glycerol 14 per cent. It is used to stain protozoa and yeasts and to stain fats in tissues.[37, 57]

NIMH   Abbreviation for National Institute of Mental Health.

NINDB   Abbreviation for National Institute of Neurological Diseases and Blindness.

ninhydrin   A compound used to stain proteins and amino acids. It is especially useful on chromatograms.

Nippostrongylus muris   A species of trichostrongylid nematodes, also known as the hookworm of rats. This parasite has been experimentally transmitted to other laboratory animals such as the hamster and rabbit. Infection usually occurs by skin penetration. It is widely used in parasitologic research.[21]

nitavirus   A name suggested to include numerous ether-sensitive, probably deoxyribonucleic acid (DNA) viruses in the size range of 100 to 200 mμ, which are morphologically similar and generally associated with single homogeneous eosinophilic bodies occupying most of the central area of the nucleus of the marginated chromatin (A-type inclusions).[39]

nitratase   A bacterial enzyme catalyzing the reduction of nitrate to nitrite.

nitrogen mustard   An alkylating agent used to suppress leukocytes, as an immunosuppressant, and as an oncolytic drug.

Nocardia   A genus of aerobic, gram-positive, weakly acid-fast microorganisms of the order Actinomycetales, with vegetative mycelium that breaks up into bacillary and coccoid elements (see table).[16]

noctiphobia   Morbid dread of night and its darkness and silence.

nodular disease   A disease of sheep, caused by the nematode *Oesophagostomum columbianum*, which infects the intestines, becoming embedded in the mucous membrane, where it forms small nodules.

nodular organ   A knot of hyphae resembling preascigerous copulation of hyphae.

nogalamycin   A cytotoxic antibiotic produced by a species of *Actinomyces* which is used against Hodgkin's disease and interferes with RNA synthesis.[36, 49]

nomo-   A combining form denoting relationship to usage or law.

nomogram   The graphic representation produced in nomography; a chart or diagram on which a number of variables are plotted, forming a computation chart for the solution of complex numerical formulae.

nonactin   One of a group of antibiotics which includes also monactin, dinactin, and trinactin, all produced by a species of *Streptomyces*. They inhibit metabolism by some

Diseases Caused by *Nocardia*

Species	Host	Disease
N. asteroides	Man	Pulmonary nocardiosis
N. braziliensis	Cat	Lesions in the submandibular lymph nodes and pleura
N. farcinica	Cattle	Farcin-du-boeuf (bovine farcy)
N. madurae	Man	Madura foot
N. pulmonalis	Cow	Infection in lungs
Other species	Dog, kangaroo, wallaby	Granuloma-like nodules in the dog; upper respiratory tract infection in the kangaroo and wallaby

mechanism associated with cation movement across mitochondrial membranes in a fashion similar to gramicidin.[36, 49]

nondisjunction　Failure of a pair of chromosomes to separate during meiosis, so that both members of the pair are carried to the same daughter nucleus, and the other daughter cell is lacking that particular chromosome.

noninclusion　See *nonoccluded*.

nonoccluded　Denoting those insect viruses in which the virions are not occluded in a dense protein crystal. Preferable to "noninclusion."

North Dakota Academy of Science　Department of Animal Science, North Dakota State University, Fargo, N.D. 58101.

Northern New England Academy of Science　5 Charles Place, Orono, Me. 04473.

Northwest Scientific Association　University of Washington, Seattle, Wash. 98105.

nosema disease　A disease of adult honeybees caused by the microsporidian *Nosema apis*. The protozoon develops mainly within the cells of the midgut epithelium. Nosema disease of the honeybee is not a serious malady, and it can be perpetually enzootic within a bee colony. The term is sometimes used in referring to diseases caused by other species of *Nosema* infecting other species of insects; *nosematosis* (q.v.) is the preferred term in these instances.[148] See also *pebrine*.

nosematosis (encephalitozoonosis)　A disease principally of rabbits caused by a small cryptosporidian parasite originally described by Levaditi and named by him *Encephalitozoon cuniculi*. While observed most commonly in rabbits, the organism has been involved as a disease agent in most laboratory species, including rats, mice, guinea pigs, and dogs, and even in man. It is also seen in insects (see *nosema disease*). This organism and its effects pose one of the classic examples of the confusion introduced by spontaneous disease in experimental animals being mistakenly interpreted as an experimentally induced disease.

The clinical disease is ordinarily mild and may even be clinically silent. Pathologically it is characterized by chronic interstitial nephritis and meningoencephalitis. Morbidity in rabbit and mouse colonies may exceed 30 per cent. Infected rabbits occasionally show signs of central nervous system involvement. Grossly discernible lesions are confined to the kidney and consist of small, depressed subcapsular scars. Lesions both in the kidney and brain consist of small granulomata (approx. 100μ in diameter) within which are the rod-shaped organisms ($2\mu \times 0.5\mu$) which can be demonstrated only with special stains (e.g., Goodpasture's carbol fuchsin or Giemsa). Because of the superficial similarity of *Nosema cuniculi* to *Toxoplasma gondii*, the table below contrasts distinguishing features of the two organisms.[142, 148] See also *toxoplasmosis*.

Nosopsyllus fasciatus　See *arthropod parasites*, under *rat*.

Notoedres muris　See *arthropod parasites*, under *rat*.

novobiocin　An antibiotic produced by a species of *Streptomyces* that is active against gram-positive and some gram-negative bacteria, some fungi, and the protozoan *Trichomonas*. Its metabolic effect is based on inhibition of cell respiration, probably related to its ability to capture magnesium ions.[10]

nuclear envelope　A double membrane which surrounds the nucleus, and which encloses a cavity known as the perinuclear cistern.[38]

nuclear polyhedrosis　See *nucleopolyhedrosis*.

nuclear transfer　Transplantation of a somatic nucleus into an enucleated egg, which in amphibians can divide and produce an entire animal.

nuclease　An enzyme or a group of enzymes which split nucleic acid into mono- and oligonucleotides. They are present as digestive enzymes in the intestinal tract and as autolytic enzymes in many cells. Similar enzymes are found in bacterial cultures.

nucleocapsid　The protein coat (capsid) of a virus together with the enclosed nucleic acid.[39, 64]

nucleocidin　An antibiotic produced by a species of *Streptomyces*, which first attracted interest because of a high degree of activity against trypanosomes. It is also active against gram-positive and gram-negative bacteria. It acts by inhibition of protein synthesis and may have considerable value as an experimental drug but very little of the substance is available.[36, 49]

nucleophosphatase　Nucleotidase.

DIFFERENTIATION OF *Nosema cuniculi* FROM *Toxoplasma gondii*

Differentiating Procedure	Nosema	Toxoplasma
H & E stain	Organisms not distinct	Organisms distinct
PAS stain	PAS negative, no capsule about the aggregate	PAS positive, a definite capsule about the aggregate
Gram stain	Gram-positive	Gram-negative
IP mouse inoculation	Never lethal	Routinely lethal on second passage
Tissue culture growth	Cultivable with extreme difficulty only in brain explants	Easily cultivable in various cell cultures and chick CAM
Sabin-Feldman dye test on suspect serum	Negative	Positive

nucleopolyhedrosis (nuclear polyhedrosis) A viral disease of insects, mainly the larvae of certain members of Lepidoptera and Hymenoptera, characterized by the formation of polyhedral inclusion bodies (polyhedra) in the nuclei of the infected cells. The virus multiplies in the epidermis, tracheal matrix, fat body, and blood cells of lepidopterous larvae. In hymenopterous larvae, the virus proliferates in the midgut epithelium. The disease is usually fatal. In the silkworm, the disease is called *grasserie* or *jaundice;* in the gypsy moth, *wilt disease;* in the nun moth, *Wipfelkrankheit* (q.v.).

nucleoprotein A substance composed of a simple basic protein, usually a histone or protamine, combined with a nucleic acid.

nucleosidase An enzyme that catalyzes the splitting of nucleosides into free sugars and bases.

nucleoside One of the glycosidic compounds into which a nucleotide is split by the action of nucleotidase or by chemical means. It is a combination of a sugar (a hexose or pentose) with a purine or a pyrimidine base.

nucleotidase (phosphonuclease; nucleophosphatase) An enzyme that splits nucleotides into nucleosides and phosphoric acid.

nucleotide One of the compounds into which nucleic acid is split by the action of nuclease.

    diphosphopyridine n. (DPN), former name for nicotinamide adenine dinucleotide.

    triphosphopyridine n. (TPN), former name for nicotinamide adenine dinucleotide phosphate.

nudomania An abnormal devotion to going naked.

nudophobia An abnormal aversion to being unclothed.

nullisomatic Lacking one pair of chromosomes.

nutria (coypu) A large aquatic rodent of the genus *Myocastor,* family Capromyidae. The single living species, *M. coypu,* inhabits central and southern South America. It looks like a large muskrat, weighs up to 25 pounds, has reddish brown fur, partially webbed hind toes, and short round ears. The mammary glands are placed along the sides of the back, which allows the young to suckle while the mother is surface swimming. It lives in shallow bank rivers and eats aquatic plants. Nutria pelts have some commercial value but require expensive processing.

nycto- A combining form denoting relationship to night or to darkness.

nyctophilia Abnormal preference for night over day.

nyctophobia Morbid dread of darkness.

nymph A stage in the life cycle of certain arthropods, as the ticks, between the larva and the adult. A nymph resembles the adult in appearance.

nympho- A combining form denoting relationship to the nymphae or labia minora.

nymphomania Exaggerated sexual desire in a female.

nystatin An antifungal antibiotic. See *polyene antibiotics.*

NZB mouse disease A disease very similar to human systemic lupus erythematosus seen in certain genetic strains of black mice. The disease is characterized by the development of a positive Coombs reaction in all affected individuals and usually the development of chronic glomerulonephritis.[47]

O

obovoid Egg-shaped, often attached by small end.

occluded Denoting insect viruses in which the virions are occluded in a dense protein crystal, large enough to be visible in the light microscope (e.g., polyhedrosis viruses, granulosis viruses).

ocellus (pl. *ocelli*) Simple eye found in many invertebrates.

ochlophobia Morbid fear of crowds.

odontoma 1. An exostosis on a tooth. 2. Any tumor of odontogenic origin; customarily used to designate a composite odontoma: adamantinoma and ameloblastoma.

odontophobia A morbid fear associated with teeth, as that aroused by the sight of teeth, or abnormal dread of dental operations.

odoratism A morbid condition produced in experimental animals by diets containing the sweet pea (*Lathyrus odoratus*) or its active principle. See *lathyrism.*

-odynia A word ending meaning pain.

oesophagostomiasis Nodular disease; an important parasitic disease in cattle and sheep. See *Oesophagostomum.*

Oesophagostomum (nodular worm) A nematode parasite of the family Strongylidae which closely resembles the hookworms, is frequently found in pigs, ruminants, and primates, and can also infect man. The larvae may be found in the intestinal wall of infected animals, where they cause abscesses or granulomata.[21] The two most common species are *O. columbianum* and *O. Apiostomum.*

Ohio Academy of Science 505 King Avenue, Columbus, Ohio 43201.

oikophobia Morbid aversion to home surroundings.

oite The female form of a bacterium.

Oklahoma Academy of Science Department of Zoology, University of Oklahoma, Norman, Okla.

oleandomycin An antibiotic of the macrolide group (q.v.) of medium antibacterial spectrum and low toxicity. Its activity and range are similar to those of erythromycin.[36, 49]

olfactophobia Morbid aversion to odors.

oligo- A combining form meaning little, scanty, or few.

Oligocene Denoting the epoch in the Tertiary period extending from 36 to 25 million years ago. See *geologic time divisions.*

oligochaete A segmented worm of the class Oligochaeta. See *annelid.*

oligomycin One of a complex of antibiotics which also includes rutamycin, isolated from a species of *Streptomyces,* and aurovertin, which is produced by a fungus. Their activity is directed against fungi with little or no inhibitory effects on bacteria. Their mechanism of action is in some phase of energy transformation associated with the terminal electron transport system.[36, 49]

olivomycin See *chromomycin.*

-oma A word termination meaning tumor or neoplasm, of the part indicated by the stem to which it is attached.

omnivorous Eating of both plant and animal matter.

omphalitis (navel-ill) Inflammation, usually of bacterial origin, of the unhealed navel and surrounding structures of newly born mammals and newly hatched birds. Such infections, especially in young calves, horses, and chickens, frequently progress to peritonitis or bacteremia. They are usually associated with parturition or hatching under conditions of defective sanitary standards, hence a variety of opportunistic bacterial pathogens, including *Spherophorous, Corynebacterium, Staphylococcus,* and streptococci, have been associated with omphalitis. Formaldehyde fumigation is a routine preventive measure used in commercial hatcheries.

Onchocerca A genus of filarial nematodes. The adults live and breed in subcutaneous fibrous nodules; the young are carried by the lymph and are found chiefly in the skin and eyes. *O. volvulus* causes onchocerciasis in man; *O. gibsoni* causes nodules in the cow; and *O. reticulata* is found in the horse. *O. armillatus* and *O. gutturosa* are also found in the cow.

onco- A combining form denoting relationship to a tumor, swelling, or mass.

oncogenic Giving rise to tumors or causing tumor formation.

oncogenic viruses A group of viral agents that are capable of causing tumors. They can be divided into two major groups, those containing RNA and those containing DNA as genetic material. See *classification,* under *virus.*

Oncogenic deoxyriboviruses include (1) papovaviruses, which are responsible for papillomas of the rabbit, dog, cow, horse, man, and other species, the papilloma being the only human tumor which has been proven to be caused by a virus; (2) polyoma virus, which produces tumors of many different types when injected into the mouse, hamster, rat, guinea pig, or rabbit; (3) simian virus 40, which produces sarcomas in the hamster and ependymomas in the rat; (4) fibroma virus, which causes fibromas in rabbits and is closely related to the virus of myxomatosis; (5) adenovirus types 3, 7, 12, 16, 18, and 31; and (6) Lucke virus, which causes renal adenocarcinoma in the frog.

Oncogenic riboviruses (oncornaviruses) form another distinctive group, and are capable of causing tumors in several species. The characteristics common to this group, while similar to those of myxoviruses, are sufficiently distinctive that they have been placed in a separate group (see *classification,* under *virus*). They possess a loose sack type of envelope, have high water content, and form particles by budding from the plasma membrane or other cell component comparable to the plasma membrane. This group of viruses is also characterized by the formation of virus particles, either within or outside the cell, which can be seen under the electron microscope. The illustration on page 146 gives a classification and description of their appearance under the electron microscope.[32, 39]

oncolytic Pertaining to or capable of causing the destruction of neoplastic cells. See *antimetabolite* for list of oncolytic substances.

oncornavirus See *oncogenic virus,* and see *leukovirus* in the *classification of viruses,* under *virus.*

oneiro- A combining form denoting relationship to a dream.

oneiroanalysis The exploration of the conscious and unconscious personality through the interpretation of pharmacologically induced dreams.

oneirology The science of dreams.

oniomania A morbid desire to make purchases.

onomatology The science of names and nomenclature.

onomatomania Mental derangement with regard to words or names, marked by persistent dwelling on some particular word, by perplexed effort to recall some word, by attaching some special significance to certain words, or by showing disgust for certain words.

onomatophobia Morbid dread of hearing a certain name or word.

oo- A combining form denoting relationship to an egg or ovum.

Oochoristica ratti See *helminth parasites,* under *rat.*

oocyst The encysted form of the ookinete found in the abdominal wall of the mosquito in malaria parasites. Also refers to zygotes of coccidia.

ookinete The fertilized form of a malarial parasite formed by fertilization of a macrogamete by a microgamete and developing into the oocyst.

operant In behavioral science, a term referring to a response or behavior identified by its consequences but for which eliciting sti-

Particle	Size Diameter mμ	Envelope	Nucleoid	Location	Tumors	Morphology
Naked A	65 - 70	No	Entire particle Electron lucent	Intracytoplasmic Occur in clusters or single	Murine mammary carcinoma Murine lymphomas Murine testicular tumor	
Enveloped A	70 - 80	Yes	Electron lucent Central	Extracellular Bud from cell membrane In vacuoles	Feline lymphosarcoma Murine lymphomas Murine mammary carcinoma	
B	80 - 110	Yes	Electron dense Eccentric	Extracellular Never bud Derived from enveloped A particles - extracellularly In vacuoles	Murine mammary carcinoma	
C	90 - 110	Yes	Electron dense Central	Extracellular In vacuoles Never bud Derived from enveloped A particles - extracellularly	Feline lymphosarcoma Murine lymphomas Avian leukosis	
Intracisternal	70 -100	Yes	Electron lucent Outer envelope close to nucleoid	Bud in cisternae from rough endoplasmic reticulum	Murine leukemias (some) Ehrlich ascites tumor Plasma cell tumor - murine Meth - A - Sarcoma - murine	

Figure 5. Nomenclature of oncogenic RNA viruses. (Adapted from E. de Harven. *In* M. A. Rich [Ed.]: Experimental Leukemia. Appleton-Century-Crofts. New York, 1968.)

muli have not been clearly determined. Operant behavior is therefore identified by its consequences rather than the stimuli which have produced it. See also *operant conditioning,* under *conditioning,* and see *vacuum activity.*

operant behavior See under *behavior.*

operant conditioning See under *conditioning.*

operant level The rate of occurrence of an operant response before the response has been experimentally reinforced. (A rat placed in a Skinner box will press the bar perhaps 10 to 12 times an hour without reinforcement. The rate will rise sharply after reinforcement.) The original rate without reinforcement is referred to as the operant level. The term is also used to describe the residual occurrence of an operant response that has previously been conditioned and then extinguished.

operant response See *operant.*

operon See *gene.*

operon network A group of operons and their associated regulator genes whose activities are interrelated in that the activity of one may initiate or repress the activity of another. See *gene.*

ophidiophobia A morbid dread of snakes.

opisthaptor The posterior disk or sucker in digenetic trematodes.

Opisthorchis A genus of trematodes of the family Opisthorchidae found in the bile ducts of fish-eating mammals, including the cat, dog, and man. Infection takes place when the definitive host eats fish containing metacercariae, which develop into adults in the bile ducts. Principal members of this group are *O. sinensis,* also known as *Clonorchis sinensis,* and *O. tonkae,* found in the muskrat. The cat and dog may be infected by *O. sinensis* and serve as a reservoir from which human infections may be acquired.[21]

opisthosoma The posterior, legless part of the body of arachnids.

opossum A small marsupial of which several genera, including *Didelphis, Marmosa,* and *Philander,* are useful in studies of embryologic development and ontogeny of antibody production because of their extreme immaturity at birth. The gestation period is about fourteen days.

opposable digit A digit capable of being held against other digits on the same limb, giving a grasping action.

orange G An acid mono-azo dye. Solubility at 15° C.: water 8 per cent, absolute alcohol 0.22 per cent, and glycerol 20 per cent. It is used with safranin and gentian violet for staining chromosomes and with thionin for infected plant tissues.[57]

orangutan   An anthropoid ape, *Pongo pygmaeus*. See *ape*.

orcein   A cytological dye.

ordinate   One of the lines used as a base of reference in graphs. See *abscissa*.

Oregon Academy of Science   Oregon State University, Department of Geology, Corvallis, Ore. 97331.

oreximania   Enormous increase in appetite and food intake due to fear of becoming thin.

organ culture   Growth of parts of or entire organs in culture.

ornithomancy   Divination from observation of the flight of birds. The words augury and auspice both owe their origin to this superstition, derived from the Latin *avis*.

Ornithonyssus bacoti   See *arthropod parasites*, under *rat*.

ornithosis   See *Chlamydia* and *psittacosis*.

Oroya fever   See *Carrion's disease*.

orthotopic graft   A graft transferred from any given site of the donor to the same site in the recipient, i.e., to a position formerly occupied by tissue of the same kind.

-osis   A word termination denoting a process, often a disease or morbid process, and sometimes conveying the meaning of abnormal increase.

osmium tetroxide (osmic acid)   A fixative commonly used in electron microscopy.

osmo-   A combining form denoting relationship to (1) odors and (2) an impulse, or to osmosis.

osmophobia   Abnormal dread of odors.

osmosis   The passage of solvent from the lesser to the greater concentration when two solutions are separated by a membrane permeable to the solvent but impermeable to the dissolved molecules, and thus is an attempt by the solution to achieve equal concentration on either side of the membrane.

Osteichthyes (bony fishes)   A class of fishes characterized by a skeleton chiefly of bone (considerable cartilage in primitive forms, e.g., sturgeons) with many distinct vertebrae although relics of the notochord may persist, and by skin with embedded dermal scales (ganoid, cycloid, or ctenoid), although some forms are without scales, some with enamel-covered scales. The mouth is usually terminal and has teeth, the jaws are well developed and articulated to the skull, the fins are both median and paired, and there are no limbs. The eyes are large and well developed, without lids. The heart is two-chambered (with atrium and ventricle) with sinus venosus and conus arteriosus, and four pairs of aortic arches. The erythrocytes are oval and nucleated. Respiration is accomplished by gills attached to bony gill arches, most forms with an air bladder. There are ten pairs of cranial nerves. The bony fishes are abundant in salt and fresh water, and some forms undergo estivation in times of drought. See table for a classification of the bony fishes.

A CLASSIFICATION OF OSTEICHTHYES

SUBCLASS	ORDER	EXAMPLES
Palaeopterygii	Archistia	No forms living
	Cladistia	– – –
	Chondrostei	Sturgeons, spoonbills
	Belonorhynchii	– – –
Neopterygii	Protospondyli	*Amia calva*, the bowfin
(Teleostei)	Gingylmodi	Gar pikes, alligator gars
	Halecostomi	– – –
	Isospondyli	Tarpon, herring, salmon, trout
	Haplomi	Pike, pickerel, muskellunge, mud minnows
	Iniomi	Lantern fishes
	Giganturoidea	– – –
	Lyomeri	Gulpers
	Ostariophysi	Electric eels, catfishes, suckers, carps
	Apodes	Eels, morays
	Heteromi	– – –
	Synentognathi	Garfishes, half beaks, flying fishes
	Cyprinodontes	– – –
	Salmopercae	– – –
	Solenichthyes	Pipefishes, sea horses
	Aanacanthini	Codfish, hake, burbot, haddock
	Allotriognathi	– – –
	Berycomorphi	Perches, fresh-water bass and sunfish, tuna mackerels
	Scleroparei	Sticklebacks
	Hypostomides	Dragonfishes
	Heterosomata	Halibut, sole, flounder, fluke
	Discocephali	Remoras
	Plectognathi	Triggerfishes, puffers
	Malacichthyes	– – –
	Xenoptergii	Clingfishes
	Haplodoci	Toadfishes
	Pediculati	Angler fishes, other deep-sea forms
	Opisthomi	– – –
Choanichthyes	Rhipidistia	– – –
	Coelacanthini	Lungfishes, mud fishes

osteoarthropathy   Any disease of the joints and bones, particularly hypertrophic pulmonary osteoarthropathy, a symmetrical proliferation of subperiosteal bone spicules near the joints of such long bones as the phalanges and long bones of the limbs, and sometimes affecting flat bones. The pathogenesis is not clearly understood but is thought to be related to circulatory disturbances of the affected areas because of pressure on certain nerve fibers (perhaps the vagus) caused by proliferative lesions within the thoracic cavity. It is nearly always accompanied by neoplastic or chronic inflammatory lesions of this area. The disease is seen in man, the dog, and the horse, and has been reported in other domestic animals.

osteoblastoma   A tumor which tends to differentiate into bone cells. The term includes osteoma and osteosarcoma.

osteochondrosarcoma   Sarcoma blended with osteoma and chondroma.

osteoclastoma   A tumor of giant cells analogous to osteoclasts.

osteodystrophia fibrosa   See *avitaminosis D*.

osteodystrophy   A defect of bone formation, particularly that seen in renal osteodystrophy, which results from chronic disease of the kidneys in which calcium is lost and phosphorus retained. There is a consequent hyperactivity of the parathyroid gland, resulting in removal of calcium from mineralized bone. This condition is common in chronic nephritis of dogs, in which it is sometimes erroneously referred to as renal rickets.

osteogenic sarcoma 342   A tumor induced in the glandular stomach of a laboratory rat of Marshall 520 strain by the injection of 20-methylcholanthrene in the laboratory of H. L. Stewart at the National Cancer Institute in 1949. The original tumor contained bone and cartilage, but these elements progressively decreased in amount with succeeding transplant generations so that subcutaneous and intraperitoneal transplants became devoid of that material. An interesting feature is that when tissues from eighteenth generation transplants were placed under the capsule of the kidney, they grew to resemble the original tumor. Subcutaneous transplants grow progressively in 100 per cent of rat hosts, killing them in about seven weeks without metastases.[150]

osteogenic sarcoma EM2   A tumor first observed in the laboratory of E. Lorenz at the National Cancer Institute in 1951 in a C3H$_f$/He mouse that was one of a group receiving 400 R total-body irradiation (with spleen protected). The tumor arose in the sternum and was transplanted with success to five nonirradiated C3H$_f$/He mice and has since been maintained by subcutaneous transplantation in others of this strain. Two sublines were selected on the basis of amount of bone formed in transplants, both of which have the same positive alkaline phosphatase reaction, and kill the host in 25 to 50 days.[150]

osteolathyrism   A skeletal disorder produced in animals by diets containing the sweet pea (*Lathyrus odoratus*) or its active substance. β-aminopropionitrile, or other aminonitriles. It is characterized in rats by hernia, dissecting aortic aneurysm, lameness of the hind legs, exostoses, kyphoscoliosis, and other skeletal deformities, apparently as the result of defective development of collagen tissue. Studies also utilize turkeys and swine.

osteoma   A benign tumor composed of bone tissue.

osteomalacia   A bone disease of adult animals similar to rickets in young animals. It consists of improper calcification of bone, which is continuously reformed by active turnover of its components. As in rickets of the young, there is an excess of osteoid tissue formed at the borders of the bone spicules. General weakening results, sometimes with distortion in weight-bearing structures. It is seen commonly in chronic nephritis of dogs because of excessive calcium loss.

osteopathy   A system of therapy founded by Andrew Taylor Still (1828-1917) and based on the theory that the body is capable of making its own remedies against disease and other toxic conditions when it is in normal structural relationship and has favorable environmental conditions and adequate nutrition. It utilizes generally accepted physical, medicinal, and surgical methods of diagnosis and therapy, while placing chief emphasis on the importance of normal body mechanics and manipulative methods of detecting and correcting faulty structure.

osteosarcoma   A sarcoma of bone, or a sarcoma containing osseous tissue.

ostreogrycin   See *streptogramin*.

ostrich   See *struthioniform birds*.

ovarian tumor IX   Luteoma IX.

ovine virus abortion   See *enzootic abortion of ewes*, under *abortion*.

oviparous   Egg-laying.

Ovis aries   The domestic sheep.

ovo-, ovi-   Combining form denoting relationship to an egg, or to ova.

ovoviviparous   Producing eggs which hatch within the mother's body before they are laid.

oxaloacetic carboxylase   An enzyme found in the glycolytic-Krebs cycle which converts oxaloacetate to pyruvate using Mg^{++} as a cofactor.

Oxford unit   That amount of penicillin which, when dissolved in 50 cc. of meat extract broth, just inhibits completely a test strain of *Staphylococcus aureus*.

oxidase   A metalloprotein that catalyzes the reduction of molecular oxygen independently of hydrogen peroxide.

oxidoreductase   An enzyme that catalyzes the reversible transfer of electrons from one substance to another (oxidation-reduction, or redox reaction).[90, 118]

oxy-   A combining form denoting (1) sharp,

quick, or sour, or (2) the presence of oxygen in a compound.

oxygenase   An enzyme that acts by the direct transference of molecular oxygen, as tryptophan oxygenase.

Oxyuris equi   A large nematode (pinworm) of horses with a life cycle which closely resembles that of *Enterobius vermicularis*[21]

oyster   A bivalve mollusk of the family Pelecypoda, with paired lateral shells.

    Malpeque disease of o's, see under *M.*

    shell disease of o's, see *maladie du pain d'épices* and *maladie du pied.*

P

Pacheco's parrot disease   Disease of psittacine birds caused by an agent thought to be a variant of the agent of psittacosis with pathogenicity for the Psittacidae but not for guinea pigs, mice, chickens, pigeons, or primates. The symptomatology in Psittacidae is similar to that of psittacosis and, although it is uncommonly reported, it should be considered in the differential diagnosis of diseases in psittacine birds.[112]

pachy-   A combining form meaning thick.

pachytene   In meiosis, the stage following synapsis in which the homologous chromosome threads shorten, thicken, and intertwine. See *meiosis.*

Pacific Coast Entomological Society   California Academy of Sciences, San Francisco, Calif. 94118.

pactamycin   An antitumor antibiotic produced by species of *Streptomyces* which is active in vitro against a variety of gram-positive and gram-negative bacteria, by interference with protein synthesis.[36, 49]

paedogenesis (pedogenesis)   Reproduction by an organism while some organs of the body are still larval in character; an extreme form of neoteny.

-pagus   A word termination denoting a fetal monster composed of symmetrical twins conjoined at the site indicated by the stem to which it is affixed, as craniopagus, pygopagus, thoracopagus.

paleo-   A combining form meaning old.

Paleocene   Denoting an epoch in the Tertiary period about 60 million years ago. See *geologic time divisions.*

Paleolithic   Denoting the period, prior to agriculture, from about 500,000 to 10,000 years ago.

Paleontological Research Institution   109 Dearborn Place, Ithaca, N.Y. 14850.

Paleontological Society   Museum of Paleontology, University of Michigan, Ann Arbor, Mich. 48104.

paleopathology   The study of disease in specimens preserved from ancient times. Most research has been limited to morphological descriptions. As suggested by Jarcho,[71] exploitation of modern technics such as electron microscopy, fluorescent antibody technics, serology, x-ray diffraction, and electrophoresis could lead to important discoveries in paleopathology.

Paleozoic   Denoting the era, extending from about 600 to 25 million years ago, during which invertebrates were the highest forms of life. See *geologic time divisions.*

palmiped   A web-footed bird.

palm vipers   See table accompanying *snake.*

Pan   A genus of anthropoid apes containing the chimpanzee and gorilla.

pan-   A prefix signifying all.

pancreatic necrosis of fish   See *infectious pancreatic necrosis.*

pancreatolipase   A lipase occurring in the pancreatic juice.

panda   See *Ailurus.*

pandemic   A disease that occurs over an entire region, or even more or less over the world.

panleukopenia (agranulocytosis; feline distemper; feline panleukopenia; cat plague; cat fever)   A highly contagious viral disease of Felidae which occurs in most parts of the world and is characterized by destruction of white blood cells. The symptoms are lassitude, inappetence, and fever; vomiting is common and many animals develop profuse diarrhea. Young cats are most susceptible and the mortality rate is high. The virus may also cause a nonfatal disease of kittens, resulting in cerebellar atrophy (see *ataxia*).[142]

papain   A proteolytic enzyme from the latex of the papaw, *Carica papaya*, which catalyzes the hydrolysis of proteins, proteoses, and peptones to polysaccharides and amino acids. It is used chiefly in medicine as a protein digestant.

papilla   A small, nipple-shaped projection or elevation; used in anatomical nomenclature as a general term to designate such a structure.

papilloma   A benign cutaneous neoplasm, frequently occurring in multiple sites on the skin (papillomatosis). It is seen in a wide range of species in association with a viral agent, but is most common in younger animals, which usually develop immunity as they mature.[142] See also *skin neoplasms,* in table accompanying *neoplasm.*

    Shope p. (rabbit papilloma, Shope papillomatosis of the rabbit, transmissible warts), a virus-induced, naturally occurring cutaneous papilloma of the rabbit, observed originally in states bordering the Mississippi River in wild species of *Sylvilagus* (cottontail rabbits), known popularly as "horned" rabbits. The papillomas were shown by Shope in 1933 to be induced by a specific viral infection, the first such demonstration in a mammalian tumor. It may be transmitted by inoculating scarified skin of either wild (*Sylvilagus*) or domestic laboratory (*Oryctolagus*) rabbits with cell-free filtrates or tumor cells derived from tumors of *Sylvilagus* rabbits. It was the first tumor transmitted by purified viral DNA. The experimental papilloma may be detected six to eighteen days after inoculation in either case. The propagation of tumors derived from *Oryctolagus* rabbits in others of the same species is not successful except under certain circumstances.

Spontaneous papillomas of *Sylvilagus* species regress in approximately 35 per cent of cases, and some 25 per cent of the remainder undergo malignant transformation after a year or more. Many benign papillomas of *Oryctolagus* rabbits carried for 200 days or longer also undergo malignant transformation, and it was from such a source that the V2 (VX2) carcinoma (q.v.) was derived. The virus is usually not demonstrable in lesion material derived from *Oryctolagus* rabbits, although other rabbits of this genus immunized with such material demonstrate complement-fixing and neutralizing antibody against the agent. It is therefore believed to be present in a masked form. The well characterized DNA virus and its derived tumors are widely used in virology and experimental oncology.[30, 53, 127, 150]

papillomatosis The development of multiple papillomas.

   oral p. of the rabbit, an infrequent disease of domestic rabbits manifested by papillomata on the mucous membranes especially on the undersurface of the tongue. These growths may be sessile or pedunculated, are discrete, and may have fungiform projections. The virus causing oral papillomatosis of *Oryctolagus* (domestic) rabbits is antigenically distinct from the Shope papilloma virus of *Sylvilagus* rabbits. The oral papilloma lesions are characterized microscopically by folded hyperplastic epithelium with eosinophilic inclusion bodies in the prickle cell layer, resembling the typical papovavirus warts of many other species.

   Shope p., see *Shope papilloma,* under *papilloma.*

papovavirus A group of ether-resistant double-stranded DNA oncogenic viruses that includes simian virus-40 (SV40), and the viruses of Shope rabbit papilloma, human papilloma (wart), polyoma bovine papilloma, canine oral papilloma, equine papilloma, and others. Shope's discovery of the rabbit papilloma was the first proof of tumor-producing virus in mammals. Later work with this virus included transmission of the tumor with pure preparations of DNA.[16, 64] See *classification* under *virus,* and see *oncogenic viruses.*

papular stomatitis See under *stomatitis.*

para- A prefix meaning beside, beyond, accessory to, apart from, against, etc. In chemistry the prefix indicates the substitution in a derivative of the benzol ring of two atoms linked to opposite carbon atoms in the ring. The abbreviation is *p-*.

parabiont See *parabiosis.*

parabiosis 1. Experimental grafting together of two or more individuals (or embryos) so that the effects of one partner upon the other(s) may be studied. Members of such unions are referred to as parabionts or parabions.[45] 2. Joined twins.

   dialytic p., the circulation of the blood of two animals through a dialyzer, separated by a membrane which permits the removal of harmful material from the recipient's blood and the contribution of essential factors from the donor's blood.

   vascular p., the crossing of the circulation between two individuals by anastomosis of blood vessels.

parabiosis intoxication An older term used to indicate the immunological attack (analogous to the graft-versus-host reaction in runt disease) by one parabiont upon the other in nonisogenic parabiosis. The condition develops eight to thirty days after the establishment of the union.

paradigm A model or design for an experimental procedure; used particularly in reference to behavioral studies.

paragnosis Diagnosis, after death, based on contemporaneous accounts of the diseases which affected historical characters.

paragonimiasis Infestation with the small reddish brown flukes of the genus *Paragonimus,* an important disease of man and animals. The two most important species are *P. westermani,* parasitic in man, and *P. kellicotti,* the adult of which may occur in the mink, dog, cat, pig, muskrat, and opossum. The adult worms are found encysted in the lung. The ova escape from the ruptured cysts and may be coughed up or enter the blood and find their way to such organs as the spleen, liver, brain, or kidney.[21]

Paragonimus A parasitic trematode (fluke). See *paragonimiasis,* and see the table of Common Trematodes, under *trematode.*

paragranuloma The most benign form of Hodgkin's disease, largely confined to the lymph nodes.

paralogia A disordered state of the reason; impairment of the reasoning power marked by illogical or delusional speech.

paralysis Loss or impairment of motor function in a part due to a lesion of the neural or muscular mechanism.

   acute p., a fatal viral disease of adult honeybees and of certain bumblebees. Affected bees are unable to feed or fly, and walk around with trembling of legs and wings. At 30° C., death occurs within one or at most two days following appearance of the symptoms. The virus particles are isometric and measure about 28 mμ in diameter.

bacillary p. (sotto disease), a disease of silkworm larvae caused by ingestion of spores and parasporal crystals of *Bacillus thuringiensis* var. *alesti* and var. *sotto*. The sudden onset of general paralysis, a few hours after ingestion of the toxin, is a pathognomonic symptom of the disease. The paralysis is usually irreversible and followed by death.

chronic p., a fatal viral disease of adult honeybees and of certain bumblebees. Affected bees are able to feed normally, but are feeble and trembly in movement. Their limbs and wings are held slightly spread. Chronically paralyzed bees, unlike acutely paralyzed bees (see *acute p.*), live for several days after appearance of the symptoms. Strongly basophilic cytoplasmic inclusions (Morison's cell inclusions) appear in the hindgut epithelium. The virus particles, which are found in large numbers in the thoracic and abdominal ganglia of the sick bees, are ovoid and occasionally irregularly shaped, with an average size of 27 by 45 mμ. It appears that queens in colonies with chronic paralysis transmit the virus or susceptibility to the disease, or both, to their offspring

guinea pig p. (Romer's paralysis), meningoencephalomyelitis, probably of viral origin, of guinea pigs manifested by paralysis of the hindquarters and urinary incontinence. It was described originally in 1911 and is still believed to occur sporadically, although it has not been reported in the literature since the original description.[60, 80]

paramutation   A mutation in which an allele changes its partner allele.

paramyxovirus   See *classification*, under *virus*.

paranemic spiral   A spiral composed of two structures coiled in opposite directions, and thus easily separated without uncoiling. Cf. *plectonemic spiral*.

paranoia   A chronic, slowly progressive mental disorder (personality disorder) characterized by the development of ambitions or suspicions into systematized delusions of grandeur and persecution which are built up in a logical form; the condition is believed to be based on unconscious homosexual conflicts.

paraphilia   Aberrant sexual activity; expression of the sexual instinct in practices which are socially unacceptable or biologically undesirable.

paraphronia   A condition of abnormal mentality marked by change in disposition or character.

parapodium (pl. *parapodia*)   The muscular projections from the side of the body in polychaete worm. Parapodia are paired and segmentally arranged.

paraprotein   An abnormal serum globulin which may be an entire immunoglobulin or a fragment, identifiable by a unique physical characteristic, such as cold insolubility, high viscosity, or high molecular weight, and by

production of a sharp, well defined peak on electrophoresis.

pararosaniline chloride   A basic tryphenylmethane dye. Solubility at 15° C.: water 1 per cent, absolute alcohol 10 per cent, and glycerol 15 per cent. It is used in the parafalg method for differential staining and grading of acidic tissue elements. It is the main component of most basic fuchsins.[37, 57]

Parascaris equorum   The common ascarid parasite of the horse; used in cytology studies because it exhibits chromosome diminution (q.v.).

parasite   A plant or animal that depends on its host for its food and habitat. It may be an ectoparasite (living on the external surface of the host) or an endoparasite (living in the body of the host).[109]

accidental p., an organism that is only occasionally parasitic.

auxiliary p., a hyperparasite that helps control a parasite.

commensal p., a parasite that derives its substance from the food of its host. See *commensalism*.

facultative p., an organism that is usually parasitic upon another but that is capable of independent existence.

intermittent p., a parasite that lives in its host only at times, being free-living during the interval.

obligatory p., a parasite that cannot live apart from its host.

spurious p., an organism that is parasitic on hosts other than man, but that occasionally passes through the human body without causing harm.

stationary p., one that spends a developmental period in the body of the host. There are several types depending on the time they spend within the host, e.g., periodic parasite such as the botflies and mermithid nematodes, and permanent parasites such as the trematodes and cestodes.

temporary p., one that stays in the host while it acquires its food and then leaves.

parasitiasis   Infestation with a potentially pathogenic parasite that does not harm the host, as when the parasites are too few in number.

parasitism   The symbiotic relationship in which one organism (the parasite) causes damage to and depends on the other (the host) for its habitat and food; parasitism is exhibited by organisms such as trematodes, cestodes, acanthocephalans, and protozoa.[109] See *symbiosis*.

parasitosis   Infection with a pathogenic parasite which harms the host.

Paraspidodera uncinata   A nematode of guinea pigs, which forms ellipsoidal eggs measuring 43 by 31 mμ and are usually found in the cecum and colon of the host.

paratuberculosis (Johne's disease)   An infection caused by an acid-fast organism, *Mycobacterium paratuberculosis*, which is known to infect cattle, sheep, and goats, and may cause disease in swine and primates. It is a granulomatous enteritis ·of chronic course.[16, 142]

parenchyma The essential elements of an organ; used in anatomical nomenclature as a general term to designate the functional elements of an organ, as distinguished from its framework, or stroma.

parhedonia Freud's name for the abnormalities of sexuality, such as the obsessive desire to see, to exhibit, or to touch the sexual organs of oneself or another. Cf. *scopophilia*.

parthenogenesis The development of an unfertilized ovum. Some invertebrate forms reproduce normally with parthenogenetic cycles. Parthenogenesis has been documented in vertebrates, particularly in galliform birds.

parthenophobia Morbid dread of girls.

partial dominance *Incomplete dominance;* see under *dominance.*

parvovirus See *classification,* under *virus.*

PAS Periodic acid-Schiff (stain).

passage A virus See *Gross leukemia virus.*

passage X virus Lymphoid leukemia virus isolated by Gross from lymphosarcoma in C3H/Bi mice induced by whole-body x-irradiation. Its relationship to passage A virus is not clear.[114]

Passalurus ambiguus A nematode (pinworm) of rabbits. The life cycle is presumably the same as that of the human pinworm (see *Enterobius vermicularis*).[21]

passeriform birds Members of the avian order Passeriformes, which includes more than a third of the recognized families and more than one half of all the recognized species of birds. Known as the perching birds and also as the song birds, the Passeriformes include the robins, sparrows, thrushes, finches, canaries, buntings, and related species. A number of species important in research are listed in the accompanying table.

PASSERIFORM BIRDS
IMPORTANT IN RESEARCH

FAMILY	SPECIES	COMMON NAME
Fringillidae	*Serinus canarius*	Canary
Estrildidae	*Phoephila castanotis*	Zebra finch
	Lonchura domestica	Bengalese finch
	Padda oryzivora	Java sparrow
Timaliidae	*Leiothrix lutea*	Pekin robin
Sturnidae	*Gracula religiosa*	Talking mynah

Pasteur effect The inhibition of glycolysis due to the presence of oxygen.[90] Cf. *Crabtree effect.*

Pasteurella A genus of microorganisms of the family Brucellaceae, order Eubacteriales, made up of small coccoid to rod-shaped, gram-negative bipolar cells that are motile or nonmotile and occur singly or in pairs, short chains, or groups. The prototype organism, *P. multocida,* was shown to be the cause of fowl cholera by Pasteur. Although many species have been named, three are distinctly separate: *P. multocida, P. pestis,* and *P. tularensis.* See *pasteurellosis.*

pasteurellosis A general designation used to refer to animal diseases associated with several organisms of the genus *Pasteurella.* The first of these diseases to be described was fowl cholera and the organism was named for Pasteur, who discovered it. Because of difficulty in differentiating the strains of the organisms isolated from diseases in a wide spectrum of animal species, the name *Pasteurella multocida* is usually applied to all regardless of their source. In addition to the disease or diseases caused by *P. multocida,* other important infections caused by organisms of this genus are plague (*P. pestis*) and tularemia (*P. tularensis*).[16, 36] Cf. *shipping fever.* See table.

enzootic p. of rabbits (snuffles; pasteurellosis; hemorrhagic septicemia; nasal catarrh), an important and clinically complex disease of laboratory and colony-reared domestic rabbits (*Oryctolagus cuniculus*). *Pasteurella multocida* (*P. lepiseptica; P. cuniculicida*) is believed by many to be the sole etiologic agent, although *Bordetella bronchiseptica* is frequently isolated. Although the disease is characteristically a chronic upper respiratory tract infection, the syndrome may be subdivided into the following categories:

Upper respiratory infection, frequently the first and only clinical sign in rabbits. There is a creamy white nasal discharge, evidence of which may be found on the medial aspect of the forepaws. This is usually mild, and many rabbits appear to be able to cope with it for long periods of time. It is believed that various stressors have the ability to lower host resistance so that progression to a more serious stage results.

Conjunctivitis, a common and mild aspect believed to result from migration of the causative bacteria up the nasolacrimal duct.

DISEASES CAUSED BY *Pasteurella*[16, 36, 142]

SPECIES	HOST	DISEASE
P. anatipestifer	Duckling	Septicemia
P. haemolytica	Sheep, cow	Pneumonia
P. multocida	Man, rabbit, cow, fowl	Respiratory or septicemic disease
P. novicida	Guinea pig, hamster, mouse	Tularemia-like infection
P. pestis	Man, rat, ground squirrel	Plague
P. pseudotuberculosis	Birds, rodents, other species	Pseudotuberculosis
P. septicaemiae	Goose	Fatal septicemia
P. tularensis	Man, rabbit, other species	Tularemia

Otitis media, believed to originate from bacterial extension up the eustachian tube to the middle, and later, the inner ear. It is a significant cause of torticollis (to the affected side) in laboratory rabbits.

Cutaneous abscesses, which may occur in the form of boils anywhere in the skin. They are invariably well encapsulated.

Genital infections, usually seen in the female in the form of a chronic pyometra resulting in sterility if bicornual, and usually terminating in peritonitis. This aspect of the syndrome is venereally transmitted by the male.

Bronchopneumonia, a common terminating end stage of the upper respiratory disease. The pneumonia may be acute and fibrinous or chronic with large pulmonary abscesses.

Septicemia, also a common terminating aspect of the syndrome. Such rabbits frequently do not have a history of chronic upper respiratory disease. The lesions of the septicemic form suggest that endotoxemia is important in the pathogenesis.

The disease is maintained and spread by carriers and most colonies have a morbidity approaching 80 per cent. It is generally held that treatment of colonies with antibiotics is useless, although identification and removal of affected and carrier rabbits dramatically reduces the opportunity for infection of new animals. Vaccination has not been advocated as a control measure. It has recently been shown that the disease is amenable to exclusion by cesarean delivery and barrier maintenance of the offspring.

patent blue   An acid triphenylmethane dye. Solubility at 15° C.: water 5 per cent, absolute alcohol 7.75 per cent, and glycerol 12 per cent.[57]

pathergy   1. A condition in which the application of a stimulus leaves the organism in a state in which it is unduly susceptible to subsequent stimuli of a different kind (Rossle). 2. The condition of being allergic to numerous antigens.

patho-   A combining form denoting relationship to disease.

pathobiology   The study of disease approached as a biological rather than a medical science and which embraces all of the basic science disciplines, such as genetics, biochemistry, physics, mathematics, etc., and places strong emphasis on comparative pathology. See *pathology.*

pathogenesis   The process by which a disease develops within a living organism; frequently a study of the mechanisms of cellular metabolic aberrations.

pathogenicity   The ability to cause disease; said of microorganisms. Cf. *virulence.*

pathognomonic   A set or sets of specifically distinctive or unique features observed biochemically and/or by tissue alterations which are characteristic of a specific disease.

pathologic physiology   (pathophysiology) The science which deals with disturbances of physiology and the means by which they express themselves as symptoms and signs in the development of disease. These abnormalities may be accompanied by morphological changes but frequently occur in the absence of anatomical deviation. For instance, they may be expressions of cellular dysfunction at the biochemical level, as in hypoglycemia as a result of a defect in gluconeogenesis, which if sufficiently severe may in turn manifest itself morphologically as fatty degeneration in the liver cells.[144]

pathology   That branch of medicine which treats of the essential nature of disease, especially of the structural and functional changes in tissues and organs of the body which cause or are caused by disease. As the complexity of biomedical research has increased during the past century, there has been an ever broadening influence of pathology and at the same time a loss of clarity in the boundaries of pathology. The accompanying diagram presents the science of pathology in a multidimensional chronological fashion, paralleled by the development of various allied sciences and technics, and illustrates the application of these ideas and technics to the interspecies study of disease as epitomized by comparative pathology. Cf. *pathobiology* and *comparative p.*

cellular p., that which regards the cells as starting points of the phenomena of disease (Virchow).

comparative p., that branch of pathology which emphasizes comparisons of disease phenomena between various species, usually with the ultimate objective of learning more about the diseases of man but at the same time with an intrinsic interest in diseases of anomen. See diagram on page 154.

clinical p., pathology as used in the diagnosis of disease in the living patient and especially that portion of pathology which emphasizes the use of laboratory methods such as those of chemistry, diagnostic microbiology, hematology, parasitology, and the application of special analytical methods to recording, filing, and recovering laboratory data.

experimental p., the study of disease in laboratory experiments frequently involving the artificial induction of disease in animals but also including the study of the spontaneous or naturally occurring diseases of anomen as a tool in comparative pathology.

general p., that which embraces the study of basic metabolic and biochemical conditions which occur in various diseases with a view to understanding their pathogenesis.

geographical p., the study of disease as related to the unique ecology of the host. This frequently includes demography, epidemiology and epizootology.

special p., the study of the pathology of particular diseases or organs.

surgical p., the study of structural alterations of tissues during the course of disease, frequently with the objective of operative intervention.

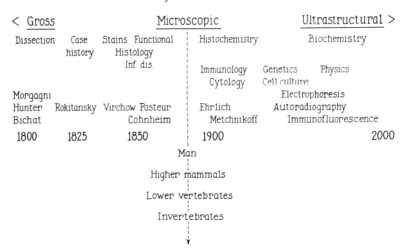

Figure 6. The evolution of comparative pathology.

pathonomia The sum of knowledge regarding the law of diseases.

pathophobia Morbid dread of disease.

pathophysiology Pathologic physiology.

pathopoiesis 1. The causation of disease. 2. The tendency of the individual to become diseased.

pathopsychology The psychology of mental disease.

-pathy A word termination denoting a morbid condition, or disease.

patroclinous Denoting an offspring that resembles the male more than the female parent. Inherited from the father.

pattern of response Topography.

pearl disease Tuberculosis of the peritoneum and mesentery of cattle.

pebrine A disease of the silkworm, *Bombyx mori*, caused by the microsporidian *Nosema bombycis*. The appearance of dark pepperlike spots on the integument of the diseased larvae is a characteristic sign of the infection. Numerous epizootic outbreaks of the disease occurred in the second half of the nineteenth century.[148]

pectin A polymer of sugars present in fruit that forms gels with sugar at the proper pH.

pectinase An enzyme present in most plants, which catalyzes the hydrolysis of pectin to sugars and galacturonic acid.

pectinate hypha Comb-shaped hyphal element.

pectose A constituent of fruits and plants from which pectin is derived.

pectosinase An enzyme that changes pectose into pectin, and pectin into various fermentable sugars.

pedal Pertaining to the foot or feet, or to a pes.

pedo- A combining form denoting relationship (1) to a child, (2) to a foot.

pedogenesis The production of offspring by young or larval forms. See *neoteny*.

pedophobia Fear or dread of children.

Pekin man An extinct human subspecies, *Homo erectus pekinensis*.

pelagic Living in midocean or in the open sea near the surface.

pelecaniform birds Members of the avian order Pelecaniformes, which includes pelicans, gannets, cormorants, darters, and frigatebirds.

pelecypod A mollusk of the class Pelecypoda. See *mollusk*.

Pelger-Huët anomaly (Pelger's anomaly) A hereditary anomaly of the nuclei of polymorphonuclear leukocytes in which there are no more than two segments in the nucleus. In the domestic rabbit, there occurs an incompletely dominant gene (Pg) which in the heterozygote is an excellent model for the Pelger-Huët anomaly of man. In this anomaly, the normal segmentation of the neutrophils is reduced, without discernible consequences, and apparently without other morphologic abnormalities. In the homozygous rabbit (the superpelger), however, the great majority die in utero, and those that are born are dwarfed and have numerous skeletal defects.[123] The anomaly has also been reported in the dog.

pelican See *pelecaniform birds*.

penetrance In genetics, the expression of the frequency with which a heritable trait is shown in individuals carrying the principal gene or genes conditioning it.

pendulous crop An exaggerated dilatation of the crop in domestic turkeys (*Meleagris gallopavo*) in which the greatly increased volume of the crop may droop nearly to the ground. The contents of the organ are watery, sour from fermentation, and static. Serious losses in some flocks are occasioned by increased water drinking during hot weather. Once thought to be an inherited weakness of the crop musculature, it is now known to be related in a complex way to the relative humidity of the environment in which rearing of the poults takes place.[11, 112]

penguin See *sphenisciform birds*.

penicillin An antibiotic substance discovered in 1929 and isolated during the early 1940's, which is produced by a mold of the penicillium group. It hinders the growth of bacteria by inhibiting the synthesis of the cell wall as a result of its interference with the cross-linkage of newly synthesized mucopeptide. Penicillin is active against a wide variety of gram-positive organisms, and less active against gram-negatives presumably because the surface materials of gram-negative bacteria impede the ability of penicillin to diffuse into the organism to reach the binding sites of substances concerned with cell wall synthesis.[36, 49]

pen mating harem mating; see under *breeding system*.

The Pennsylvania Academy of Sciences The Pennsylvania State University, University Park, Pa. 16802.

Pennsylvanian Denoting an epoch in the Carboniferous period extending from about 310 to 270 million years ago. See *geologic time divisions*.

pent-, penta- Combining form meaning five.

pentadactyl Having five digits, the typical limb of amphibians and higher vertebrates.

pentastomid mite A member of the phylum Arthropoda, subphylum Pentastomida (Linguatulida). These organisms are greatly modified for parasitic life, being soft and wormlike, with a short cephalothorax, two pairs of ventral retractile hooks beside the mouth, and with no circulatory, respiratory, or excretory organs. They are organized into two orders: (1) Cephalobaenida, which is characterized by direct development, without an intermediate host. Examples are *Cephalobaena tetrapoda*, infesting South American snakes, and *Reighardia*, infesting gulls and terns. (2) Porocephalida, in which development is indirect, the larvae developing in a different host than the adults. An example is *Linguatula serrata*, the larval form of which is found in the liver or lungs of rabbits, horses, and cows, and the adult of which is found in the nasal cavity of carnivores and man. See also *arthropod*.

pentosuria A congenital metabolic error involving the breakdown of glucose through the glucuronic acid (q.v.) pathway and which is characterized by the absence of the enzyme that catalyzes the reaction of L-xylulose to xylitol. Sugars are present in the urine, but the disorder is harmless. See also *inborn errors*, under *metabolism*.

pepsin The proteolytic enzyme of the gastric juice that changes the native proteins of the food into proteoses and peptones (molecular weight not above 1000), by breaking the peptide linkages, particularly those of tyrosine and phenylalanine.

pepsinase One of a class of enzymes that split native proteins to peptides in acid solution.

peptidase One of a class of proteolytic enzymes that catalyze the hydrolysis of peptide linkages.

peptide One of a class of compounds of low molecular weight, yielding two or more amino acids on hydrolysis. Formed by reaction of the NH_2 and COOH groups of adjacent amino acids, they are known as di-, tri-, tetra- (etc.) peptides, depending on the number of amino acids making up the molecule.

peptidoglycan See *glycopeptide*.

peptone A derived protein, or a mixture of split products, produced by the hydrolysis of a native protein either by an acid or by an enzyme. Peptones are readily soluble in water, are levorotatory, and are not precipitated by heat, by ammonium sulfate, or by the action of alkalis or acids. They include amphipeptone, antipeptone, hemipeptone, and propeptone.

per- 1. A prefix meaning throughout, in space or time, or completely or extremely. 2. A prefix used in chemical terms to denote a large amount or to designate combination of an element in its highest valence.

peracute Excessively acute or sharp.

perception 1. The conscious mental registration of a sensory stimulus. 2. In behavioral science, a term referring to the complex sensory control of behavior inferred from the appearance of that behavior, and thought to be a hypothetical internal event of unspecified and complex nature controlled largely by external stimuli.

performance A measure of observed behavior.

peri- A prefix meaning around.

perianal gland (circumanal gland) Any of numerous glands in the vicinity of the anal orifice that are both sebaceous and nonsebaceous in type and open into the hair follicles. They frequently become neoplastic in the dog (see *perianal gland tumor*). Cf. *anal sac*.

perianal gland tumor A neoplasm of the dog that arises from the sebaceous perianal glands. It is nearly always an adenoma, rarely an adenocarcinoma, and is composed of large polyhedral eosinophilic epithelial cells supported by a basement membrane. The cells are sometimes alluded to as "hepatoid."

periarteritis nodosa of the rat (polyarteritis nodosa) A naturally occurring disease of uncertain etiology of aging rats. The arteries most frequently involved are the spermatic, mesenteric, and pancreatic, less frequently the hepatic, coronary, and ovarian. Grossly the lesions are nodular thickenings distributed along the adventitial aspect of the artery. Microscopically the lesions include focal inflammation and degeneration of the media and adventitia of the medium-sized and small arteries, followed by fibrinoid necrosis of the intima and media, with fragmentation of elastic lamellae and thrombosis. Late stages include a granulomatous cuff around a fibrotic nodule. The lesions are histologically consistent with hypersensitivity, but no convincing evidence for the pathogenesis has yet emerged.[27] See *arteritis*.

peridial hyphae Thick, claw-like hyphae that entangle to form the cleistothecia.

periodic acid-Schiff stain (PAS stain) A method that depends on selective oxidation by periodic acid which attacks 1,2-glycols and 1,2-amino alcohols, oxidizing the adjacent groups to aldehydes, and breaking the carbon chains. The aldehydes form a reddish purple color with Schiff's reagent. The polysaccharides, glycoproteins, or glycolipids stain varying shades from bright red to pink.[37, 153]

peripheral body Mesosome.

perisarc The chitinous or horny covering of the soft parts in hydrozoans.

Perissodactyla An order of ungulates possessing an odd number of toes, including the horse, tapir, and rhinoceros.

peritonitis See *infectious feline peritonitis*.

Permian Denoting the most recent of the Paleozoic periods. See *geologic time divisions*.

pero- A combining form meaning maimed or deformed.

peromelia Congenital deformity of the limbs.

peroxidase An enzyme that catalyzes the transfer of oxygen from hydrogen peroxide or an organic peroxide to a suitable substrate and thus brings about oxidation of the substrate. It causes breakdown of peroxide only in the presence of a suitable oxidizable substrate.

perseverative See under *error*.

persona Jung's term for the assumed personality which the individual takes on to mask his real individuality.

-petal A word termination meaning directed or moving toward, the point of reference being indicated by the word stem to which it is affixed, as centripetal (toward a center), corticipetal (toward the cortex), etc.

petechia A pinpoint, nonraised, perfectly round, purplish red spot caused by intradermal or submucous hemorrhage. Cf. *ecchymosis*.

petrel See *procellariiform birds*.

-pexy A word termination meaning fixation.

peyote A drug obtained from the Mexican cactus, *Anhalonium*, used by the natives to produce a state of intoxication marked by feelings of ecstasy.

phage Bacteriophage.

phage cross Multiple infection of a single bacterium with bacteriophages of differing genotype. Recombination with progeny of mixed genotype occurs upon lysis.

phage induction Manipulation of a bacterial culture containing prophage so that the bacteriophage enters the vegetative state. It is accomplished by exposing lysogenic cultures to x-ray, ultraviolet radiation, or other inducing agent.

phago- A combining form denoting relationship to eating or consumption by ingestion or engulfing.

phagocyte Phagocytic cell.

phagocytic cell (phagocyte) Any of the ameboid cells produced in the bone marrow from stem cells, their primary function being to engulf, and sometimes to digest, foreign material and thus to provide the host with natural resistance against microbial invaders. The main types of phagocytic cells are neutrophils, eosinophils, and macrophages (q.v.). The last type transform into epithelioid cells under the influence of certain types of irritants.

phagocytin A bactericidal substance contained in neutrophilic leukocytes.

phagocytosis The engulfment by a cell of bacteria or other foreign materials. See *phagocytic cell*. Cf. *endocytosis, pinocytosis,* and *ropheocytosis*.[165]

phagolysosome A cytoplasmic vacuole containing ingested foreign material into which lysosomal enzymes have been discharged.[33]

phagosome A phagocytic or endocytic vacuole of a cell containing foreign material. After lysosomes discharge their enzymes into these structures, they are known as phagolysosomes.[33]

phalanger See *marsupial*.

phallus 1. The penis. 2. The primordium of the penis or clitoris before the definitive organ is established in the developing embryo.

pharmacogenetics The study of genetic factors which cause variation in the reaction of individuals to drugs.

pharmacology The science that deals with the study of drugs.

pheasant See *galliform birds*.

phenocopy 1. An individual whose phenotype mimics that of another genotype but whose character is determined by the environment rather than heredity. 2. The simulated trait in a phenocopy individual. 3. The simulation by an individual of traits characteristic of another genotype.

phenolphthalein A chemical used in biology as a dye and indicator of pH.

phenotype The outward, visible expression of the hereditary constitution of an organism.

pheromone A body secretion that affects the behavior of other members of the same species, as sex attractants, territorial markers, etc.

Philadelphia chromosome See under *chromosome*.

-philia A word termination designating notable or abnormal fondness or attraction for the subject indicated by the stem to which it is affixed.

philopatridomania Uncontrollable desire to return to one's native land.

philopatry The desire of an individual to return to or stay in its home region.

Philosophy of Science Association Department of Philosophy, Michigan State University, East Lansing, Mich. 48823.

phlebo- A combining form denoting relationship to a vein or veins.

Phlebotomus A genus of blood-sucking flies which transmit oriental sore, kala-azar, leishmaniasis, and Oroya fever.[105, 159]

phleomycin An antibiotic produced by a species of *Streptomyces,* which is effective against a variety of bacteria. It acts by inhibition of DNA synthesis. Although in HeLa cell cultures there is marginal inhibition of DNA synthesis, the almost complete blockage of cell division indicates that the sensitive step follows DNA synthesis.[36, 49]

phlogo- A combining form denoting relation to inflammation.

phlogocyte A cell characteristic of tissue in an inflamed state; a plasma cell.

phlogogenic Causing inflammation.

phloxin B An acid dye of the xanthene group. Solubility at 15° C.: water 10.5 per cent, absolute alcohol 0.5 per cent, and glycerol 9 per cent. It is used with methyl green and glycerol jelly as a differential stain and mordant, and with trypan blue as a differential stain for virus inclusions in plant tissues.[57]

phocomelia A developmental anomaly characterized by absence of the proximal portion of a limb or limbs, the hands or feet being attached to the trunk of the body by a single small, irregularly shaped bone. This abnormality became of particular interest following the tragic disclosure that thalidomide could cause such defects when ingested by pregnant females.

phono- A combining form denoting relationship to sound, often specifically to the sound of the voice.

phonopathy Any disease or disorder of the organs of speech.

phonophobia Morbid dread of sounds or of speaking aloud.

phosphatase An enzyme that hydrolyzes monophosphoric esters, with liberation of inorganic phosphate, found in practically all tissues, body fluids, and cells, including erythrocytes and leukocytes.

    acid p., a phosphatase most active in acid pH and found in mammalian erythrocytes and yeast (optimal activity at pH 6), prostatic epithelium, spleen, kidney, blood plasma, liver, and pancreas, and in rice bran (optimal activity at pH 5), and taka-diastase (optimal activity at pH 3 to 4).

    alkaline p., a phosphatase most active in an alkaline pH and found in blood plasma or serum, bone, kidney, mammary gland, spleen, lung, leukocytes, adrenal cortex, and seminiferous tubules (optimal activity at about pH 9.3).

    serum p., the phosphatase of the blood serum.

phosphocreatinase An enzyme which in the presence of adenosine triphosphate splits phosphocreatine into creatine and phosphoric acid.

phosphoenolpyruvic carboxylase kinase An enzyme found in the glycolytic-Krebs cycle that converts oxaloacetate to phosphoenol-pyruvate.

1-phosphofructokinase An enzyme of the Embden-Meyerhof glycolytic pathway that catalyzes the conversion of D-fructose-1-phosphate into D-fructose-1,6-diphosphate, using ATP and Mg^{++} as co-factors.

6-phosphofructokinase An enzyme of the Embden-Meyerhof pathway that catalyzes the conversion of D-fructose-6-phosphate to D-fructose-1,6-diphosphate, using ATP and Mg^{++} as co-factors.

phosphoglucoisomerase An enzyme of the Embden-Meyerhof pathway that catalyzes the interconversion of fructose-6-phosphate to glucose-6-phosphate.

phosphoglucomutase An enzyme active in glycogenesis that catalyzes the interconversion of D-glucose-1-phosphate and D-glucose-6-phosphate, using glucose-1,6-diphosphate and Mg^{++} as co-factors.

3-phosphoglyceric-1-kinase An enzyme of the Embden-Meyerhof pathway that converts 1,3-diphospho D glycerate to 3-phospho-D-glycerate, using ADP and Mg^{++} as co-factors.

phosphoglyceric mutase An enzyme of the Embden-Meyerhof pathway that converts 3-phospho-D-glycerate to 2-phospho-D-glycerate, using 2,3-diphosphoglycerate and Mg^{++} as co-factors.

phosphohexoisomerase An enzyme found in muscle extract that catalyzes the interconversion of glucose-6-phosphate and fructose-6-phosphate.

phosphoketopentoepimerase An enzyme of the hexose-monophosphate shunt that converts D-ribulose-5-phosphate to D-xylose-5-phosphate.

phospholecithinase An enzyme found in the kidneys and the intestinal mucosa that splits phosphoric acid from lecithin and some other phospholipids.

phosphomannoisomerase An enzyme of the Embden-Meyerhof pathway that catalyzes the interconversion of fructose-6-phosphate to mannose-6-phosphate.

phosphonuclease *Nucleotidase.*

phosphoriboisomerase An enzyme of the hexose-monophosphate shunt that converts D-ribulose-5-phosphate to D-ribose-5-phosphate.

phosphoribomutase An enzyme of the hexose-monophosphate shunt that catalyzes the conversion of D-ribose-5-phosphate to α-D-ribose-1-phosphate, using ribose-1,5-diphosphate as a co-factor.

phosphorylase An enzyme which, in the presence of inorganic phosphate, is able to catalyze the depolymerization of glycogen into glucose-1-phosphate or the Cori ester.

phosphotransacetylase An enzyme that catalyzes the transfer of an acetyl group between acetylphosphate and acetyl coenzyme A.

phosphotransferase An enzyme that catalyzes the transfer of a phosphate group. See *kinase* (def. 1).

photo-   158   pigeon

photo- A combining form denoting relationship to light.

photobiology That department of biology which deals with the effect of light on living organisms.

photobiotic Living in the light only.

photochromogen A microorganism whose pigmentation develops as a result of exposure to light, specifically *Mycobacterium kansasii* (pathogenic for man), which is yellow-orange if grown in the light, and almost colorless if grown in the dark. See also *atypical acid-fast bacteria,* under *acid-fast bacteria.*

photomicrograph The photograph of a minute object as seen under the light microscope, produced by ordinary photographic methods.

photoperiodicity The regularly recurring changes in the relation of light and darkness in various areas of the world, noted in the annual passage of the earth about the sun; applied also to the rhythm of certain biological phenomena as determined by those changes.

photoperiodism The physiologic response of animals and plants to variations of light and darkness.

photophilic Loving light; fond of light.

photophobia Abnormal intolerance to light.

photosensitization Severe inflammation and necrosis of the skin caused by the activity of sunlight on certain types of fluorescent pigments which may accumulate in superficial tissue cells. Two such pigments are porphyrin (q.v.) and phylloerythrin, a breakdown product of chlorophyll. In herbivores, this latter pigment is ordinarily detoxified by the liver, but hepatotoxins can cause secondary photosensitization because of the rise in the level of phylloerythrin in the blood. See also *porphyria.*

phren- A combining form denoting relationship to the diaphragm or to the mind.

phrenopathy Any mental disease or disorder.

phrenoplegia 1. A sudden attack of mental disorder. 2. Loss or paralysis of the mental faculties. 3. Paralysis of the diaphragm.

phyco- A combining form denoting relationship to seaweed.

Phycological Society of America, Inc. Department of Biological Sciences, Dartmouth College, Hanover, N.H. 03755.

phycology The scientific study of algae.

phylloerythrin A fluorescent pigment resulting from the breakdown of chlorophyll, found in the ruminant stomach. See *photosensitization.*

physiology The science which treats of the functions of the living organism and its parts.

  comparative p., the study of organ functions in various types of animals, vertebrate and invertebrate, in an effort to find fundamental relations in the physiology of members of the entire animal kingdom. Cf. *comparative pathology.*

  general p., the science of the general laws of life and functional activity.

  hominal p., the physiology of human beings.

  pathologic p., the study of disordered function or of function in diseased tissues.

  special p., the physiology of particular organs.

  vegetable p., the physiology of plants.

phyto- A combining form denoting relationship to a plant or plants.

phytohemagglutinin A substance of plant origin that agglutinates blood cells. It usually refers to material derived from the bean *Phaseolus vulgaris.* Phytohemagglutinins are often potent stimulators of protein synthesis and mitotic division in lymphocytes. They are used in experimental immunology and cytogenetic studies. See also *mitogen, pokeweed mitogen, concanavallin.*

phytophagous Plant-eating organisms.

phytotron A group of laboratories designed to study plants under carefully controlled, reproducible environments.

pica (allotriophagia) Craving for and ingestion of materials other than normal food. It may occur in animals suffering from dietary deficiency or in closely confined animals who become bored.

piciform birds Members of the avian order Piciformes, which includes the jacamars, puffbirds, toucans, and woodpeckers.

pico- A combining form used in naming units of measurement to indicate one-trillionth (10^{-12}) of the unit designated by the root with which it is combined.

picogram A unit of mass (weight) of the metric system, being 10^{-12} gram. Abbreviated pg. Called also *micromicrogram* (abbreviated $\mu\mu$g.).

picornavirus A group of extremely small viruses comprising those readily isolated from intestinal sources as well as the rhinoviruses, which are isolated from the upper respiratory tract. The name is derived from pico (small), RNA, and virus. This group comprises enteroviruses, poliovirus, Coxsackie A and B viruses, echovirus, rhinovirus, and the picornaviruses of anomen.[16, 39, 64] See table, and see *classification,* under *virus.*

picric acid An acid dye of the nitro group. Solubility at 15° C.: water 1.2 per cent, absolute alcohol 9 per cent, and glycerol 5 per cent. It is used as a substitute for phosphotungstic acid in Mallory's aniline blue for staining collagen and for quenching fluorescence of mounting media. It is an important ingredient of several fixatives and also can be used as a mordant.[37, 57, 153]

picro- A combining form meaning bitter.

pigeon See *columbiform birds.*

  domestic p., any of several breeds of the genus *Columbia,* including the homing pigeon, carneaux, dragon, etc. Some of these are of great value in studying the pathogenesis of atherosclerosis (q.v.).

pigeon-feeder's disease See *aspergillosis.*

DISEASES CAUSED BY PICORNAVIRUSES

AGENT	HOST	DISEASE
Coxsackie virus Group A	Monkey, man	Poliomyelitis-like lesions in monkeys; possibly paralytic poliomyelitis and aseptic meningitis in man
Coxsackie virus Group B	Man	Aseptic meningitis and epidemic myalgia (Bornholm disease); myocarditis or encephalomyocarditis in early childhood
Echovirus, types 1 to 24	Cattle	Infertility in bulls
Poliovirus, types 1, 2, 3	Man	Poliomyelitis
Porcine picornavirus	Swine	Stillbirth; embryonic death; infertility; Teschen disease

pigeon milk   A secretion of the adult crop on which the nestlings of all pigeons (columbiform birds) are fed for the first few days of life. In pigeons, the crop is a well developed, two-chambered sac used for food storage. In both sexes, during the last days of egg incubation, the stratified lining epithelium of the two dorsolateral planes of the crop enlarges and assumes a honeycomb-like appearance. From this region cells are sloughed off that contain the milk, a substance that looks and smells like whey cheese, is very rich in proteins and fats, and much resembles mammalian milk (water 65 to 81 per cent, protein 13 to 18 per cent, fat 7 to 13 per cent, ash 1 to 5 per cent; no carbohydrate but active amylase and invertase, and rich in vitamin A and B complex; the ash rich in sodium but lacking calcium). As with mammals, milk production is under the control of pituitary prolactin.

pigeonpox   A disease of pigeons that produces lesions in the mouth and may affect the eyelids and produce blindness.[16]

pilo-   A combining form denoting relationship to hair; resembling or composed of hair.

pinocytosis   The endocytosis or engulfment of liquid droplets by a cell.

pinosome   A membrane-bound cytoplasmic vacuole containing recently engulfed fluid.

pinworm (seatworm)   An intestinal nematode parasite of the superfamily Oxyuroidea, species of which infest invertebrates as well as vertebrates, including *Enterobius vermicularis* (man), *Aspicularis tetraptera* (mouse), *Oxyuris equi* (horse), *Passalarus ambiguus* (rabbit), *Skrjabinema ovis* (sheep), and *Syphacia obvelata* (rat and mouse).

piscivorous   Fish-eating.

Pithecanthropus erectus   Currently known as *Homo erectus*, the immediate predecessor of *Homo sapiens*.

pituitary tumor of Furth (thyrotrophin-secreting pituitary tumor of Furth)   A functionally active, hormone-secreting tumor induced in the anterior lobe of the pituitary gland of a C57B1 mouse radiothyroidectomized by[131] I in the laboratory of J. Furth in 1949. One transplant subline (JB2014) is dependent, growing only in radiothyroidectomized hosts, while the other (JB2005) is autonomous, growing in untreated hosts. Both of the variants (dependent and autonomous) have descended from line 3 of the original thyrotrophin-secreting tumor. Mice bearing the autonomous tumor show changes in a variety of endocrine organs, including the adrenals, pancreas, and thyroid, but not the gonads.[150]

pit viper   See table accompanying *snake*.

plantigrade   Characterized by walking with the metacarpal (plantar) or metatarsal (volar) surface making contact with the ground, as in the bear and man.

plasmablast   A name given to the cell of origin of plasma cells (plasmacytes), although the exact cell type from which plasma cells originate is not completely understood; sometimes referred to as an immunoblast (q v) or less specifically as a pyroninophilic cell.

plasmapheresis   The removal of blood, the separation of plasma from cells by centrifugation, and the reinjection of the cells into the donor. The plasma can then be used for scientific studies or for clinical treatment of disease.

plasmid   A generic term for all types of intracellular inclusions that can be considered as having genetic functions, including bioblasts, endosymbionts, plasmagenes, plastids, viruses, etc.

plasmin   The active portion of the fibrinolytic or clot-lysing system, a proteolytic enzyme with a high specificity for fibrin, with the particular ability to dissolve formed fibrin clots but also having a similar effect on other plasma proteins and clotting factors.

plasminogen (profibrinolysin)   The inactive precursor of plasmin.

plasmo-   A combining form denoting relationship to plasma, or to the substances of a cell.

Plasmodium   A genus of blood protozoa of class Sporozoa which infect mammals, birds, and other animals. Several species of *Plasmodium* are etiologic agents of malaria. There are two stages in the life cycle of plasmodia: the sexual cycle, known as sporogony, which occurs in the intermediate host (i.e., the *Anopheles* mosquito), and during which are produced sporozoites infective for the definitive host, and the asexual cycle, known as schizogony, which occurs without fertilization by the division of the plasmodia in the definitive host.

After the infective mosquito injects the sporozoites, they are carried through the blood stream to the parenchymal cells of the liver, where they develop into cryptozoites. This is known as the exoerythrocytic stage.

After this stage, the metacryptozoic mero-zoites escape and enter the erythrocyte and become trophozoites. This is the youngest form found in the red blood cell, and it continues to develop into an immature schizont and finally a mature schizont. When the erythrocyte ruptures, it releases the mero-zoites, which after five generations form the gametocytes or sexual forms, which are then ready for transmission by the mosquito.

Species of *Plasmodium* infective for man are *P. vivax*, *P. ovale*, *P. malariae*, and *P. falciparum*.

Species infective for monkeys are *P. knowlesi*, *P. cynomolgi*, and *P. inui*. See also table of *Plasmodium* parasites, under *primate*.

Species pathogenic for birds are *P. galli-naceum*, *P. cathemerium*, *P. lophurae*, *P. paddae*, *P. fallax*, *P. oti*, *P. polare*, *P. vau-ghani*, *P. nucleophilum*, and *P. relictum*, which is commonly used for life cycle and experimental animal studies. *P. vassali* is found in the squirrel.[21, 109]

-plasty　　A word termination meaning the shaping or the surgical formation of.

platy-　　A combining form meaning broad or flat.

plectonemic spiral　　A spiral composed of two structures coiled in the same direction and which must be uncoiled and rotated to be separated. Cf. *paranemic spiral*.

-plegia　　A word termination meaning paraly-sis, or a stroke.

pleiotropy　　That property of a single gene by which it is responsible for more than one distinct phenotypic manifestation.

Pleistocene　　Denoting the epoch extending from approximately 10,000 to 1 million years ago. See *geologic time divisions*.

pleopod　　The flattened appendage on the ab-domen of an arthropod used in swimming.

pleuropneumonia　　An infectious pneumo-nia and pleurisy of cattle caused by *Myco-plasma mycoides*. This disease was studied extensively in the United States during the nineteenth century, and the Bureau of Ani-mal Industry was established to eliminate it. *M. mycoides* was the first species of *Myco-plasma* to be cultured, a feat accomplished in 1898. See also *mycoplasmosis*.[62]

pleuropneumonia-like　　Denoting a group of organisms now known as the genus *Myco-plasma* (q.v.), originally named from the dis-ease pleuropneumonia of cattle. Members of this genus are now known to cause pri-mary atypical pneumonia in man, arthritis in swine, rodents, and sheep, abortion in cattle, and chronic respiratory disease in rodents and poultry. See also *mycoplasmosis*.

Pliocene　　Denoting the epoch in the Tertiary period lasting from 13 to 1 million years ago. See *geologic time divisions*.

ploidy　　The status of the chromosome set in the karyotype. Used also as a word termina-tion denoting the condition in regard to the degree of multiplication of chromosome sets, as aneuploidy, diploidy, haploidy, etc.

pluramycin　　An antibiotic obtained from a species of *Streptomyces*, which inhibits growth of bacteria and tumor cells by inhibi-tion of DNA and RNA polymerase reac-tions.[36, 49]

pneumo-　　A combining form denoting rela-tionship to the lungs, or to air or to the breath

Pneumocystis carinii　　See *protozoan para-sites*, under *rat*.

pneumoencephalitis (avian)　　Newcastle disease.

pneumoenteritis　　See *calf pneumonia*, under *pneumonia*.

pneumonia　　Inflammation of the lungs, which takes a variety of forms.

calf p. (enzootic p. of calves; pneumoenter-itis), an acute infectious disease that af-fects primarily the respiratory tract of calves. The etiologic agent is possibly a vi-rus, but the condition is usually complicated by secondary bacterial invaders such as *Cor-ynebacterium pyogenes* and *Pasteurella multocida*. The disease is manifested by loss of appetite, high fever, prostration, a nasal discharge, and rapid breathing. Transmis-sion usually occurs through inhalation of in-fective droplets projected into the air.[16]

giant cell p. of monkeys (measles), an infection with measles virus that has respir-atory manifestations. Although most sus-ceptible imported nonhuman primates acquire immunity to measles virus from a clinically silent infection, occasional isolated cases or even epizootics are reported. In these cases, respiratory manifestations, in-cluding rhinitis and pneumonia, as well as conjunctivitis and facial edema, are seen. The key microscopic lesions are the forma-tion of inclusion bodies and syncytial (giant) cells which line and thicken the alveolar walls. The disease typifies the measles sub-group of myxovirus infections, and the le-sions are similar to those seen in measles of man, rinderpest of cattle, and distemper of dogs. The inapparent acquisition of immu-nity to measles frustrated the early efforts of experimenters to pass human measles virus into subhuman primates, although they were later successful.

The giant cells seen in this disease prob-ably constitute an in vivo example of hybrid cell formation, a phenomenon occurring with considerable frequency in myxovirus infections of many species. It provides a mo-del to study the biological implications of cell fusion in terms of aberrant functions and altered antigenic nature of the cells, as well as possible latency of virus infections. See also *heterokaryon, slow virus*, and *Dawson's encephalitis*.[3, 44, 59, 114]

wild rat p. (WRP), a disease caused by a viral agent isolated by Nelson during a sur-vey of respiratory disease in wild rats (*Rat-tus norvegicus*). It was transmitted to labo-ratory mice, in which it regularly produced death in seven to fourteen days. Lungs of infected mice displayed red, patchy consolidation with marked edema. There were occasional cases of otitis media. Contact transmission between infected and noninfected rats or mice was irregular. The virus has been isolated from naturally infected laboratory rats, but not from laboratory mice despite their susceptibility. Its role in the epizootiology of chronic murine pneumonia is uncertain, but is not generally considered to be significant.[27]

pneumonia virus of mice (PVM) A pneumotropic virus of laboratory mice (*Mus musculus*). The lung is the only organ from which the virus can be recovered in either spontaneous or experimental infections, and intranasal inoculation of mice is the only effective route by which animals can be infected. Lesions are not associated with spontaneous infections (detected serologically), although blind passages of material makes for selection of more virulent variants, with pulmonary lesions being observed by the third to fifth passage. PVM infections are quite prevalent in conventional stocks, and serologic evidence indicates that it is not passed transplacentally, is not harbored as a latent infection by young mice, and does not persist in the presence of antibody.[27, 63]

pneumonitis A condition of localized acute inflammation of the lung without toxemia.

    feline p., a highly contagious respiratory infection of domestic cats due to an agent of the *Chlamydia* group. The lesions are confined to the respiratory tract and the conjunctival membranes. Recent research has disclosed that herpesviruses cause similar clinical syndromes in cats.[16] See *feline respiratory disease*.

    mouse p. (Nigg pneumonitis), an infection of laboratory mice with an agent of the *Chlamydia* (psittacosis-lymphogranuloma venereum) group which causes pneumonitis similar to that caused by related agents in cats and man. Although the agent is susceptible to sulfonamides and tetracycline, its significance in the epizootiology of murine respiratory disease is uncertain. It is not a common isolate and is not currently considered to be important as a cause of spontaneous pulmonary disease in mice.[27, 114]

pneumotropic virus A group of viruses which affect the lungs of mice. The pneumonia virus of mice, mouse pneumonitis (Nigg pneumonitis) virus, and K virus are included in this group.

podiatry (formerly *chiropody*) The diagnosis and treatment of disorders of the feet.

podicipediform birds Members of the avian order Podicipediformes, with legs located far back on the body and a reduced tail, typified by the grebes.

podo-, pod- Combining form denoting relationship to the foot.

podophyllotoxin An antimetabolite isolated from *Podophyllum peltatum* which inhibits mitosis and is used to treat warts.

poikilo- A combining form meaning varied or irregular.

poikilocytosis Presence in the blood of erythrocytes showing abnormal variation in shape.

poikiloploidy The state of having varying numbers of chromosomes in different cells.

poikilothermy 1. The exhibition of body temperature which varies with the environmental temperature. 2. The ability of organisms to adapt themselves to variations in the temperature of their environment.

poison Any substance which when ingested, inhaled, or absorbed, or when applied to, injected into, or developed within the body in relatively small amounts may by its chemical action cause damage to structure or disturbance of function.

pokeweed mitogen An extract of the pokeweed *Phytolacca americana* which stimulates protein synthesis and mitosis in lymphocytes in vitro. When berries of this plant are ingested, a transient plasmacytosis is produced in the blood.

poly- A combining form meaning many or much.

polyandrous Having more than one mate; said of females. See also *polygamous* and *polygynous*.

polyarteritis nodosa See *periarteritis nodosa*.

polychaete A worm of the class Polychaeta; see *annelid*.

polyembryony The development of multiple embryos from a single zygote by its division at an early developmental stage, as monozygotic twins, triplets, etc. Certain species of wasps produce thousands of embryos from a single zygote.

polyene antibiotic Any of a group of antibiotic materials that are active against fungi and ineffective against bacteria. This selective toxicity is probably due to interaction of a unique component present in the membranes of the fungi that is not present in bacteria. This component is probably a sterol. The principal use of the polyenes is against such infections as blastomycosis, cryptococcosis, and histoplasmosis. Those used most commonly are nystatin and amphotericin B.[36, 49]

polygamous Having more than one mate. See also *polyandrous* and *polygynous*.

polygenic Pertaining to or influenced by several different genes.

polygynous Having more than one mate; said of male animals. This situation is more common in nature than polyandrous matings. See also *polygamous*.

polyhedron A crystal-like inclusion body (enclosing a number of polyhedrosis-virus particles) produced in the cells of tissues affected by certain insect viruses. Ordinarily the polyhedrosis-virus particles formed in the nuclei of the host cells are rod-shaped, while those formed in the cytoplasm are polyhedral or approximately spherical. See *polyhedrosis*.

polyhedrosis A viral disease of certain insects characterized by the formation of polyhedral inclusions in the tissues of the infected insect. If the inclusion bodies (poly-hedra) are formed in the nuclei of the infected cells, the disease is known as nu-clear polyhedrosis or nucleopolyhedrosis. If the inclusions are formed in the cytoplasm, the disease is known as cytoplasmic poly-hedrosis. It is not correct to speak of "poly-hedral disease" since this literally means "a many-sided disease."

polykaryon A giant cell containing several nuclei. See *heterokaryon.*

polymerase A remarkable class of enzymes that assemble specific polynucleotide base sequences employing a preexisting polynu-cleotide as a template and nucleotide triphos-phate as substrate. Polymerases have been described which assemble RNA from DNA templates, DNA from DNA templates, and RNA from RNA templates. Recently an RNA-dependent DNA polymerase has been isolated from virus-infected cells and may be of great importance in working out mechanisms of virus replication and onco-genic transformation.[90, 118]

polymyxin A group of peptide antibiotics produced by *Bacillus polymyxa.* They are active against most gram-negative bacteria but lack effect against gram-positive organ-isms and pathogenic gram-negative cocci and mycobacteria. They act on the cyto-plasmic membrane of bacteria owing to their properties as cationic surface-active com-pounds. They have a high level of nephrotox-icity and must be used systemically with great care. They are, however, virtually unabsorbed from the intestine and are fre-quently used to sterilize the digestive tract. Closely related antibiotics are circulin and colistin.[36, 49]

polyoma A tumor caused by an oncogenic virus of broad host range, originally isolated from parotid gland tumors of mice inocu-lated with Gross leukemia virus. The isolate, which grew without cytopathogenic effect (CPE) in monkey kidney cultures, was called polyoma virus. The agent, when injected into mice, induced malignant tumors of the parotid gland and other organs. Polyoma is now known to have a characteristic CPE in mouse embryo cell cultures and these cul-tures, when injected into a variety of labora-tory animals, cause the formation of at least twenty histologically distinct neoplasms, in-cluding sarcomas and hemangiomas in neo-natal hamsters, rats, and guinea pigs, fibro-matous nodules in rabbits, and various tumors in ferrets and *Mastomys.* In general, oncogenic susceptibility varies inversely with host age and directly with virus dose concentration. The agent, classified as a pap-ovavirus, was one of the first mammalian tumor viruses from which infectious DNA was extracted.

Infection with this agent is widely distrib-uted in conventional mouse stocks, but natu-rally acquired infections are usually clini-cally silent, although they may be detected by the hemagglutination-inhibition test in sus-pect serum or by the use of the MAP test.[53, 114, 127]

polyphenoloxidase An enzyme that oxi-dizes phenols and their amino compounds, but not tyrosine.

Polyplax serrata See *arthropod parasites,* under *rat.*

Polyplax spinulosa See *arthropod para-sites,* under *rat.*

polyploid 1. Having more than two full sets of homologous chromosomes. There may be three (triploid), four (tetraploid), five (pen-taploid), six (hexaploid), seven (heptaploid), eight (octaploid), etc. 2. An individual or cell having more than two full sets of ho-mologous chromosomes.

polyploidy The state of having more than two full sets of homologous chromosomes. See *polyploid.*

polyribosome (polysome) A structure con-taining several ribosomes usually in a spiral shape within the cytoplasm of a cell.

polysomaty The state of having redupli-cated chromatin in the nucleus. The term is applied both to an increase in chromosome number resulting from a previous endomito-tic cycle and to an increase in the amount of chromatin per chromosome (polyteny).

polysome Polyribosome.

Polysorbate 80 Trademark for a sorbitan polyoxyalkalene derivative used as an emul-sifier.

polyspermy Fertilization of the ovum by more than one sperm.

polyteny Replication of chromosomal strands within the chromosome without separation into a distinct daughter chromo-some.

ponceau An acid dye of the mono-azo group. Solubility at 15° C.: water 3 per cent, abso-lute alcohol 1.2 per cent, and glycerol 20 per cent. It is used with trypan blue for plant tissues.[57]

Pongidae The family of primates compris-ing the anthropoid apes. See *primate.*

ponophobia 1. Abnormal dread of pain. 2. Dread of work; morbid laziness.

Population Association of America, Inc. Office of Population Research, Princeton University, Princeton, N.J. 08540.

porcine influenza A viral disease of swine closely related to human influenza. It was shown by Shope that the virus can be har-bored for long periods of time in the eggs and larvae of the swine lungworm, *Metas-trongylus apri,* of which the earthworm is the intermediate host.

porcine rhinitis Atrophic rhinitis.

porfiromycin See *mitomycin.*

poriferan (sponge) Any member of the phy-lum Porifera, comprising multicellular ani-mals, some symmetrical and some asymmet-rical. Individual members are composed of two germ layers with cells imperfectly ar-ranged as tissues. Known as the sponges, most poriferans are marine, found in depths ranging from the low tide line to $3\frac{1}{2}$ miles. All are sessile, being attached to solid objects. The body surface is porous, allowing water to move through a system of canals and chambers that perforate an internal skeleton of mineralized fibers. Three classes are distinguished: Calcarea, the calcareous sponges; Hexactinellida, the glass sponges (silaceous skeleton); and Desmospongiae (some with silaceous skeletons, others with no skeleton).

porphyria   The occurrence of excessive amounts of porphyrins in the blood, seen in man as a familial disease. Large quantities are deposited in bones, teeth, and skin, resulting in red fluorescence under ultraviolet light. Porphyria has also been seen in Holstein-Freisian, Hereford, and Shorthorn cattle as a mendelian recessive trait, in which there is discoloration of teeth and urine, and marked photosensitivity of the lighter colored areas of skin. This condition has not been shown to be an exact metabolic counterpart of human congenital porphyria. Porphyria occurs in swine as a dominant trait. Although the teeth and urine contain fluorescent pigment, there does not appear to be any accompanying photosensitivity. The Florida fox squirrel (*Sciurus niger*) produces high levels of porphyrin, and its teeth, feces, and urine contain fluorescent pigment, but this condition appears to be a normal metabolic characteristic not accompanied by disease.[76]

porphyrin   Any of a group of iron-free or magnesium-free pyrrole derivatives that occur universally in protoplasm. They form the basis of the respiratory pigments of animals and plants. The porphyrins are protoporphyrin, mesoporphyrin, hematoporphyrin, deuteroporphyrin, etioporphyrin, coproporphyrin, uroporphyrin, rhodoporphyrin, pyrroporphyrin, pyrroetioporphyrin, chlorophyllin, and chlorophyll. See *porphyria.*

porpoise   See *cetacean.*

porpoise sonar   See *echolocation.*

Portuguese man-of-war   A coelenterate of the genus *Physalia;* see *coelenterate.*

-posia   A word termination denoting relationship to drinking, or to intake of fluids.

Pott's disease   Osteitis or caries of the vertebrae, usually of tuberculous origin. It is marked by stiffness of the vertebral column, pain on motion, tenderness on pressure, prominence of certain of the vertebral spines, and occasionally abdominal pain, abscess formation, and paralysis. With the elimination of tuberculosis of bovine origin by rigid control of cattle health, this disease has virtually disappeared from the human population.[136]

poult   A prepubertal domestic turkey (*Meleagris gallopavo*).

Poultry Science Association   Texas A & M College, College Station, Tex. 77843.

pox   A group of similar diseases of many species caused by agents known as poxviruses (q.v.). Lesions usually consist of papules and pustules in the skin. There is a marked tendency for epithelial cells infected by poxviruses to proliferate, which led to

early speculation that they might be involved in the pathogenesis of neoplasms. The virus of Shope fibroma of rabbits and the Yaba virus of monkeys are in this group.

poxlike disease (Yaba-like pox disease)   A spontaneous poxvirus skin disease first observed at the Oregon Regional Primate Center in an epizootic of monkeys (*Macaca fuscata*) and their human caretakers. The lesions consist of circular, firm, flat, initially papular, later vesicular pocks 1 to 3 mm. in diameter. There is a central crust, and the late lesions umbilicate. Typical poxvirus intracytoplasmic inclusions are seen in epithelial cells. The typical course runs six to eight weeks, with no fatalities. The virus is antigenically unrelated to monkeypox or vaccinia virus. Recovered animals are immune for periods exceeding six months.[3]

poxvirus   Any member of an important group of animal viruses whose basic attributes are as follows: large, complex, brick-shaped particles (300 by 200 by 100 mm.) which contain DNA, essential lipid or lipid-containing envelopes, sensitivity to pH 3.0, multiplication in the cytoplasm of susceptible cells, and a common internal nucleoprotein antigen. The sixteen known poxviruses are divided into three antigenic subgroups and a fourth group unrelated antigenically. They are listed in the accompanying table on page 164.[39] See also *classification* under *virus.*

PPLO   Pleuropneumonia-like organisms. See *mycoplasmosis.*

practice   1. The utilization of one's knowledge in a particular profession.   2. The repeated occurrence of a specified pattern of behavior; the greater number of occurrences the greater the amount of practice.

   massed p., in behavioral science, an experimental procedure in which a very small time interval is allowed between successive trials in relation to the duration of the trial being performed.

   spaced p., in behavioral science, an experimental procedure in which the interval between successive trials is large compared to the duration of the trial.

prairie dog   A small rodent of the genus *Cynomys,* family Seiuridae. There are five species and four subspecies found in North and South Dakota, Nebraska, Kansas, Oklahoma, Texas, Montana, Wyoming, Colorado, New Mexico, Utah, and Arizona. They are not dogs, but heavy-bodied burrowing squirrels which weigh 2 pounds, measure 16 inches in length, and bark (the only resemblance to the dog).

pre-   A prefix signifying before.

Precambrian   Denoting the geological period which ended about 600 million years ago. See *geologic time divisions.*

precocial animals   Those that are active and well-developed as soon as they are delivered or hatched. See also *nidifugous birds.*

preconditioning   See *sensory conditioning,* under *conditioning.*

Diseases Caused by Poxviruses

Subgroup	Disease	Host (Natural Disease)
Vaccinia	Vaccinia	None known
	Rabbitpox	Rabbit
	Smallpox (variola)	Man
	Cowpox	Cow, man
	Monkeypox	Subhuman primates
	Mousepox (ectromelia)	Mouse
Avian	Fowlpox	Chicken
	Pigeonpox	Pigeon
	Canarypox	Canary
	Turkeypox	Turkey
	Sparrow pox	Sparrow
	Juncopox	Junco
Myxoma	Myxoma	Rabbit
	California myxoma	Rabbit
	Fibroma (Shope)	Rabbit
	Squirrel fibroma	Squirrel
Ungrouped	Molluscum contagiosum	Man
	Milker's nodule (pseudocowpox)	Cow, man
	Monkey tumor (Yaba poxvirus)	Subhuman primates
	Bovine papular stomatitis	Cow
	Contagious pustular dermatitis (orf)	Sheep
	Sheep pox	Sheep
	Swinepox	Swine
	Raccoon pox	Raccoon
	Mouse papular virus	Mouse
	Fishpox (?)	Carp

primary feathers Flight feathers borne on the parts of a bird's wing corresponding to the mammalian carpus, metacarpus, and phalanges. See also *remiges*.

primate Any member of the mammalian order Primates. The order Primates, widely used in research, contains a large number of taxonomically complex families and is replete with confusing synonymy. In everyday speech, any primate can be called a monkey, but it is useful to divide the order into three groups: (1) man, (2) apes (anthropoids) and monkeys (simian primates), and (3) prosimian primates. Terms such as "infrahuman," "subhuman," and "nonhuman" have been used to distinguish groups (2) and (3) from (1), with the latter term being generally preferred. Simian primates are further divided into two geographic groups. Those native to Africa, Asia, and the South Pacific are called "Old World monkeys," and those native to Central and South America are called "New World monkeys."

In general, Old World monkeys lack prehensile tails and have ischial tuberosities (callosities), cheek pouches, and a narrow nasal septum; hence the name "catarrhine" has been applied to them. In addition, Old World monkeys are quite susceptible to tuberculosis, may be carriers of herpesvirus B, and utilize dietary sources of vitamin D_2.

New World monkeys may have prehensile tails, lack ischial callosities, are resistant to tuberculosis, and have a wide nasal septum, suggesting the name "platyrrhine" monkeys. New World monkeys do not carry herpesvirus B, and they require dietary sources of vitamin D_3.

Most of the primates used in research are trapped in the country of origin, collected at holding centers and then air-freighted to the country of import. Among the stresses of this period, they are sensitive to changes in environment and nutrition, are often heavily parasitized, and are prone to bacterial and viral infections, particularly of the digestive and respiratory tracts. Before being used for research purposes, they must be quarantined and conditioned not only for the health of the monkey, but also because many of the diseases they may carry constitute major zoonotic hazards for man.[41] The system of classification of the order Primates given in the accompanying table has been adapted from that of Simpson, but it must be recognized that the order is subject to frequent taxonomic revision, and the obsolescence of taxons is an ever present (and vexing) problem to nontaxonomic primatologists.[10, 103, 139] For this reason, a second table is given, listing the common names in alphabetical order (p. 166).

arthropod parasites of nonhuman p's, the arthropod parasites of nonhuman primates appear to have diverged more completely from those of man than have the helminth or protozoan parasites. Few are important as zoonotic agents, although the sucking lice (*Anoplura*) of man, anthropoid apes, and New World simians may be regarded as interchangeable. Old World primates appear to have a group-specific anopluran louse (see table, p. 167). None of the arthropod parasites is important as a cause of disease in laboratory primates, but appear as sporadic problems in certain shipments or individuals. Although clinically insignificant, many of these parasites are widely distributed; indeed it has been said that *Ma-*
(Text continued on p. 168)

FAMILY	GENUS	No. of SPECIES (APPROXIMATE)	COMMON NAME	ORIGIN
(A) Suborder Prosimii (the prosimians or subprimates)				
Tupaiidae	Tupaia	12		
	Anathana	1		
	Dendrogale	3	Tupaia or tree shrew	Southeast Asia
	Tana	5		
	Urogale	2		
Lemuridae	Lemur	6		
	Hapalemur	1		
	Lepilemur	2	Lemur	Madagascar
	Cheirogaleus	3		
	Microcebus	2		
	Phaner	1		
Indriidae	Indri	1	Indris	
	Avahi	1	Indris	Madagascar
	Propithecus	2	Sifaka	
Daubentoniidae	Daubentonia	1	Aye-aye	Madagascar
Lorisidae	Loris	1	Loris	Asia
	Arctocebus	1	Angwantibo	Africa
	Nycticebus	1	Slow loris	Asia
	Perodicticus	1	Potto	Africa
	Galago	3		
	Euoticus	1	Bush baby or galago	Africa
	Galaguides	1		
Tarsiidae	Tarsius	3	Tarsier	South Pacific
(B) Suborder Anthropoidea				
Callithricidae	Callithrix	(12)	Marmoset	
(= Hapalidae)	(= Hapale)	10	tufted-eared	
	(= Mico)	1	naked-eared	
	(= Cebuella)	1	pigmy	
	Saguinus	(20)	Tamarin	South and
	(= Tamarin)	3	black-faced	Central
	(= Tamarinus)	13	white-faced	America
	(= Marikina)	2	bald	
	(= Oedipomidas)	2	Pinches	
	Leontideus	(3)	Golden lion-tamarin	
	(= Leontocebus)	3		
Cebidae	Cebus	3	Capuchin	
	Saimiri	4	Squirrel monkey	
	Alouatta	6	Howler monkey	
	Aotus	1	Night monkey	
	Ateles	5	Spider monkey	South and
	Brachyteles	1	Wooly spider	Central
	Iagothrix	2	Wooly monkey	America
	Callicebus	7	Titi	
	Pithecia	2	Saki	
	Cacajao	4	Uakari	
	Chiroptes	3	Sakis	
Cercopithecidae	Cercopithecus	11	Guenon or grivet	Africa
	Cercocebus	4	Mangabey	Africa
	Cynopithecus	1	Black ape	Asia
	Macaca	12	Macaque	Africa, Asia
	Papio	7	Baboon	Africa
	Theropithecus	1	Baboon	Africa
	Colobus	3	Leaf-eater	Africa
	Nasalis	1	Proboscis monkey	
	Presbytis	5	Langur or	
	Pygathrix	2	Leaf monkey	Asia
	Rhinopithecus	2	Snub-nosed monkey	
	Simias	1	Langur	
Pongidae	Pongo	1	Orangutan	South Pacific
	Pan	2	Chimpanzee	Africa
	Gorilla	1	Gorilla	Africa

A Classification of the Order Primates (Continued)

Family	Genus	No. of Species (Approximate)	Common Name	Origin
(B) Suborder Anthropoidea (Continued)				
Hylobatidae	Hylobates	6	Gibbon	Asia
	Symphalangus	1	Siamang	Asia
Hominidae	Homo	1	Man	Worldwide
Totals 12	61	115		

A Guide to Scientific Names of Nonhuman Primates

Common Name	Scientific Name
Angwantibo	Archtocebus
Avahi	Avahi
Aye-aye	Daubentonia
Baboon, Guinea or Western	Papio papio
Chacma	P. comatus
yellow	P. cynocephalus
anubis or dog-faced	P. doguera
Hamadryas	P. hamadryas
Gelada	Theropithecus gelada
Barbary ape	Macaca sylvana
Bush baby, greater	Galago crassicaudatus
lesser	G. senegalensis
dwarf	Galagoides demidovii
Capuchin, white fronted	Cebus albifrons
black capped	C. apella
white-throated	C. capucinus
Cai weeper	C. griseus
Celebes black ape	Cynopithecus niger
Chimpanzee, greater	Pan troglodytes
lesser	P. paniscus
Cinammon ringtail	Cebus albifrons
Colobus, red	Colobus badius
Cynomologous	Macaca irus
Diana monkey	Cercopithecus diana
Douroucouli	Aotus trivirgatus
Drill	Papio leucophaeus
Gibbon, black	Hylobates, concolor
dark-handed	H. agilis
Kloss	H. klossi
Sunda Island	H. moloch
Gorilla	Gorilla gorilla
Green monkey	Cercopithecus aethiops
Guenon	Cercopithecus spp.
Guerza	Colobus spp.
Howler, rufous-handed	Alouatta belzebul
brown, ursine	A. guariba
mantled	A. palliata
red	A. seniculus
Guatemalan	A. villosa
Indris, babakoto	Indri spp.
wooly	Avahi laniger
Langur, purple-faced	Presbytis senex
Pagai Island	Simias spp.
Leaf monkey, Sunda Island	Presbytis aygula
silvered	P. cristatus
maroon	P. rubicunda
Lemur, ringtailed	Lemur catta
brown	L. fulvus
black	L. cacaco
mongoose	L. mongoz
red-bellied	L. rubriventer
ruffed	L. variegatus
gentle	Hapalemur griseus
sportive	Lepilemur
weasel	L. mustelinus
red-tailed	L. ruficaudatus
greater dwarf	Cheirogaleus major
fat-tailed	C. medius
hairy-eared dwarf	C. trichotis
Coguerels mouse	Microcebus coguereli
Millers mouse	M. murinus
fork-marked mouse	Phaner furcifer
Loris, slender	Loris tardigradus
slow	Nycticebus coucang

Common Name	Scientific Name
Macaque, bonnet	Macaca radiata
crab-eating	M. irus
Assamese	M. assamensis
Formosan	M. cyclopis
Celebes or Moor	M. maurus
liontailed	M. silenus
Japanese	M. fuscata
pig-tailed	M. nemestrina
stump-tailed	M. speciosa
Mandrill	Papio sphinx
Mangabey, black-peaked	Cercocebus aterrimus
sooty	C. atys
agile	C. galeritus
red-headed	C. torquatus
Marmoset, tufted-eared	Callithrix (=Hapale)
white-necked	C. albicollis
white-eared	C. aurita
yellow-legged	C. chrysoleucos
buff-headed	C. flaviceps
white-shouldered	C. humeralifer
common	C. jacchus
white-fronted (Geoffroy's)	C. leucocephala
black-penciled	C. penicillata
elegant	C. petronius
santarem	C. santamarensis
pygmy	C. (=Cebuella) pygmaeus
Goeldi's	C. (=Callimica) goeldii
golden lion	Leontideus spp.
silvery	Callithrix argenatus
Mona monkey	Cercopithecus mona
Moustached monkey	C. cephus
Night monkey	Aotus trivergatus
Orangutan	Pongo pygmaeus
Patas monkey	Cercopithecus (=Erythrocebus) pe
Pinche, cottontop	Saguinus oedipus
spix's	S. spixi
Potto	Perodicticus potto
Proboscis monkey	Nasalis larvatus
Rhesus	Macaca mulatta
Saki, pale headed	Pithecia pithecia
hairy	P. monacus
bearded or cuxius	Chiropotes spp.
red-backed	C. chiropotes
white-nosed	C. albinasa
black	C. satanas
Siamang	Symphalangus syndactylus
Sifaka, diademed	Propithecus diadema
verreaux's	P. verreauxi
Spider monkey, long haired	Ateles belzebuth
brown headed	A. fusciceps
black	A. paniscus
red-bellied	A. rufiventris
wooly	Brachyteles arachnoides
Squirrel monkey, black-headed	Saimiri boliviensis
red-backed	S. oerstedi
common	S. sciurea
short-tailed	S. usta
Sykes monkey	Cercopithecus mitis
Talapoin	Cercopithecus spp.
Tamarin, silky	Leontideus rosalia
bare-faced (bald)	Marikina spp.
pied	M. bicolor
Martin's	M. martinsi
hairy-faced (black-faced)	Saguinus (=Tamarin) spp.

Common Name	Scientific Name	Common Name	Scientific Name
Negro	S. tamarin	Titi, ashy	Callicebus cinerascens
red-handed (Lacepede's)	S. midas	red	C. cupreus
white-faced	S. (=Tamarinus) spp.	grey	C. gigot
brown-headed	S. fusicollis	orabassu	C. molloch
Rio Kapo	S. graillsi	Ollala's	C. ollalae
red-mantled	S. illigeri	masked	C. personatus
Emperor	S. imperator	collared or yellow-handed	C. torguatus
red-bellied, white-lipped	S. labiatus	Toque monkey	Macaca sinica
white-footed	S. leucopus	Tree shrew (tupaia)	Tupaia sp., Anathana sp.,
white	S. melanoleucus		Dendrogale sp., Tana sp.,
moustached	S. mystax		Urogale sp.
black and red	S. nigricollis	Uakari, bald	Cacajao calvus
red-capped (bonneted)	S. pileatus	black	C. roosevelti
Lonnberg's	S. pluto	black-headed	C. melanocephalus
Golden-mantled	S. triparitus	red	C. rubicundus
Weddell's or Deville's	S. weddelli	Vervet	Cercopithecus aethiops
Tarsier, western	Tarsius bancanus	Wooly monkey, Humboldt's	Lagothrix lagotricha
Eastern	T. spectrum	gray or smoky	L. cana
Philippine	T. syrichta		

Arthropod Parasites of Nonhuman Primates

Species	Common Name	Location on Host	Principal Host or Geographic Distribution
Insecta: Anoplura			
Pedicinus longiceps	Sucking louse	Skin	Old World simians
Docophthinus acionctus	Sucking louse	Skin	Tree shrews
Phthropediculus propitheci	Sucking louse	Skin	Lemurs
Lemurphthirus galagos	Sucking louse	Skin	Galagos
Pediculus lobatus pseudohumanus	Sucking louse	Skin	New World
Harrisonia uncinata	Sucking louse	Skin	New World
Gliricola pintoi	Sucking louse	Skin	New World
Pediculus humanus friedenthali	Sucking louse	Skin	Orangutan
Phthirus pubis	Sucking louse	Skin	Chimpanzee
P. gorillae	Sucking louse	Skin	Gorillas
P. schaffi	Sucking louse	Skin	Chimpanzee
Insecta: Mallophaga			
Trichodectes armatus	Chewing louse	Skin	New World
T. colobi	Chewing louse	Skin	Colotus monkey
T. mjoebergi	Chewing louse	Skin	Loris
T. semiarmatus	Chewing louse	Skin	Howler monkey
Trichophilopterus babakotophilus	Chewing louse	Skin	Lemurs
Tetragynopus aotophilus	Chewing louse	Skin	Douroucouli
Arachnida			
Sarcoptes scabei	Mange mite	Skin	Universal
Audycoptes greeri	Sinus hair follicle mite	Skin	New World
A. lawrenci	Sinus hair follicle mite	Skin	New World
Mortelmansia longus	Nasal cavity mite	Nose	New World
M. brevis	Nasal cavity mite	Nose	New World
M. duboisi	Nasal cavity mite	Nose	New World
Fonsecalges saimirii	– – –	Skin	New World
Pneumonyssus simicola	Lung mite	Lung	Old World
P. duttoni	Lung mite	Trachea	Cercopithecus
P. congoensis	Lung mite	Lung	Old World
P. dinolti	Lung mite	Lung	Old World
P. stammeri	Lung mite	Lung	Lagothrix
P. oudemansi	Lung mite	Lung	Chimpanzee
P. vitzthumi	Lung mite	Lung	Orangutan
Armillifer armillatus	Pentastomid larva	Connective tissue	New World
Porocephalus cercopitheci	Pentastomid larva	Connective tissue	Old World
P. clavati	Pentastomid larva	Connective tissue	Old World
Linguatula serrata	Pentastomid larva	Connective tissue	Old World

167

(*Text continued from p. 164*)

caca mulatta is universally infested with species of the lung mite, *Pneumonyssus*.[21, 41, 126, 128]

helminth parasites of nonhuman p's, nonhuman primates are hosts for a large variety of helminth parasites, some of which have followed their simian hosts in diverging from man and the anthropoid apes sufficiently to be considered strictly parasites of the lower genera of primates. Many of the parasites, however, are sufficiently nonspecific in choice of hosts to embrace both higher and lower primates, including man. Most of the helminth parasites of anthropoid apes also infect man. The most important parasites are listed in the accompanying table.[21, 41, 66, 126, 128]

HELMINTH PARASITES OF NONHUMAN PRIMATES

PHYLUM	SPECIES	LOCATION IN HOST	PRINCIPAL HOST OR GEOGRAPHIC DISTRIBUTION	COMMENT
Trematoda	*Watsonius watsoni*[3]	Gut	Baboons	– – –
	Asthesmia foxi[3]	Bile ducts	New World	– – –
	Eurytrema brumpti	– – –	Anthropoids	– – –
	Controrchis biliophilus[3]	Gallbladder	New World	– – –
	Dicrocelium spp.[3]	Liver	New World	– – –
	Phaneropsolus orbicularis[3]	– – –	New World	– – –
	Gastrodiscoides hominis[3]	Gut	Macacs	– – –
	Schistosoma magna[3]	Blood	Anthropoids	– – –
	S. mansoni[1, 3]	Blood	Africa, New World	– – –
	S. hematobium[1, 3]	Blood	Baboons	– – –
Cestoda	*Diphyllobothrium (spargana)*[1, 4]	Connective tissue	Worldwide	Sparganosis
	Raillietina alouattae[1, 3]	Gut	New World	– – –
	R. multitesticulata[3]	Gut	New World	– – –
	Hymenolepsis diminuata[1, 3]	Gut	Old World	– – –
	H. nana[1, 3]	Gut	Old World	– – –
	Bertiella cercopitheci[1, 3]	Gut	Worldwide	– – –
	B. conferta[1, 3]	Gut	Worldwide	– – –
	B. fallax[1, 3]	Gut	Worldwide	– – –
	B. mucronata[1, 3]	Gut	Worldwide	– – –
	B. polyorchis[1, 3]	Gut	Worldwide	– – –
	B. satyri[1, 3]	Gut	Worldwide	– – –
	B. studeri[1, 3]	Gut	Worldwide	– – –
	Monieza rugosa[3]	Gut	New World	– – –
	Atriotaenia megastoma[3]	Gut	New World	– – –
	Taenia solium[4]	Connective tissue	Worldwide	*Cysticercus cellulosae*
	T. tenuicollis[4]	Connective tissue	Worldwide	*Cysticercus tenuicollis*
	Multiceps serialis[4]	Connective tissue	Worldwide	*Coenurus*
	Echinococcus granulosus[1, 4]	Connective tissue	Worldwide	Hydatid
Acanthocephala	*Prosthenorchis spirula*[2, 3]	Gut	Old World	– – –
	P. elegans[2, 3]	Gut	Worldwide	– – –
Nematoda	*Oesophagostomum apiostomum*[1, 2, 3]	Gut	Worldwide	Nodular worm
	O. stephanostomum[1, 2, 3]	Gut	Old World	Black disease
	Ancylostoma duodenale[1, 3]	Gut	Worldwide	Hookworm
	Necator americanus[1, 3]	Gut	Worldwide	Hookworm
	Ternidens deminutus[1, 3]	Gut	Old World	Hookworm
	Strongyloides cebus[2, 3]	Gut	New World	– – –
	S. stercoralis[1, 2, 3]	Gut	Old World	– – –
	S. fulleborni[1, 2, 3]	Gut	Old World	– – –
	Nochtia nochti[3]	Stomach	Old World	Tumor-inducing
	Trichuris trichiura[1, 3]	Cecum	Old World	– – –
	Capillaria hepatica[1, 3]	Liver	– – –	– – –
	Trichinella spiralis[1, 3]	Gut	Worldwide	– – –
	Enterobius vermicularis[1, 3]	Colon	Worldwide	Pinworm
	Protospiura muricola[3]	Stomach	New World	– – –
	Gnathostoma[3]	Colon	New World	– – –
	Gongylonema minimum[3]	Esophagus	Old World	– – –
	Oslerus cynopitheci[3]	Lungs	Old World	Lungworm
	O. barretoi[3]	Lungs	New World	Lungworm
	Dipetalonema gracile[2, 3]	Connective tissue	New World	– – –
	D. caudispina[2, 3]	Peritoneum	New World	– – –
	Tetrapetalonema parvum[2, 3]	Peritoneum	New World	– – –
	T. atalensis[3]	Peritoneum	New World	– – –
	T. digitata[3]	Peritoneum	Old World	– – –
Colum	*Loa loa*[1, 3]	Connective tissue	Old World	– – –

Key: 1. An agent also found in man. 2. A significant disease agent. 3. Adult parasite. 4. Larval form.

Plasmodium parasites of nonhuman p's, see *Plasmodium,* and see accompanying table.[159]

pristinamycin See *streptogramin.*

pro- A prefix signifying before or in front of.

proband See *propositus.*

proboscis monkey Any member of species *Nasalis larvatus;* see *primate.*

Probstmayria vivipara A nematode (pinworm) of the horse.[21]

procarboxypeptidase The inactive precursor of carboxypeptidase, which is converted to the active enzyme by the action of trypsin.

procellariiform birds Members of the avian order Procellariiformes, having webbed feet, long narrow wings, and tubular nostrils, and including the albatross and petrel.

process 1. A prominence or projection. 2. A series of operations leading to a specific result. 3. In behavioral science, a change in response strength related to experimental manipulation.

proctodeum See *cloaca (avian).*

profibrinolysin Plasminogen.

progenesis The maturation of the gametes within an organism before it has reached physical maturity in other respects. See also *neoteny* and *pedogenesis.*

progeny test The study of certain characteristics of offspring, such as eye color, blood type, or performance, under specified conditions in order to determine the genotype of the parent.

prognathism The condition of having marked projection of the jaw.

prolegs Short, unjointed appendages borne on the abdomen of caterpillars.

prolidase An intestinal enzyme that catalyzes the hydrolysis of peptide bonds between the ring nitrogen of proline and the CO of an adjacent α-amino acid.

proliferative stomatitis See *papular stomatitis,* under *stomatitis.*

pronase A proteolytic enzyme that digests mucoproteins.

pronotum The chitinous covering of the dorsal surface of the first segment of an insect's thorax.

prophage The genome of a bacteriophage in a lysogenic bacterium which carries the information necessary to produce a complete bacteriophage under the proper stimulus. See *phage induction.*

prophase The first stage in mitosis or meiosis, including all the processes up to the metaphase or separation of the chromosomes. See *mitosis* and *meiosis.*

propositus (proband) The original individual observed with a mental or physical disorder and whose case serves as the stimulus for a hereditary or genetic study.

prosoma The anterior, leg-bearing portion of the body of arachnids.

prostaglandin Any of several fatty acid derivatives found in extracts of many tissues, so named because von Euler first isolated them from seminal fluid. They stimulate smooth muscle and have the ability to lower blood pressure, among other biologically active properties.

prosthetic group A nonprotein co-factor that must be bound very tightly to enzyme protein (apoenzyme) in order to form a complete enzyme (holoenzyme). Cf. *coenzyme.*[90]

protandry In hermaphrodite animals, the condition of producing first male and then female gametes.

protease A general term for a proteolytic enzyme, such as peptidase.

Protista A term proposed by Haeckel for a third kingdom to contain all the microorganisms, thus to include some from the plant and animal kingdoms as well as other more primitive forms. The Protista are commonly divided into three groups: (1) viruses are acellular, totally host-dependent, minute intracellular parasites; (2) lower protists are organisms with very simple cell structure and primitive locomotor apparatus, comprising some free-living and some parasitic

Plasmodium (MALARIA) PARASITES OF THE ORDER PRIMATES

CLASSIFICATION	MAN	ANTHROPOID APES	MONKEYS
Quartan (malariae) malaria	P. malariae [P. knowlesi]*	P. rodhaini [P. malariae] P. hylobati	P. knowlesi – – – – – –
Benign tertian (vivax) malaria	[P. brasilianum] P. vivax [P. cynomolgi bastianelli] [P. schwetzi] – – – – – – – – –	P. schwetzi [P. vivax] – – – – – – – – –	P. brasilianum P. gonderi P. cynomolgi P. cynomolgi bastianelli P. inui P. osmaniae P. fieldi
Ovale malaria	P. ovale [P. simium]	P. ovale – – –	P. ovale P. simium
Malignant tertian (falciparum) malaria	P. falciparum	P. reichenowi	– – –

*Brackets indicate known susceptibility of an unnatural host.

forms, including the blue-green algae, bacteria, rickettsiae, *Chlamydia,* spirochetes, and others; (3) higher protists have a more complex cell structure and may even be multicellular, are relatively large, and occur both in the free-living and parasitic states, including the algae above the blue-green, the fungi, and the Protozoa.[159]

proto-, prot- Combining form meaning first.

protoanemonin An antibiotic produced by plants of the family Ranunculaceae, active against certain gram-positive and gram-negative bacteria. Its mechanism of activity is not well understood.[49]

protoplast The inner part of the plant cell, which is metabolically active and is surrounded by a cytoplasmic membrane different from the rigid cell wall.

bacterial p., a transformed bacterial body which lacks a cell wall, does not readily multiply but retains the physiological characteristics of the parent bacterial cell, and may revert if the external integument of the cell retains some glycopeptide fragments. See also *L-form.*

Protozoa The lowest division of the animal kingdom, comprising unicellular organisms. Protozoa are usually separated into four classes: Sarcodina, having pseudopodia; Mastigophora, having flagella; Sporozoa, having no locomotor organs in the adult stages and reproducing by sporulation; and Infusoria, having cilia. See also *protozoan parasites,* under *rat.*

provirus A latent stage of an animal virus, equivalent to prophage.

psammo- A combining form denoting relation to sand or to sandlike material.

psammocarcinoma Carcinoma containing calcareous matter.

psammoma A tumor, especially a meningioma, that contains psammoma bodies; formerly sometimes called *Virchow's psammoma.*

pseudo- A combining form signifying false or spurious.

pseudoconditioning See under *conditioning.*

pseudocowpox A viral disease of cattle that closely resembles cowpox.[16]

pseudocyst An aggregation of organisms of the species *Toxoplasma gondii.* See also *toxoplasmosis.*

Pseudomonas A genus of gram-negative, aerobic microorganisms capable of forming water-soluble fluorescent (fluorescein) and bluish-green (pyocyanin) pigments.[36] *P. aeruginosa,* the type species, is pathogenic for many species (see table).

pseudorabies See *Aujezsky's disease.*

pseudotuberculosis A bacterial disease seen with diminishing frequency in laboratory animals, but still of importance in their feral counterparts. In rodents and lagomorphs, the etiologic agent is *Pasteurella pseudotuberculosis* and in sheep *Corynebacterium pseudotuberculosis,* but regardless of the agent the clinical course of progressive loss in condition, with caseous nodules generally disseminated in most lymph nodes and internal organs, is similar in all species. Infection is by the oral route, and bacteria are passed in the feces. Terminal signs include cachexia, anorexia, and dyspnea. In addition, the lesions may include arthritis. Microscopic lesions comprise caseous, well-encapsulated abscesses with Langhans-type giant cells and lymphocytes about the periphery. The infection spreads slowly in colonies, and no treatment is recommended other than destruction of affected individuals.[27, 142]

murine p., an infectious disease of laboratory rats and mice caused by *Corynebacterium kutscheri.* Many conventionally derived rats and mice can apparently carry the organism in a latent (clinically silent) phase from which symptomatic evidence of infection can be elicited by exposure to a nonspecific array of stressors known to include x-irradiation, pantothenate deficiency, steroid treatment, and virus infections.

Symptomatology is related to focal abscessation in various organs, chiefly those involved in bacteremic filtering, the kidney, lungs, and liver, in that order. Diagnosis is based on cultural demonstration of the specific organism. The corynebacteria can be excluded by gnotobiotic derivation, but no other control measure, save destruction of affected colonies, is advocated.[27]

psicofuranine An antibiotic produced by a species of *Streptomyces,* which has considerable activity against *Staphylococcus* and which acts by inhibition of the enzyme xanthosine-5'-phosphate aminase.[36, 49]

psittacine birds Members of the avian order Psittaciformes. The single family Psittacidae comprises the parrots, parakeets, macaws, lorikeets, and cockatoos, including a number of important research and fanciers' species. Some are listed in the accompanying table.[112]

DISEASES CAUSED BY *Pseudomonas aeruginosa*

HOST	DISEASE
Swine, cattle	Necrotic pneumonia, necrotic enteritis, spleen abscess
Cattle	Pericarditis, abortion, mastitis
Calf	A form of scours
Poults, turkey, chicken, duck	Diarrhea (?)
Mare	Genital infection
Dog	Otorrhea, eye infection
Mink	Hemorrhagic pneumonia

SOME IMPORTANT SPECIES OF PSITTACINE BIRDS

SPECIES	COMMON NAME	HABITAT
Melopsittacus undulatus	Parakeet, budgerigar	Worldwide in southern latitudes
Agapornis spp.	Lovebirds	Africa, Madagascar
Nymphicus hollandicus	Cockatiel	Australia
Psittacus erithacus	African gray parrot	Africa
Amazona ochrocephala	Yellow-headed Amazon	South and Central America
Ara spp.	Macaws	South America
Andorhynchus spp.	Macaws	South America

psittacosis A generalized infection of man derived from birds, including parrots, parakeets, lovebirds, pigeons, ducks, and turkeys. See *Chlamydia.*

psittacosis-lymphogranuloma organisms See *Chlamydia.*

Psoregates simplex See *arthropod parasites,* under *rat.*

psycho- A combining form denoting relationship to the psyche, or to the mind.

psychobiology That branch of biology which considers the interactions between body and mind in the formation and functioning of personality; the scientific study of the personality function.

psychology That branch of science which treats of the mind and mental operations, especially as they are shown in behavior.

  abnormal p., the study of derangements or deviations of mental functions.

  analytical p., psychology by introspective methods, as opposed to experimental psychology.

  animal p., the study of the mental activity of animals. See also *ethology.*

  behavioristic p., see *behaviorism.*

  child p., the study of the development of the mind of the child.

  cognitive p., that branch of psychology which deals with the human mind as it receives and interprets impressions from the external world.

  comparative p., the study of the mental action of animals. See also *ethology.*

  constitutional p., the relation of the psychology of the individual to the morphology and physiology of his body.

  criminal p., the study of the mentality, the motivation, and the social behavior of criminals.

  depth p., the psychology of the unconscious; psychoanalysis.

  dynamic p., psychology which stresses the element of energy in mental processes.

  experimental p., the study of the mind and mental operations by the employment of experimental methods.

  genetic p., that branch of psychology which deals with the development of mind in the individual and with its evolution in the race.

  gestalt p., see *gestaltism.*

  hormic p., psychology which asserts that active striving toward a goal is a fundamental category of psychology.

  physiologic p., psychology which applies the facts taught in neurology to show the relation between the mental and the neural.

  social p., psychology which treats of the social aspects of mental life.

psychopathology The pathology of mental disorders; the branch of medicine which deals with the causes and nature of mental disease.

psychosis Formerly, a generic name for any mental disorder. Specifically, the deeper, more far-reaching and prolonged behavior disorders, as schizophrenia and manic-depressive psychosis.

  affective p., a functional emotional psychosis; manic-depressive psychosis.

  alcoholic p., mental disorder in which excessive use of alcohol is the chief etiologic factor. See *Korsakoff's p.*

  Cheyne-Stokes p., a condition resembling cardiac asthma, with intense motor agitation, sometimes seen along with the onset of Cheyne-Stokes respiration in chronic heart disease.

  circular p., properly, the circular type of manic-depressive psychosis, that type in which there is no free interval between the manic and depressive reactions.

  depressive p., a psychosis characterized by states of mental depression, melancholy, despondency, inadequacy, and feelings of guilt.

  drug p., a toxic psychosis due to the ingestion of drugs.

  epileptic p., psychosis occurring in a person suffering from epilepsy.

  exhaustion p., mental disorder due to some exhausting or depressing occurrence, as an operation.

  functional p., a psychosis in which organic disease or dysfunction does not play a part.

  gestational p., a psychosis developing during pregnancy.

  idiophrenic p., organic p.

  involutional p., mental disorder occurring in or about the middle years of life, believed to be associated with the climacteric changes, and characterized by agitation, depression, self-condemnatory trends, and sometimes by paranoid reactions.

  Korsakoff's p., a psychosis which is usually based on chronic alcoholism, and which is accompanied by disturbance of orientation, susceptibility to external stimulation and suggestion, falsification of memory, and hallucinations. The signs of polyneuritis (wristdrop, etc.) are usually present. Called also polyneuritic psychosis, cerebropathia psychia toxaemica, and chronic alcoholic delirium.

manic p., a psychosis characterized by marked emotional instability.

manic-depressive p., an essentially benign, affective psychosis, chiefly marked by emotional instability, striking mood swings, and a tendency to recurrence. It is seen in the manic, depressed, circular, mixed, perplexed, and stuporous types.

organic p., a psychosis due to a lesion of the central nervous system, such as general paresis.

paranoic p., a psychosis in which the patient has delusions that others are plotting to injure him.

periodic p., a condition in which intermittent periods of depression or hypomania recur regularly in a seemingly mentally healthy or nearly healthy individual.

polyneuritic p., Korsakoff's p.

prison p., any psychosis for which prison environment has been a precipitating factor.

puerperal p., any psychotic state occurring during pregnancy or following childbirth.

purpose p., a psychotic state motivated by a clear-cut wish, such as a wish to appear insane and therefore not responsible.

schizoaffective p., a psychotic state characterized by mixed schizophrenic and manic-depressive symptoms.

senile p., one of the several forms of mental deterioration in old age in which the patient shows a tendency to confabulation, loss of memory of recent events, irritability, and assaultiveness.

situational p., a transitory mental disorder caused by an unbearable situation over which the patient has no control.

toxic p., a psychosis due to the ingestion of toxic agents (e.g., alcohol, opium) or to presence of toxins within the body.

zoophil p., a psychosis marked by abnormal affection for or interest in animals.

psychrophilic Fond of cold; said of bacteria which develop best between 15° and 20° C. See also *mesophilic,* and *thermophilic.*

psychrophobia Abnormal dread of cold.

pterygote Belonging to the group of insects Pterygota, which are either winged, or have winged ancestors. See also *insect.*

puberty See table of reproductive data, under *mammal,* for the age at which various animals reach puberty.

puff adder See table accompanying *snake.*

pullet A young female chicken (*Gallus gallus*).

pullorum (bacillary white diarrhea of chicks) An intestinal disease of chicks and poults characterized by diarrhea and septicemia and caused by *Salmonella pullorum.* The disease is highly contagious, and death causes severe losses in flocks of young birds. It is vertically transmitted through the egg.

pulmonary adenocarcinoma See under *adenocarcinoma.*

pulmonary nematodiasis See under *nematodiasis.*

punishment In behavioral science, the presentation of an aversive stimulus following the occurrence of a conditioned response.

puromycin An antibiotic produced by a species of *Streptomyces,* which inhibits protein synthesis because of its activity as a structural analog of aminoacyl-sRNA. Because puromycin inhibits protein synthesis at a step probably shared by all living cells, it has a broad range of activity and as expected is far too toxic for use as a systemic antibiotic. It is highly nephrotoxic, and the lesion seen in the kidneys of rats is of interest as a model for the study of the nephrotic syndrome of man.[36, 49]

purple brood A condition of the unsealed brood of honeybees that have foraged on the southern leatherwood, *Cyrilla racemiflora,* in which the brood turns purple and dies. Poisoned purple brood usually appears in early summer.

purple-faced langur *Presbytis senex.* See *primate.*

purposive See under *behavior.*

PVM Pneumonia virus of mice.

pygmy goat A small goat of about 26 kg. used in studies of reproduction and cardiovascular physiology.

pyo- A combining form denoting relationship to pus.

pyocyanine A blue pigment produced by *Pseudomonas aeruginosa,* which was described as long ago as 1899 and found to inhibit the growth of gram-positive and gram-negative bacteria. It has a complex mode of action but appears to act primarily on oxidative metabolism by interference with the terminal electron transport system because of its high affinity for reduced flavoprotein.[36, 49]

pyro- A combining form meaning fire or heat or, in chemistry, produced by heating.

pyrolagnia Sexual gratification from witnessing or making fires.

pyroninophilia A marked affinity for pyronine, observed in cells with active endoplasmic reticulum because of the staining characteristics of the RNA contained in ribosomes. Examples of pyroninophilic cells are plasma cells, fibroblasts, and other actively growing cells.

pyronin Y A basic dye of the xanthine group. Solubility at 15° C.: water 9 per cent, absolute alcohol 0.5 per cent, and glycerol 3 per cent. It is used with methyl green for staining gonococci, as a differential stain for DNA, and with alphanaphthol for staining granules in blood cells.[57]

pyrrolopyrimidin riboside A class of cytotoxic antibiotics produced by species of *Streptomyces,* which include tubercidin, toyocamycin, and sangivamycin. Their mechanism of activity is not well understood but they appear to be incorporated into cellular RNA and perhaps DNA, where they may function as competitive analogs of the normal components of nucleotides.[36, 49]

pyruvic kinase An enzyme of the Embden-Meyerhof pathway that converts phosphoenolpyruvate to pyruvate, using ADP, Mg^{++}, and K^+ as co-factors.

Q

quail   See *Japanese quail.*
quartan malaria   See *malaria.*
Quaternary   Denoting the most recent of Cenozoic periods. See *geologic time divisions.*

quotidian malaria   See *malaria.*

R

rabbit   A mammal of the order Lagomorpha, family Leporidae. The family consists of nine genera and fifty species, which inhabit the major land masses and some islands. They were also introduced by settlers into Australia and New Zealand. Rabbits are not sharply separated from hares, and the terms are used as though they were synonymous. But rabbits are born naked, blind, and helpless in a fur-lined nest, whereas hares are born fully haired, with open eyes.

The typical rabbit is the European *Oryctolagus cuniculus*, also known as the Belgian hare or domestic laboratory rabbit. It was originally from Central Europe (north of the Mediterranean), Ireland, Western Russia, and North Africa. There are many domesticated varieties of the European rabbit, such as the Flemish giant, New Zealand white, silver gray, chinchilla, Havana, American blue, Polish, Dutch belted, and Angora.

The cottontail rabbit, *Sylvilagus*, is found in North and South America. The marsh cottontail (*S. palustris*) and the swamp cottontail (*S. aqualticus*) are found in southeastern United States, *S. floridanus* in the United States east of the Rockies southward to Costa Rica, Nutall's cottontail (*S. nuttallii*) from southern Canada to central Arizona, and Audubon's cottontail (*S. aubonii*) from Montana to central Mexico.

Rabbits are of economic importance: their fur is used in the fur industry; their flesh, which is low in cholesterol, has an excellent taste; and they are easily reared in captivity.

They are widely used in research, especially *Oryctolagus cuniculus;* some of the more favored breeds are the New Zealand white, New Zealand red, and Dutch belted rabbit.

Parasites of rabbits: The accompanying tables list the more common arthropod and helminth parasites of the domestic laboratory rabbit.

rabbit papilloma   See *Shope papilloma,* under *papilloma.*

rabbit pox (rabbit plague)   A highly infectious poxvirus infection of laboratory rabbits seen clinically in two forms: a peracute fulminating disease without significant gross lesions, and a milder, acute disease with skin lesions (pocks) typical of poxvirus infections. The peracute form is seen in highly susceptible rabbits and is associated with high morbidity and mortality. Death comes before secondary and tertiary crops of virus reach the skin, hence it has been called pockless rabbit pox, or in Europe, rabbit plague. Spontaneous infections are confined to the rabbit, but experimental infections can be induced in the guinea pig foot pad, chick embryo CAM, and tissue cultures.

The milder form is characterized by enlargement of superficial lymph nodes, a macular rash followed by the development of papules, subcutaneous edema, and keratitis with ulceration of the cornea. Vesicles and pustules do not form. In both the peracute and the acute form, pneumonia is the usual cause of death and is the sole constant lesion in pockless rabbit pox. Inclusion bodies are

COMMON ARTHROPOD PARASITES OF THE DOMESTIC LABORATORY (*Oryctolagus*) RABBIT

COMMON NAME	SPECIES	TYPE	LOCATION ON HOST
Sticktight flea	*Echidnophaga gallinacea*	Insect	Face
Wolves or warble	*Cuterebra cuniculi*	Larval insect	Subcutaneous tissue
Ear mange mite	*Psoroptes cuniculi*	Acarid	External auditory meatus
Ear mange mite	*Chorioptes cuniculi*	Acarid	External auditory meatus
Body mange mite	*Sarcoptes scabei (cuniculi)*	Acarid	In the skin
Body mange mite	*Notoedres minor (cuniculi)*	Acarid	In the skin
Louse, rabbit	*Haemodipsus rentricosus*	Insect	On body surface
flea, rabbit	*Spilopsyllus cuniculi*	Insect	On body surface
Fur mite	*Cheyletiella parasitovorax*	Acarid	On hairs
Fur mite	*Listrophorus gibbus*	Acarid	On hairs

Common Helminth Parasites of the Domestic Laboratory (*Oryctolagus*) Rabbit

COMMON NAME	SPECIES	LOCATION IN HOST
	NEMATODES	
Stomach worm	*Obeliscoides cuniculi*	Stomach
Pinworm	*Passalurus ambiguus*	Cecum and colon
Whipworm	*Trichuris lipuris*	Cecum
Lungworm	*Synthetocaulus* spp.	Bronchi
Stomach worm	*Graphidium strigosum*	Stomach
Trichostrongylid	*Trichostrongylus retortaeformis*	Duodenum
	CESTODES	
– – –	*Cysticercus pisiformis* (larval form of *Taenia pisiformis*)	Serosal peritoneum
– – –	*Coenuris serialis* (larval form of *T. serialis*)	Subcutaneous tissue
Tapeworm	*Cittotaenia denticulata*	Small intestine
Tapeworm	*C. pectinata*	Small intestine
Tapeworm	*Hymenolepis diminuata*	Small intestine

seen infrequently in rabbit infections, although they occur in abundance on chick embryo CAM preparations.

Diagnosis is based on clinical signs supported by serologic detection of antibody against vaccinia. The virus is a typical member of the antigenic subgroup of poxviruses that includes variola (smallpox), mouse ectromelia, vaccinia, and rabbit pox. Rabbits may be immunized against rabbit pox with vaccinia virus. Epizootics in the United States in the 1930's were typically of the milder form; those since World War II have been of the peracute pockless type.

rabbit syphilis (vent disease)   Spirochetosis.

rabies (hydrophobia)   A viral disease with an extremely wide spectrum of susceptible hosts, including man and all species of domestic animals. The species most commonly affected in the United States are the dog, the fox, and the skunk. It is transmitted in the saliva, usually from the bite of an infected animal, although aerosol transmission has been demonstrated experimentally in bat caves. Many species of bats are able to harbor the rabies virus without severe illness, but can transmit it to man and anomen. This was first noted in cattle of Trinidad, which became infected from the bites of blood-sucking vampire bats.[114, 116, 142]

racemase   An enzyme in various bacteria that catalyzes the racemization of a mixture of dextro- and levo-lactic acid.

Radfordia affinis   See *arthropod parasites*, under *rat*.

Radiation Research Society   The American University, Washington, D.C. 20016.

radio-   A combining form denoting relationship to radiation; sometimes used with specific reference to the emission of radiant energy, to radium, or to the radius. It is also affixed to the name of a chemical element to designate a radioactive isotope of that particular element, as radiocarbon, radioiodine, etc.

radioautography   Autoradiography.

radiobiology   That branch of science which is concerned with the effect of light and of ultraviolet and ionizing radiations upon living tissues or organisms.

radiocarcinogenesis   Cancer formation caused by exposure to radiation.

radiochroism   The capacity of a substance to absorb certain radioactive and roentgen rays.

radioisotope   An isotope which is radioactive, produced artificially from the element or from a stable isotope of the element by the action of neutrons, protons, deuterons, or alpha particles in the chain-reacting pile or in the cyclotron. Radioisotopes are used as tracers or indicators by being added to the stable compound under observation, so that the course of the latter in the body can be detected and followed by the radioactivity thus added to it. The stable element so treated is said to be "labeled" or "tagged."

radiolesion   A lesion caused by exposure to radiation.

radiology   The science of radiant energy and radiant substances, especially that branch of medical science which deals with the use of radiant energy in the diagnosis and treatment of disease. Cf. *roentgenology*.

radiolucent   Permitting the passage of radiant energy, such as x-rays, yet offering some resistance to it, the representative areas appearing dark on the exposed film.

radiomimetic   Exerting effects similar to those of ionizing radiation; said of a chemical or infectious agent that mimics effects of radiation such as destruction of lymphoid tissue and leukopenia. These agents include chemicals such as nitrogen mustards and purine analogs, and infections such as feline panleukopenia and hog cholera.

radiomutation   Change in the genetic character of cells caused by exposure to radiation.

radionecrosis   Destruction of tissue or ulceration caused by radiant energy.

radiopaque   Not permitting the passage of

radiant energy, such as x-rays, the representative areas appearing light or white on the exposed film.

radioparent Radiotransparent.

radiopathology Pathology having to do with the effects of radiation on tissues.

radiophobia Morbid anxiety about the damaging effects of x-rays and radium.

radiotransparent (radioparent) Permitting the passage of roentgen rays or of other forms of radiation.

radula The horny strip in the mouth of a mollusk used for rasping food.

random breeding See *breeding system.*

ranikhet See *Newcastle disease.*

raptorial Predatory, or adapted for seizing prey.

rat A small rodent of the genus *Rattus* and related genera of the family Muridae. There are about 570 named forms which are widely distributed throughout the world, but the majority live in tropical southeastern Asia and in Africa. There are two common types: the Alexandrine black rat (*R. rattus*), which inhabits Asia Minor and the Orient and weighs 115 to 350 gm., and the Norway rat (*R. norvegicus*), which is usually brown, inhabits Europe, the United States, Japan, and possibly eastern Asia, and weighs from 200 to 485 gm.

Rats are aggressive, omnivorous, adaptable, and very successful as biological organisms. The standard research rats are albino mutants of *R. norvegicus* that have been laboratory bred since the early 1900's. Breed names (now called stocks) are generally assigned to the various original sources, e.g., Sprague-Sawley, Wistar, Holtzman, etc. Long-Evans rats, piebald or hooded mutants of *R. norvegicus*, are also widely used in research. A number of characterized inbred strains are available.

Another family, Cricetidae, also includes many rodents which are called rats, e.g., the cotton rat, rice rat, brush rat, bamboo or root rat, and the kangaroo rat.

Arthropod and helminth parasites. Arthropods and helminths are among the parasites whose life cycles are most easily interrupted by gnotobiotic technology, and for this reason they are unimportant as parasites of SPF rodent colonies. They are, however, important in conventional rodent colonies. In the accompanying two tables, the rat and mouse are considered together as hosts of these parasites because of the considerable degree of overlap in specificity.[21, 27]

Protozoan parasites. See table on page 176 for the more common protozoan parasites of the rat (*Rattus norvegicus*) and the mouse (*Mus musculus*), which are considered together because of the overlap in specificity.

African white-tailed r., a species of rat, *Mystomys albicaudatus,* which has the longest life-span (four years) of any common laboratory rodent. It is relatively free of disease and adapts well to cage environment.

rat mammary fibroadenoma See *mammary fibroadenoma R2737,* under *fibroadenoma.*

rattlesnake See table accompanying *snake.*

rat unit The highest dilution of an estrus-producing hormone (estrin) which, when given to a mature spayed rat in three injections at four-hour intervals, during the first day will produce cornification and desquamation of the vaginal epithelium.

Rauscher leukemia virus A lymphoid leukemia virus originally found in spontaneous leukemia in a BALB/c mouse. When subjected to passage, it induced lymphoid leukemia and an erythrocytic disease in both young and adult BALB/c, DBA/2, Swiss, C3H, CFW, PRI, C57B1, and AKR mice, and in Osborne-Mendel rats. Young mice injected intraperitoneally develop symptoms as early as six days after inoculation, a palpable spleen in 12 days, and die in 25 to 50 days in 80 to 100 per cent of cases. The virus may be carried, without cytopathogenic effect, in BALB/c cell cultures.[114]

ray A cartilaginous fish of the chordate class Chondrichthyes. All forms are marine. Examples include the eagle ray, *Myliobatus freminvellei,* the butterfly ray, *Pteroplatea,* the electric ray, *Torpedo californica,* the round sting ray, *Urolophus halleri,* and the giant manta ray, or devilfish, *Manta.* See also *cartilaginous fish.*

ARTHROPOD PARASITES OF THE RAT AND MOUSE

PARASITE	COMMON NAME	HOST	LOCATION IN HOST
Leptopsylla segnis	Flea	Mouse	On skin
Nasopsyllus fasciatus	Flea	Rat, mouse	On skin
Ctenophthalmus agyrtes	Flea	Rat, mouse	On skin
Xenopsylla cheopis	Indian rat flea	Rat	In skin
*Polyplax serrata**	Sucking louse	Mouse	On skin
*P. spinulosa**	Sucking louse	Rat	On skin
Hoplopleura eonomydis	Sucking louse	Rat	On skin
Echinolaelaps echidninus	Mite	Rat	On skin
*Myobia musculi**	Fur mite	Mouse	On hairs
Psorergates simplex	Follicle mite	Mouse	Sudermal cysts
Radfordia affinis	Fur mite	Mouse	On hairs
*Myocoptes musculinus**	Fur mite	Mouse	On hairs
M. romboutsi	Fur mite	Mouse	On hairs
Notoedres muris	Mange mite	Rat	In skin
Ornithonyssus bacoti	Tropical rat mite	Rat, mouse	On skin (for feeding)

Helminth Parasites of the Rat and Mouse

Parasite	Common Name	Host	Location in Host
	CESTODES		
Hymenolepis diminuata*	Tapeworm	Rat, mouse	Ileum
Hymenolepis nana*	Dwarf worm	Rat, mouse	Ileum
Oochoristica ratti	Tapeworm	Rat, mouse	Ileum
Cysticercus (Taenia) fasciolaris	Bladder worm†	Rat, mouse	Liver
Coenurus (Taenia) serialis	Bladder worm†	Rat, mouse	Subcutaneous tissue
	NEMATODES		
Heterakis spumosa	Pinworm	Rat,	Cecum, colon
Aspicularis tetraptera*	Pinworm	Rat, mouse	Cecum, colon
Syphacia obvelata*	Pinworm	Rat, mouse	Cecum, colon
Trichinella spiralis	– – –	Rat	Muscle
Capillaria hepatica	– – –	Rat, mouse	Liver
Trichosomoides crassicauda*	Bladder worm	Rat	Urinary bladder
Nippostrongylus muris	Strongyle	Rat, mouse	Small intestine
Angiostrongylus cantonensis	Lung worm	Rat	Pulmonary arteries
Gongylonema neoplasticum	– – –	Rat, mouse	Tongue, esophagus
	ACANTHOCEPHALA		
Moniliformis moniliformis	Thorny-headed worm	Rat, mouse	Small intestine

*Most common as parasites of conventional rodent colonies.
†Larval forms.

Protozoan Parasites of the Rat and Mouse

Species	Host	Size	Location in Host
	NONPATHOGENIC		
Balantidium coli	Rat, mouse	30–200 μ	Cecum, colon
Cryptosporidium muris	Mouse	7 μ	Stomach
C. parvum*	Mouse	4 μ	Small intestine
Chilomastix bettencourti	Rat, mouse	10–15 μ	Colon
Endolinas nana	Rat	8–10 μ	Colon
Entamoeba muris	Rat	9–19 μ	Cecum
Giardia muris	Rat, mouse	– – –	Small intestine, cecum
Hexamita muris	Rat, mouse	4.8 μ	Small intestine, cecum
Isodamoeba buetschlii	Rat	7–15 μ	Colon
Klossiella muris*	Mouse	– – –	Kidney
Sarcocystis muris	Rat, mouse	15 μ	Muscle
Trypanosoma duttoni	Mouse	25 μ	Blood
T. lewisi	Mouse	25 μ	Blood
	PATHOGENICITY UNKNOWN		
Eimeria carinii	Rat	– – –	Small intestine, cecum, colon
E. halli	Rat	– – –	Small intestine, cecum, colon
E. hasei	Rat	– – –	Small intestine, cecum, colon
E. hindlei	Mouse	– – –	Small intestine, cecum, colon
E. keilini	Mouse	– – –	Small intestine, cecum, colon
E. krijgsmanni	Mouse	– – –	Small intestine, cecum, colon
E. musculi	Mouse	– – –	Small intestine, cecum, colon
E. nochti	Rat	– – –	Small intestine, cecum, colon
E. ratti	Rat	– – –	Small intestine, cecum, colon
E. schueffneri	Mouse	– – –	Small intestine, cecum, colon
E. separata	Rat	– – –	Small intestine, cecum, colon
	PATHOGENIC		
Eimeria falciformis	Mouse	– – –	Small intestine, cecum, colon
E. miyarii	Rat	– – –	Small intestine, cecum, colon
E. nieschulzi	Rat	– – –	Small intestine, cecum, colon
Eperythrozoon coccoides*	Rat, mouse	0.5 μ	Erythrocytes, RES
Hepatozoon muris	Rat, mouse	30 μ	Liver
Nosema cuniculi*	Rat, mouse	2–3 μ	CNS, kidney
Pneumocystis carinii	Rat	– – –	Lung
Toxoplasma cuniculi	Rat, mouse	4–7 μ	CNS, reticuloendothelial system (RES)

*Important parasites of laboratory animals.

176

reaction   See *response.*

recapitulation   The theory, first propounded by Haeckel, that during embryonic development each individual passes through the stages of its evolution, i.e., ontogeny recapitulates phylogeny.

recombination   Random independent assortment of genes which results in progeny with a mixture of parental characters.

recovery   See *spontaneous recovery.*

red blood cell count   Determination of the number of red blood cells in a measured volume of blood. See *hemogram.*

red muscardine   This term has been used to denote various mycoses of insects, caused by species of hyphomycetous fungi and characterized by the appearance of pink to brick-red colors on the body of the dying or dead hosts. Certain strains of *Beauveria bassiana* are responsible for red muscardine of silkworm larvae. *Sorosporella uvella* causes red muscardine of cutworm larvae (*Noctuidae*) as well as other insects. Unlike the true muscardine fungi (see *muscardine*), *S. uvella* does not produce fruiting bodies and spores on the exterior of the insect.

reductase   An enzyme that has a reducing action on chemical compounds; a dehydrogenase.

    acetaldehyde r., an enzyme that catalyzes the reduction of acetaldehyde to alcohol. It consists of a protein and a prosthetic group, nicotinamide adenine dinucleotide.

    cytochrome r., an enzyme that catalyzes the simultaneous oxidation of nicotinamide adenine dinucleotide phosphate and the reduction of cytochrome C.

    Schardinger's r., a reductase in milk that reduces methylene blue, especially in the presence of formaldehyde.

reductionism   The attitude now so common that biological phenomena can be thoroughly explained by molecules, valence bonds, and pathways, an idea which must be tempered by an appreciation of the interplay of all the complexities of chemistry and environment as they are reflected in cellular and organismal events.

refaunation   Reintroduction of mutualistic fauna in a host deprived of such fauna. See also *mutualism, defaunate, infaunate,* and *transfaunation.*

reflex   1. A reflected action or movement; the sum total of any particular involuntary activity. 2. In behavioral science, any correlation between a stimulus and a response; stimulus-response correlation. Also a stimulus-response correlation that is observable in all members of a species under a given set of conditions.

reflex response   The occurrence of a reflex (q.v.).

reflex sensitization   A reflex response which occurs as a reaction to a stimulus other than that which had originally elicited it and with which the reflex stimulus had not been paired.

regional enteritis   Regional ileitis; see under *ileitis.*

regional ileitis   See *regional ileitis* and *terminal ileitis of hamsters,* under *ileitis.*

registry   A central agency for the collection of pathologic material and related clinical, laboratory, x-ray, and other data in a specified field of pathology, so organized that the data can be properly processed and made available for study.

Registry of Comparative Pathology   A section of the American Registry of Pathology at the Armed Forces Institute of Pathology, Washington, D.C., for the collection and documentation of animal diseases, especially as they relate to the study of human disease.

regression   1. A return to a former or earlier state. 2. A subsidence of symptoms or of a disease process. 3. In biology, the tendency in successive generations toward mediocrity. 4. In behavioral science, the reappearance, during experimental extinction, of responses which had been extinguished prior to the introduction of the conditioned response undergoing extinction. Also the occurrence of a previously acquired conditioned response after punishment for a conditioned response more recently induced.

regulator gene   A gene that controls the rate of synthesis of other genes. See *gene.*

reinforcement   In behavioral science, the presentation of a reinforcing stimulus such as food to an animal after it has made a response, provided that it can be demonstrated that the use of the reinforcement produces a modification in behavior under the stated conditions. See *reinforcing stimulus,* under *stimulus.*

    aperiodic r., see *schedules of r.*

    continuous r., see *schedules of r.*

    differential r., the reinforcement of a response when it occurs in the presence of one stimulus and the withholding of reinforcement when the response occurs in the presence of another stimulus. See *discrimination training.*

    fixed interval r., see *schedules of r.*

    fixed ratio r., see *schedules of r.*

    heterogeneous r., the phenomenon in which a reinforcing stimulus evokes a response other than that being reinforced.

    homogeneous r., reinforcement in which the reinforcing stimulus evokes a response identical with the response being reinforced.

    irrelevant r., reinforcement in which a reinforcing stimulus is presented that is not directly related to, nor involved in, the drive-reducing operations antecedent to reinforcement (e.g., when food is removed from the subject animal and the response being conditioned is followed by the presentation of water).

    intermittent r., see *schedules of r.*

    partial r., see *schedules of r.*

    periodic r., see *schedules of r.*

    primary r., the use of a reinforcing stimulus that is effective when presented to any animal of a given species without special training.

    random r., see *schedules of r.*

regular r., see *schedules of r.*

relevant r., the employment of a reinforcing stimulus that is directly related to the drive-reduction operation antecedent to conditioning.

schedules of r., specific plans utilized by the experimenter to determine which of a series of responses will be reinforced. Some of the most common reinforcement schedules are: (1) continuous or regular reinforcement: the procedure of reinforcing a response each time it occurs; (2) intermittent (partial) reinforcement: any of several procedures in which a response is reinforced only on some of its occurrences; (3) fixed interval (periodic) reinforcement: a schedule of intermittent reinforcement in which reinforcement stimuli are delivered or withheld according to a regular time schedule; (4) variable interval (aperiodic or random) reinforcement: a schedule in which reinforcement stimuli are delivered according to a predetermined but irregular time schedule; (5) fixed ratio reinforcement: a schedule in which every *n*th instance of the response is reinforced; (6) variable ratio reinforcement: a schedule in which the response, on the average every *n*th instance of occurrence, is reinforced; (7) multiple schedule: a schedule in which reinforcement stimuli are programmed according to two or more schedules in alternation (e.g., a certain schedule is followed through an interval during which a discriminative stimulus is presented; at the end of this interval the first schedule is followed but with a different reinforcement presented in association with a different discriminative stimulus. This second stimulus is then used for a period of time and then there is a return to the first discriminative stimulus.); (8) tandem schedule: a schedule in which single reinforcements are delivered according to two schedules acting in succession.

secondary r., reinforcement which, initially ineffective, becomes effective when the stimulus is presented contiguously in time with another reinforcing stimulus that is effective.

variable interval r., see *schedules of r.*
variable ratio r., see *schedules of r.*
reinforcer A reinforcing stimulus.
reinforcing stimulus See under *stimulus.*
releaser A sign stimulus (q.v.) produced by the physical structure or behavior of an animal that releases or stimulates a particular species-specific response in another animal. Often referred to as a social response.
releasing mechanism See *innate releasing mechanism.*
remiges The large flight feathers of a bird's wing, including both primaries and secondaries.
renal adenocarcinoma See under *adenocarcinoma.*
reovirus A double-stranded ribovirus which measures about 75 mμ in diameter and was originally classified as echovirus.[64] See *classification*, under *virus.*

reovirus-3 (encephalomyocarditis virus, EMC virus, Mengo virus) A virus that causes an important and apparently widespread infection in laboratory mouse stocks, originally called the encephalomyocarditis virus and also the AHA, or ascites hepatitis agent of Nelson. Spontaneous epizootics are common in breeding colonies, in which mice 10 to 14 days of age are found to be stunted, diarrheal, occasionally jaundiced, and with oily hair. These outbreaks are most commonly associated with first-litter dams, which may also become stained with the steatorrheic feces. Lesions include peritoneal exudate, pneumonia, hepatitis, pancreatitis, myocarditis, and encephalitis. Degeneration of islets of Langerhans and diabetes have also been reported. While morbidity is high, mortality is low. Adult mice are resistant to symptomatic expression. Diagnosis is established by the characteristic clinical signs, lesions, and serologic evidence of reovirus-3 infection. It must be differentiated from EDIM and LIVIM virus infection (see *infantile diarrhea of mice*). The virus may also cause conjunctivitis in cats.[27, 63]

replication 1. Repetition of an experiment to ensure accuracy. 2. The multiplication of organisms and cells by asexual means, as replication of virus within cells. See under *virus.*

repressible enzyme An enzyme the production of which can be repressed by certain metabolites.

repression See *enzyme repression.*

reproduction See table of reproductive data, accompanying *mammal.*

reservoir host See under *host.*

residual body A membrane-bound cellular inclusion containing undigested residues such as membrane fragments and ferritin-like particles. It can develop from either autophagic or heterophagic vacuoles.[33]

resolving power The degree to which a magnifying system is able to distinguish two adjacent objects as being separate. The light microscope can resolve about 0.2μ (2000 Å) and the electron microscope about 0.5 mμ (5 Å).

respiratory disease Any disease of the respiratory system.

chronic r. d. of chickens (CRD), an infectious respiratory disease of chicks caused by *Mycoplasma gallisepticum* and characterized by tracheal rales, nasal discharge, and coughing.

chronic r. d., murine (CRD), a clinical syndrome of laboratory rats and mice with a complex etiology, characterized by slow insidious onset and a protracted course. It embraces pulmonary disease (enzootic bronchiectasis or chronic murine pneumonia), upper respiratory infection (infectious catarrh), and middle ear involvement (murine otitis media or labyrinthitis). The weight of experimental evidence appears to indict both a respiratory virus and a species of *Mycoplasma* (either of which is necessary and sufficient) as the triggering agents in the pulmonary aspects, and several Mycoplasma species as the incitants of the upper respiratory and middle ear symptomatology.

Several genera of bacteria have been associated with CRD as secondary invaders and are considered important in the expression of the disease. These bacteria include *Corynebacterium kutscheri, Streptobacillus moniliformis, Bordetella bronchiseptica,* and *Pasteurella pneumotropica,* as well as streptococci and a variety of unidentified gram-negative rods.

This disease more than any other—because of its prevalence in rat and mouse colonies and the degree to which it has impeded research workers using them—provided the impetus that culminated in the large-scale application of gnotobiotic technology for disease exclusion that now characterizes most modern rodent production and research facilities. The implicit assumption, which has proved so successful, is that if the neonates are removed by hysterectomy, taken directly to pathogen-free quarters, and maintained within them, they will remain free of infectious disease. In practice, however, it is still not possible to eliminate completely mycoplasma and viruses from these animals.[27, 86] See also *mycoplasmosis* and *gnotobiote.*

feline r. d., respiratory disease of cats. Respiratory diseases pose one of the most serious obstacles to successful maintenance of laboratory cats. Several agents, none of which is well characterized, appear to be involved. These are (1) picornaviruses of several serotypes, which may eventually be placed in the rhinovirus group; (2) herpesviruses, one serotype of which causes recurrent feline rhinotracheitis (FVR) of Crandell; (3) reoviruses, which cause conjunctivitis; and (4) *Miyagawanella* (Chlamydia group), a possible cause of pneumonia.

respondent Those parts of behavior for which eliciting stimuli are identified.

respondent behavior See under *behavior.*

respondent response See *respondent.*

response In behavioral science, any of those types of behavior or parts of behavior that can be observed to vary together systematically as a function of time or other environmental variables. In order to be placed in a particular class or identified as an instance of a given response, they must be objectively identified and measured, so that appropriately trained observers can recognize them without disagreement when they occur. Some responses are identified in terms of specific movements (topography) and others in terms of their effect on the environment.

amplitude of r., a quantitative measure of one dimension of a response, such as quantity of saliva or amplitude of an eye blink.

backward conditioned r., see *conditioned r.*

conditioned r., a response that appears or is modified because of conditioning. Several types of conditioned responses have been observed, including *backward conditioned r.:* a conditioned response stimulated by classical conditioning when the unconditioned stimulus precedes the conditioned stimulus (there is some controversy as to whether this is possible); *delayed conditioned r.:* that which is stimulated by classical conditioning when the interval between the conditioned stimulus and the unconditioned stimulus is greater than several seconds; *simultaneous conditioned r.:* that which is developed by classical conditioning when the interval between the conditioned stimulus and the unconditioned stimulus ranges from zero to several seconds, and when the conditioned and unconditioned stimuli overlap in time; *trace conditioned r.:* that which is stimulated by classical conditioning when an interval of several seconds intervenes between the conditioned stimulus and the unconditioned stimulus.

consummatory r., see *consummatory act.*

delayed conditioned r., see *conditioned r.*

equivalence r. (response generalization), a response that is the equivalent of another response but is not identical in its manifestations; even though the responses differ topographically, they have the same result on the environment (e.g., a rat may press a bar with the nose or with the foot; although the responses differ topographically, they are subclasses of the same response).

goal r., the response given to a reinforcing stimulus.

incompatibility r., if the occurrence of one response makes impossible or highly improbable the simultaneous occurrence of a second response the two are considered mutually incompatible.

intensity of r., the degree of change in magnitude or topography of a response to a constant stimulus which has been increased in intensity. Thus a response may be called a low-intensity response when in actuality it is an incomplete response (e.g., a light shined in the eye may stimulate a response of blinking, but if a brighter light is then used, the response may be more intense or may differ in topography, as in squinting, secretion of tears, etc.).

latency of r., the time elapsed between the beginning of a stimulus and the commencement of the response to it.

learning r., see under *learning.*

magnitude of r., any of several descriptive measures of a response instance, including amplitude or duration, velocity, and frequency.

measurement of r., assignment of quantitative value to responses or response instances, including such measurements as extinction, resistance, amplitude of response, intensity of response, latency of response, magnitude of response, etc.

operant r., see *operant.*

pattern of r., topography.

probability of r., the relative frequency of a response measured over a number of trials in situations in which one of several responses may be given.

rate of r., the number of response instances occurring within a specified unit of time.

reflex r., the occurrence of a reflex (q.v.).

respondent r., see *respondent.*

ritualized r., a response that appears in most members of a species, is relatively constant in topography, and is usually a social releaser.

simultaneous conditioned r., see *conditioned r.*

species-specific r., a response that is part of species-specific behavior; see under *behavior.*

strength of r., a measure of a response as compared to measures of the same response at other times and under other conditions.

superstitious r., see *superstition.*

threshold of r. (threshold of reaction), minimal value of a stimulus that will evoke a response. See *threshold stimulus.*

topography of r., see *topography.*

trace conditioned r., see *conditioned r.*

unconditioned r., a regular and measurable response elicited by an unconditioned stimulus.

Reticuloendothelial Society   Department of Biology, Bryn Mawr College, Bryn Mawr, Pa. 19010.

reticulum cell sarcoma 8469 (transferable liver neoplasm; polymorphous-celled sarcoma; reticuloendotheliosis; monocytoma; histiocytoma)   A spontaneous tumor arising in the abdominal organs (exclusive of the spleen) of an 18-month-old female hybrid (C57 × A) mouse in the laboratory of Dunn at the National Cancer Institute in 1948. It was transplanted subcutaneously into other F_1 mice of the same cross and has since been propagated in them with an average transplant interval of 100 days. Subcutaneous transplants generally become disseminated to various organs, especially the liver, in which it causes enlargement and ascites. It has since been seen to arise spontaneously in various mouse strains.[150]

retinoblastoma   A tumor arising from retinal germ cells; glioma of the retina.

retrices   The large flight feathers of a bird's tail.

reward   An alternative term for positive reinforcing stimulus.

token r., a reinforcing stimulus that was itself once a conditioning stimulus, as an object such as a poker chip which elicits manipulative behavior. If conditioning can be demonstrated as a result of the use of this object as a reinforcing stimulus, the object is termed a token reward.

rhabdo-   A combining form meaning rod-shaped or denoting relationship to a rod.

rhabdomyosarcoma   A malignant tumor containing cells which indicate it has originated from striated muscle.

r. H668, a tumor that arose spontaneously in the intercostal muscles of an untreated BALB/c mouse in the laboratory of K. Hummel at the Jackson Memorial Laboratory. It has been maintained in BALB/c mice, in which the tumor grows without regression in 100 per cent of animals inoculated, becoming palpable in seven days and killing the host within 50 days.[150]

-rhaphy   A word termination meaning joining in a seam, or suturation.

rhea   See *rheiform birds.*

-rhea   A word termination meaning flow.

rheiform birds   Members of the avian order Rheiformes, comprising the rheas, large flightless birds with an unkeeled sternum.

rhesus   A member of *Macaca mulatta;* see *primate.*

-rhexis   A word termination meaning bursting forth or breaking; the rupture of an organ or a vessel.

Rh factor   A red blood cell antigen which can cross the placenta from an Rh-positive fetus and sensitize an Rh-negative mother, resulting in anti-red blood cell antibodies which cause hemolytic anemia in the fetus. A similar condition occurs in the horse, pig, and dog.[76] See also *hemolytic anemia of newborn,* under *anemia.*

rhinitis   See *atrophic rhinitis.*

rhino-, rhin-   Combining form denoting relationship to the nose, or a noselike structure.

rhinocephalia   A developmental anomaly characterized by the presence of a proboscis-like nose above eyes partially or completely fused into one.

rhinoceros viper   See table accompanying *snake.*

rhinopneumonitis   Inflammation of the mucous membranes of the nose and lung.

equine r. (equine virus abortion; equine influenza), a viral disease of horses which usually occurs as a mild acute respiratory infection unless complicated by secondary bacterial invaders. In pregnant mares, however, the virus enters the fetus and causes abortion at about the eighth to eleventh month of gestation. Lesions consist of necrotic foci in the liver, and intranuclear inclusions in liver, lung, spleen, and lymph nodes. The agent is a herpesvirus.[142]

rhinotracheitis   Inflammation of the nasal cavity and trachea.

feline r., see *feline respiratory disease,* under *respiratory disease.*

infectious bovine r. (IBR; necrotic rhinotracheitis; "red nose" disease), an acute contagious respiratory disease of cattle caused by a virus of the herpes group. Infection usually begins with high fever, depression, anorexia, and nasal discharge. The nasal mucous membranes become very inflamed, resulting in the name "red nose."[16]

rhinovirus   Any of a group of viral agents isolated in Salisbury, England, and considered to be etiologically related to the common cold. Several immunological types occur. See also *classification,* under *virus.*

Rhodesian man A fossil subspecies of man who lived in the Pleistocene Epoch.

ribonuclease An enzyme that catalyzes the depolymerization of ribonucleic acid.

ribonucleic acid (RNA) A nucleic acid originally isolated from yeast, but later found in all living cells; on hydrolysis it yields adenine, guanine, cytosine, uracil, ribose, and phosphoric acid. It is usually single stranded except in certain viruses (see *reovirus*). Recently, small amounts of double-stranded RNA have been found in mammalian cells. *Messenger RNA* is an RNA fraction of intermediate molecular weight, with a base ratio corresponding to DNA of the same organism, which transports information from DNA to the protein-forming system of the cell. *Soluble RNA,* or *transfer RNA,* is of low molecular weight (S = 4), existing as 20 species, each of which combines with one amino acid species, transferring it from activating enzyme to ribosome. *Ribosomal RNA* translates the information into protein synthesis.[32, 61, 90] See *gene.*

ribonucleoprotein A macromolecule composed of protein and RNA. An example is the core material of myxovirus (q.v.).

ribonucleotide A compound of a purine or pyrimidine base with ribose and a phosphate group. Ribonucleotides are the monomers that form ribonucleic acid.

ribosome One of the minute granules about 100 to 200 Å in diameter, seen in the cytoplasm of cells. They are the sites of translation in protein synthesis. Ribosomes may be attached to the membrane of the endoplasmic reticulum, which is then called rough ER, may be free in the cytoplasm (free ribosomes), or may be formed into aggregates (polyribosomes or polysomes). They consist of two unequal subunits with sedimentation constants of about 30S and 50S and, when bound together by magnesium ions, have a sedimentation constant of about 70S. Poly-somes, which contain several ribosomes, have sedimentation constants from 100S to much larger values. Ribosomes are about 60 per cent RNA and 40 per cent protein.[90]

ribovirus A group of viruses containing ribonucleic acid as their genetic material. See also *oncogenic RNA viruses,* and see *replication of viruses,* under *virus.*

Rickettsia A group of pleomorphic, coccobacillary organisms which can be seen with the light microscope but which resemble viruses, since they multiply only within certain cells of susceptible species. Classified between the viruses and bacteria, rickettsiae occur in various arthropods under natural conditions. See table. For a comparison of rickettsiae and other microscopic forms, see *microorganism.*

rictal Pertaining to the mouth of a bird.

rifamycin A group of antibiotics produced by species of *Streptomyces,* which are active against gram-positive bacteria, including *Mycobacterium tuberculosis,* and have limited activity against gram-negative organisms. The primary site of activity appears to be in the inhibition of protein synthesis.[90, 10]

Rift Valley fever An acute viral disease which in nature affects primarily sheep and cattle, although man is also quite susceptible. Goats, monkeys, ferrets, mice, rats, and several other species can be experimentally infected. The disease is characterized by a short incubation period and high mortality rate in lambs and calves, and by abortion in pregnant cows and ewes. The etiologic agent is an arbovirus, probably transmitted by mosquitoes.[2, 136]

Riley's LDH virus See *lactic dehydrogenase virus.*

rinderpest (cattle plague, Oriental cattle plague) An acute, contagious disease of ruminants, especially cattle. The disease is caused by a viral agent and usually starts

DISEASES CAUSED BY *Rickettsia*

AGENT	VECTOR	HOST	DISEASE
R. akari	Allodermanyssus sanguineus, Mus musculus	Man	Rickettsialpox
R. (Ehrlichia) bovis	Tick	Cattle	Tickborne disease
R. (Coxiella) burnetii	Contaminated dust	Man	Q fever
R. (Ehrlichia) canis	Tick	Dog	Tickborne disease
R. conjunctivae	Mechanical means	Goat	Conjunctivitis
R. mooseri (typhi)	Xenopsylla cheopis	Rat	Murine typhus
R. (Ehrlichia) ovina	Tick	Sheep	Tickborne disease
R. phagocytophila	Tick	Sheep, cattle, goat	Tickborne disease
R. prowazeki	Pediculus humanus corporis, P. humanus capitis, P. vestimenti	Man	Typhus fever
R. quintana	Pediculus humanus	Man	Trench fever
R. rickettsii	Dermacentor variabilis (dog tick)	Man	Eastern form of Rocky Mountain fever
	Dermacentor andersoni (sheep tick)	Man	Fatal form of Rocky Mountain fever
	Amblyomma cajemmese	Man	Brazilian Rocky Mountain fever
R. tsutsugamushi	Trombicula akamushi	Man	Scrub typhus
Neorickettsia	Nanophyetus salmincola	Dog, fox	Salmon disease; may be similar disease of man in Japan

with a high temperature, followed by congestion of the buccal mucosa, suspension of rumination, and severe diarrhea. Mortality in European and American cattle is between 90 and 100 per cent. The causative agent is a member of the paramyxovirus group and is closely related to the influenza and canine distemper viruses. Because of its rapid spread, high rate of mortality, and the fact that North American cattle are highly susceptible, this disease could cause disaster to the cattle population of the United States if an infected animal were to escape quarantine and be imported.[2, 16, 39, 142]

ringtail A disease of uncertain etiology seen in laboratory rats (*Rattus norvegicus*) and certain strains of mice, principally C57B1. The lesions consist of severe necrotic rings involving the dermis, subcutis, and underlying musculature at the base of the tail, and in severe cases, the hind legs as well. Distal to the necrotic (and inflammatory) zone there frequently is dry gangrene. The disease is seen most frequently in young rats in cages with suspended wire floors, leading to the present concept of impaired circulation owing to low relative humidity. In addition, the strain of rat, the type of bedding, and caging conditions influence expression of the disease.[24]

ristocetin An antibiotic that interferes with bacterial cell wall synthesis. It is specific for gram-positive bacteria, including mycobacteria, and is inactive against gram-negative organisms, yeast, fungi, or protozoa.[36, 49]

ritualized response See under *response*.

RNA Ribonucleic acid.

RNA polymerase An enzyme that catalyzes the formation of RNA from ribonucleotide triphosphates. Actinomycin D is thought to inhibit the production of messenger RNA by displacing RNA polymerase.

roentgenology That branch of radiology which deals with the diagnostic and therapeutic use of roentgen rays.

roentgen ray (x-ray) Electromagnetic emissions of short wavelength (below 5 Å.), produced when electrons moving at high velocity strike various materials, especially heavy metals. They are able to penetrate most substances to some extent, some more so than others, and this variable ability to penetrate plus their ability to affect a photographic emulsion in a fashion similar to that of light rays makes it possible to use them in making radiographs of various parts of the body.

Romer's paralysis See *guinea pig paralysis*, under *paralysis*.

rooster Mature male chicken (*Gallus gallus*).

ropheocytosis Endocytosis of small molecules by a cell, e.g., ferritin.

ropy brood See *American foulbrood*, under *foulbrood*.

rosaniline A basic dye that is the parent compound of triphenylmethane dyes.

Rose chamber A closed vessel in which media can be changed to allow long-term observation of cell cultures under phase microscopy.

roundworm Nematode.

Rous sarcoma See under *sarcoma*.

royal jelly A nutrient secreted by nurse bees which when fed to larvae produces queen bees. Unusual powers of healing and preservation of youth have occasionally been attributed to this material by medical quacks.

-rrhage, rrhagia, -rrhea Word termination denoting excessive flow or discharge.

Rubarth's disease See *infectious canine hepatitis*, under *hepatitis*.

rubella (German measles) A viral disease which may occur as a mild acute exanthematous response, as usually seen in an adult, or as a slowly progressive and persistent infection of the fetus. If the disease occurs in the fetus during critical periods, many abnormalities of development can occur.

runt disease An instance of graft-versus-host reaction in which there is gross retardation of the development of the recipient of immunologically competent cells, frequently with a fatal termination.

runway In behavioral science, a straight pathway usually without interruption, along an elevated rail or through an enclosure, and leading from a starting box to a goal box in which food or water is placed.

Russell body A spherical or crystalloid structure within the cytoplasm of plasma cells, probably consisting of gamma globulin which has become impacted within the cavity of the endoplasmic reticulum. Russell bodies are seen in chronic inflammatory conditions, in multiple myeloma, and in some other kinds of neoplasms. Among animen, they are particularly common in Aleutian disease of mink.

Russell's viper See table accompanying *snake*.

Russell's viper venom See under *venom*.

rutamycin See *oligomycin*.

S

sacbrood A lethal viral disease of the larval honeybee. Infected larvae die in the propupal stage after they have spun their cocoons. The infection appears to disturb the endocrine balance, resulting in accumulation of an unusual amount of fluid between the last larval skin and the prematurely darkened pupal skin, which causes a flabby, saclike appearance. The isometric virions which replicate in the cytoplasm of the fat-body cells have a diameter of 28 mμ. The disease is prevalent in the spring, and has been reported from Europe, North America, New Zealand, and Australia.

saccharase Invertin.

sacculinization A condition occurring in decapod crustaceans, usually crabs, manifested by abnormal or underdeveloped gonads and secondary sex characteristics as a result of infestation by species of *Sacculina*, a genus of small rhizocephalan crustaceans.

sacrifice See *euthanasia.*

sadism Sexual perversion in which satisfaction is derived from the infliction of cruelty upon another.

safranin O A basic dye of the azine group. Solubility at 15° C.: water 4.5 per cent, absolute alcohol 3.5 per cent, and glycerol 15 per cent. It is used as a counterstain in Weigert's elastica stain and the leuco-patent blue method for erythrocyte peroxidase, in Harman's method for mitochondria in tissue sections, in the Gram stain method, and with cimline blue for plant tissues, cell walls, and chromosomes.[57, 153]

Saimiri sciureus See *squirrel monkey.*

saki Any member of several genera of South American monkeys, including *Pithecia* and *Chiropotes.* See *primate.*

salamander A kind of lizard-like animal. Species of the genus *Ambystoma* are used in various types of experiments. See *axolotl.*

salivary gland virus disease See *cytomegalovirus infection.*

salmon disease A disease of dogs, foxes, and coyotes caused by *Neorickettsia helminthoeca,* an intracellular parasite. It is noncontagious and transmitted by a fluke, *Nanophyetus salmincola,* which carries the infection in metacercariae encysted in the flesh of fish of family Salmonidae. Animals become infected by eating uncooked fish.[142] In Japan, a similar disease called sennetsu occurs in man.

Salmonella A genus of gram-negative motile microorganisms which characteristically fail to ferment lactose and sucrose, and are the causative agents of typhoid and paratyphoid fevers and food poisoning. Identification of members of this group is based on their somatic and flagellar antigens, most animal types falling into four somatic types, designated B, C, D, E.[36.] See table.

salmonellosis Infection with salmonellae. It is caused by ingestion of the organisms or their products and may be marked by violent diarrhea, with cramps and tenesmus.

Previously regarded as the most serious and prevalent disease in the colony husbandry of laboratory mice (*Mus musculus*), salmonellosis (mouse typhoid) has diminished in importance as laboratory rodent health standards have risen through gnotobiotic

DISEASES CAUSED BY *Salmonella*

AGENT	HOST	DISEASE
S. abortus-equi	Horse	Abortion
S. abortus-ovis	Sheep	Abortion
S. anatum	Duckling	Salmonellosis
S. bareilly	– – –	Salmonellosis
S. bredeney	Anomen	Septicemia
S. choleraesuis	Swine	Secondary invader in hog cholera
S. derby	Anomen, man	Septicemia in anomen; gastroenteritis in man
S. dublin	Cattle	Salmonellosis
S. enteritidis	Rodents, man	Gastroenteritis
S. gallinarum	Adult birds	Fowl typhoid
S. montevideo	Man	Gastroenteritis
S. muenchen	– – –	– – –
S. newport	Poult	Salmonellosis
S. oranienburg	Fowl	Salmonellosis
S. pullorum	Young chicks	Pullorum disease or bacillary white diarrhea
S. typhimurium	Birds, mammals (including man)	Mouse typhoid; food poisoning in man
S. typhisuis	Swine	Secondary invader in hog cholera
S. typhosa	Man	Typhoid fever

technology and the increasing awareness of intercurrent disease in laboratory animals.

Salmonellae may be truly regarded as comparative pathogens because of their non-selectivity in the choice of hosts; thus most species, including domestic farm livestock and primates (including man), have a well characterized typhoid or paratyphoid syndrome. The comparative thread is exemplified by the dysentery-like symptomatology of the acute enteric phase, the dependence on endotoxicosis for systemic symptomatology, and a latent carrier (or "shedder") stage in asymptomatic and recovered animals. Although various lesions, e.g., focal hepatic necrosis in the mouse, and pulmonary phlebothrombosis in the hamster, are considered as characteristic for a species, enteritis and reticuloendotheliosis are common to all. See also *pullorum*.

Similarly each species is usually associated with a more or less common spectrum of *Salmonella* species or serotypes. In the mouse the two most frequent isolates are *S. typhimurium* and *S. enteritidis*. Diagnostic methods include an agglutination test and standard fecal cultures for enteric bacteria. In laboratory rodents, control methods usually resolve themselves to destruction of the affected colony.

salt fractionation A method for the separation of immunoglobulins based on the solubility of proteins. It employs high concentrations of neutral salts, such as ammonium sulfate or sodium sulfate, to precipitate proteins from solution. It is useful for large volumes of material but does not provide a pure precipitate.

sand vipers See table accompanying *snake*.

sapro- A combining form meaning rotten or putrid, or designating relationship to decay or to decaying material.

saprophagous Feeding on dead or decaying organic matter.

saprophyte Any vegetable organism, such as a bacterium, living upon dead or decaying organic matter. Cf. *parasite*.

sarco- A combining form denoting relationship to flesh.

Sarcocystis muris See *protozoan parasites*, under *rat*, and see *sarcosporidiosis*.

sarcoid 1. Resembling flesh; fleshy. 2. A sarcoma-like tumor.

s. of Boeck, a type of multiple benign granuloma of unknown cause, showing predilection for the face, arms, and shoulders, although it may involve internal organs.

equine s., a cutaneous growth in members of Equidae which consists of multiple eroded areas of skin surrounded by intact epithelium that is markedly hyperplastic, and accompanied by extreme hyperplasia of the underlying dermis. This growth of immature fibroblastic tissue has resulted in the name sarcoid (sarcoma-like), although it is referred to by some as fibropapilloma. It in no respect resembles sarcoid of Boeck in man. The lesion is transplantable and possibly is caused by the bovine papilloma virus.[142]

sarcoma A malignant tumor made up of connective tissue elements.

s. 37 (S-37; 375), a rapidly growing undifferentiated tumor derived from a spontaneous mammary adenocarcinoma (carcinoma 37) observed in the laboratories of M. Haaland at the Imperial Cancer Research Fund, London, in 1906. Although not strain-specific, it grows better in certain strains (in over 99 per cent of BALB/c, DBA/2, ABc, ZBc, and [BALB/c × A] F hybrids). Because of its broad strain adaptability, this tumor is widely used in screening cancer chemotherapeutic agents. Subcutaneous transplants generally kill the host within three weeks.[150]

Jensen s. (Jensen rat sarcoma; Jensen tumor; JRS), a sarcoma of rats first observed when two rats injected with acid-fast bacilli from pseudotuberculous cattle by B. Bang were necropsied by C. O. Jensen in his laboratory, in Copenhagen in 1907. They were bacteriologically negative, but both rats were found to have sarcomas of both the abdominal and thoracic organs. It was not recorded which tumor of the two was subsequently subjected to serial passage in a variety of rat stocks in Jensen's laboratory. Presently the tumor can be transplanted with progressive growth in nearly 100 per cent of Sherman, Wistar, or Sprague-Dawley rats, but regresses in about 18 per cent. It invades adjacent tissue but rarely metastasizes, killing the host in 17 to 56 days.[150]

Rous s., a virus-induced neoplasm of fibroblasts discovered by Rous in 1911 in a chicken. It has been profitably studied by many investigators in cell cultures, in chickens, and in other species. The agent was referred to by Rous as a "do-all" virus.[53, 127] See also *oncogenic virus*.

sarcosporidiosis A condition characterized by microscopic cysts containing crescent-shaped tubular organisms of uncertain classification known as *Sarcocystis*. They are very common within the cells of skeletal and cardiac muscle of birds and mammals, particularly in herbivores, but have rarely been reported in man.[142]

sarkomycin An antitumor agent possessing weak antibacterial activity produced by a species of *Streptomyces*. It appears to interfere with the adenylic acid system by inhibition of the rate of formation of ATP, and also interferes with DNA synthesis.[36, 49]

satellite In genetics, a segment of condensed chromatin at the distal end of the short arm of a chromosome, being attached by a thin strand of chromatin.

Saunders' myositis See *myositis of guinea pig*.

scaly face See *scaly leg*.

scaly leg Descriptive term for a skin disease of birds caused by sarcoptic mites of the genus *Cnemidocoptes* (*Knemidocoptes*). These mites tunnel and burrow through the epidermal layer of the skin, like typical sarcoptic mites, but have a predilection for highly cornified skin in birds, as on the legs and cere, and where the beak joins the face. The skin reacts with a scaly dermatitis (hence the names scaly face and scaly leg), which in chronic cases results in bizarre thickened encrustations of the skin and malformation of claws and beak. *C. mutus* is associated generally with gallinaceous birds and *C. pilae* with psittacine and passerine birds. *C. jamaicensis* and *C. fossor* have been associated with passerine birds. *C. gallinae* causes a typical sarcoptiform mange ("depluming itch") in gallinaceous birds affecting the soft skin.[11, 112]

scarlet R A non-ionic dis-azo dye. Solubility at 15° C.: water nil, absolute alcohol 0.6 per cent, and insoluble in glycerol. It is used for staining fat in plant tissues, for staining proteins, and in Masson's trichrome stain.

schedule See *schedules of reinforcement*, under *reinforcement*.

Schiff's reagent A chemical that attaches to and colors compounds containing dyglycol or aldehyde groups. This compound is used in periodic acid-Schiff and Feulgen stains (q.v.).

schisto- A combining form meaning split or cleft.

Schistosoma A genus of trematodes (blood flukes), family Schistosomatidae, which contains three species that infect humans. *S. mansoni* forms a nonoperculated egg with a large posterolateral spine and measures 114 to 175μ by 45 to 68μ. It also infects monkeys and rodents. *S. haematobium* parasitizes the bladder, and its eggs resemble those of *S. mansoni* but possess a terminal spine. Monkeys and other rodents may also be infected. *S. japonicum* parasitizes the superior and inferior mesenteric and caval system. The eggs have a small lateral spine. The cow, goat, pig, cat, shrew, and weasel may be infected.

The cercaria of blood flukes of ducks and muskrats infect people swimming in contaminated waters and cause the syndrome known as swimmer's itch, or cercarial dermatitis.

Schistosomatium douthitti, a related species found in the blood of field voles and muskrats, has been used for experimental studies.

Other schistosomes are *S. bovis*, found in the cow, and experimentally in the guinea pig; *S. indicum* in the horse, cow, goat, and buffalo; *S. nasale* in cattle in India; and *S. suis* in the pig and dog in India.[21]

Schistosomatium A genus of trematodes (blood flukes) of the family Schistosomatidae. *S. douthitti*, found in the blood of field voles and muskrats, has been used for experimental studies.

schistosomiasis Infection with worms of the class Trematoda, principally of the genus *Schistosoma* (q.v.). It has been known since the beginning of recorded history in ancient Egypt. The worms are small trematodes which live in the blood vessels of the host. Their ova circulate as emboli, and lodge in tissue as foreign bodies, producing severe irritation. They have been linked to possible development of tumors of the urinary bladder.[21]

schizo- A combining form meaning divided, or denoting relationship to division.

schizochroism The loss of one pigment such as melanin or carotenoid in an organism, particularly birds, which normally has more than one such pigment located in separate areas, or which has one pigment overlying another. The resultant depigmentation is known as schizochroism. Since the two most common melanins in birds are controlled by separate genes, it is possible for birds to lack one or the other in cells that normally have both. The latter condition results in *melanic schizochroism* of two forms: *gray variants*, which have lost phaeomelanins, and *fawn variants*, which have lost eumelanins. In *melano-carotenoid schizochroism*, either the melanin or the carotenoid normally found in the same cell is lost, unmasking the single pigment remaining; e.g., in green budgerigars the loss of melanin yields a yellow plumage, and the loss of the carotenoid yellow yields blue.[112]

schizogony Asexual reproduction of sporozoa by fission, which takes place in the vertebrate host.[109, 159]

Schmorl's disease (necrobacillosis of rabbits) Progressive ulceration and subcutaneous swelling of the skin, especially about the face, in domestic rabbits (*Oryctolagus cuniculus*). *Spherophorous necrophorous* (Schmorl's bacillus) can usually be isolated, along with many secondary invaders. The ulceration is common about the lips and inside the oral cavity, with edema and sloughing of necrotic areas. When deeper tissues become abscessed, the capsule is very thick and contains creamy, white pus. The draining ventral cervical lymph nodes may be inflamed. Affected animals have difficulty eating. Diagnosis is made by physical examination and isolation of the organism. Individuals may be treated by incising the abscesses and supporting with penicillin, but the usual practice is to destroy the affected animal.

schwannoma A neoplasm of the nerve sheath.

Schwartz leukemia virus A lymphoid leukemia virus isolated by Schwartz from brain tissues of a leukemic Swiss mouse. With repeated passage in Swiss mice, leukemia developed in as short a time as three weeks following inoculation. Extracts of the lymphoid tissue did not induce leukemia. When brain extracts were passed into BALB/c inbred mice, 5 to 40 per cent developed lymphoid leukemia after a period of four months.[114]

Scientific Research Society of America University of California, Los Angeles, Calif. 90024.

scopophilia   1. The derivation of sexual pleasure from looking at genital organs (active s.). 2. A morbid desire to be seen (passive s.).

scopophobia   A morbid dread of being seen.

scorpion   See *arachnid.*

-scopy   A word termination meaning the act of examining.

scours   Diarrhea in newborn animals. See *calf scours.*

scrapie   A neurological disease of sheep which gets its name from the principal clinical manifestation, which involves scraping of the wool against gates or fenceposts, because of intense pruritus. The disease has been known in Europe and the British Isles for nearly 200 years but only recently has spread to Canada and the United States. It can be transmitted by intracerebral inoculation of filtered brain tissue from sheep into other sheep or into goats, mice, hamsters, rats, and other laboratory animals. It is characterized by prolonged incubation period (as long as two years) and by marked predilection for certain families or breeds of animals. No gross lesions can be detected but mild degenerative changes in the medulla, pons, midbrain, and spinal cord are characteristic. The most striking and diagnostic lesions consist of proliferation of astrocytes and formation of large vacuoles or bubbles in the cytoplasm of neurons.

Recently, the disease has been described as being very similar to a chronic central nervous system degeneration known as kuru, which affects certain families of natives in New Guinea (see *kuru*). This relationship between a slow degenerative disease caused by a virus in sheep and one possibly caused by a virus in man, has opened a new area of study in the entire field of chronic degenerative diseases of the central nervous system, including such diseases as multiple sclerosis, amyotrophic lateral sclerosis, Creutzfeldt-Jakob disease, and subacute sclerosing panencephalitis, among others.[14, 44]

screw-worm   See *Callitroga hominivoras.*

scrub typhus   (tsutsugamushi)   A self-limited febrile disease of two weeks' duration, caused by *Rickettsia tsutsugamushi*, transmitted by chiggers. It is characterized by sudden onset of fever with a primary skin lesion (eschar) and development of a rash about the fifth day.

scurvy   A syndrome resulting from deficiency of ascorbic acid (vitamin C) in the diet of guinea pigs, all primates, and several species of lesser importance. Deficiency of the vitamin appears to be reflected in failure to produce normal collagen or osteoid tissue, which in turn results in the formation of defective connective tissue. The bones and teeth are affected first, but other important lesions include hemorrhages in almost any part of the body (due to increased capillary fragility), weakness of tissues, and stiffening of the legs (hindlegs in the guinea pig). It is generally believed that guinea pigs and primates in research animal facilities require dietary supplementation with ascorbic acid even though prepared diets contain adequate amounts, because the vitamin is so easily destroyed by oxidation.[80, 117, 144]   See *ascorbic acid.*

sea anemone   See *coelenterate.*

sea cucumber   See *echinoderm.*

seal   An aquatic mammal of any of three families of the suborder Pinnipedia: Otariidae (sea lions and fur seals), Odobenidae (walruses), and Phocidae (true seals). Among seals, sea lions are the most agile on land, and it is members of this group that perform as trained seals in circuses and zoos. Seals and sea lions have proved useful in the pursuit of several biomedical problems, as in studies of the diving reflex (as it relates to several aspects of shock and acid-base balance), the underwater echolocating mechanism, cataracts, and blood clotting factors.

sea snakes   See table accompanying *snake.*

sea spider   A small marine arthropod.

sea squirt   See *ascidian.*

sea urchin   See *echinoderm.*

secondary feathers   Flight feathers borne on the parts of a bird's wing corresponding to a mammalian forearm. See also *remiges.*

sedimentation coefficient (S)   The rate at which a given molecule sediments in a centrifugal field. The sedimentation coefficient is the rate of sedimentation per unit centrifugal field. See *density gradient,* under *centrifugation.*

semidominance   See *incomplete dominance,* under *dominance.*

seminoma   See *testicular neoplasm,* under *neoplasm.*

Sendai virus   A paramyxovirus causing an important and widespread respiratory infection of laboratory mice. Sendai virus was first isolated from an epidemic of fatal pneumonitis in Japanese children. It was also first found in laboratory mouse stocks in that country. Subsequent isolates of Sendai virus from both Japan and Russia indicate that human and murine Sendai isolates may be antigenically related but biologically different. Sendai virus infection is widely disseminated in conventionally maintained mouse stocks in the United States as a clinically silent enzootic.

The virus is not carried as a latent infection, and it disappears in the presence of antibody. Diagnosis is established by serologic (hemagglutination-inhibition) detection of specific antibody and virus isolation.[27, 63] The virus is used in experimental work in the study of genetic regulation because it has been shown that animal cells in culture can be rapidly fused together by high concentrations of this virus (see *heterokaryon*).

sensory   See under *adaptation.*

septicemia   The presence in the blood of multiplying bacteria and their toxins.

sericulture   The culture of silkworms.

serology   The study of antigen-antibody reactions in vitro.

serotonin   An organic compound (5-hydroxy-tryptamine) present in blood platelets, enterochromaffin cells, and mast cells, which acts as a smooth muscle contractant and increases capillary permeability. It probably plays a part in allergic reactions and also in the metabolism of the central nervous system.

Sertoli cell tumor   See *testicular neoplasm,* under *neoplasm.*

sessile   Fixed and immobile.

sex chromatin   Material of which the sex chromosomes are composed, seen as a small dark mass at the periphery of the nucleus. Often used as a synonym for *Barr body* or *leukocyte drumstick.* See also *late-replicating X chromosome,* under *chromosome,* and see *Lyon hypothesis.*

sex chromosome   See *chromosome.*

sexduction   The process in which a fragment of genetic material, e.g., that controlling lactose fermentation, is transferred from one bacterium to another, owing to its association with factor F.[32]

sex linkage   Location of a gene on a sex chromosome; the situation in which a gene that produces a certain phenotypic expression is transmitted by the sex chromosomes. Examples of genes located on the X chromosome of mammals are those responsible for hemophilia (in man and dog), anhidrotic ectodermal dysplasia (in man and cow), structure of glucose-6-phosphate dehydrogenase (in man, hare, and horse), and Xg blood group antigens (in man and gibbon).

sexual dimorphism   The property of developing physical traits that distinguish male from female. See also *autosexing.*

sexual skin   Areas of skin about the genitalia and over the buttocks that show a marked reddening in sexually active adult primates of several species (especially the rhesus, *M. mulatta*). The color and extent of skin involved is much more pronounced in females than in males; in the former it may extend up the back as far as the crest of the ilium. The reddening is often accompanied by dramatic swelling of the skin, more in younger than older females, and is most marked in the middle of the menstrual cycle, blanching out during menstrual flow. The reddening is due to engorgement of a plexus of thin-walled blood vessels beneath the epithelium, and not to skin pigmentation.

SGOT   Serum glutamic oxaloacetic transaminase.

shaping   See *approximation conditioning,* under *conditioning.*

shark   See *cartilaginous fish.*

Shay's leukemia   Chloroleukemia 123.

sheep pox   A generalized eruption of the skin and occasionally of the trachea and pharynx of sheep.[16]

shell disease   Disease of the shell of an animal.

s. d. of lobsters, softening of the exoskeleton, caused by chitinivorous bacteria; reported in *Homarus americanus* in artificial holding ponds.

s. d. of oysters, see *maladie du pain d'epice,* and *maladie du pied.*

Shigella   A genus of slender, nonmotile, gram-negative, nonlactose-fermenting bacteria which produce bacillary dysentery in man. *Shigella* organisms may be found in primates fed an inadequate diet, and dogs may be transient excreters in highly endemic areas of shigellosis.[36]

shigellosis   An important enteric disease of the order Primates caused by bacteria of the genus *Shigella.* In nonhuman primates, the most frequent isolates are *S. flexneri, S. sonnei,* and *S. schmitzii.* They are also important zoonotic agents for man. But the major isolate in human bacterial dysentery is *S. dysenteriae,* which does not appear to be an important pathogen of nonhuman primates. Shigellae can apparently be carried as latent agents by most nonhuman primates, causing disease when host resistance is reduced through such stresses as shipping, nutritional deprivation, or experimentation, and is therefore especially important in recently transported animals.

Symptoms, which are related to colonic infection and endotoxicosis, include profuse bloody diarrhea, fever, tenesmus, and depression. Congestion of the colon, mucosal ulcers, and colitis are the typical post-mortem findings. Prompt treatment with fluids and antibiotics is usually satisfactory. The diagnosis must be established by isolation of shigellae from rectal or fecal cultures.[41, 128]

shipping fever (shipping pneumonia)   A febrile disease of cattle characterized by pneumonia or septicemia. The disease is probably the result of a combined infection with the virus of infectious bovine rhinotracheitis and organisms of the genus *Pasteurella.* A myxovirus belonging to the parainfluenza group has also been isolated from typical cases of shipping fever. However, the true role of each of these agents of bovine respiratory diseases remains to be determined.[16, 142] Cf. *pasteurellosis.*

Shope fibroma   See under *fibroma.*

Shope papilloma (Shope papillomatosis)   See under *papilloma.*

shrimp   See *crustacean.*

sib   A blood relative; one of a group of persons all of whom are descendants of a common ancestor. See also *sibling.*

sibling   Another offspring of the same parents as the person of reference; a brother or sister.

sickle cell   See *sickling.*

sicklemia   See *sickling.*

sickling   The formation of oat- or sickle-shaped erythrocytes, seen in hereditary sicklemia. The shape of the erythrocyte is due to stretching of the red blood cells when the hemoglobin molecules form tactoids. It has been shown that the molecular defect consists of the substitution of one amino acid (valine) of the 580 in the chain for glutamine. Tactoid formation occurs as a result of reduced oxygen concentration both in vivo and in vitro. This induces decreased permeability to phosphate, predisposes the cell to metabolic death, and lowers its resistance to hemolysis.

Multiple and polymorphic hemoglobins have also been identified in anomen, including adult sheep, in which hemoglobin C can be induced by establishing severe anemia; the horse and stump-tailed macaque monkey, in which there are differences in concentration of slow and fast hemoglobins; and salmon, which change hemoglobin type when migrating from salt to fresh water. The erythrocytes of most species of deer can be caused to sickle in vitro under increased oxygen concentration. Although this does not appear to have any pathological significance, the phenomenon is related to polymorphic hemoglobin types.[76, 162]

sidero- A combining form denoting relationship to iron.

sideromycin A group of iron-containing antibiotics produced by species of *Streptomyces*. Some are active against gram-positive and gram-negative bacteria, others against gram-positive organisms only. Included in the group are griesin and albomycin. Their precise mechanism of action is not known, but they probably impair carbohydrate metabolism, perhaps by inhibition of thiamine.[36, 49]

sigma virus The agent which causes carbon dioxide sensitivity (q.v.) in various species of fruit flies. The virion is cylindrical, with one hemispherical end, and is about 70 by 180 mμ long.

sign An indication of the existence of something; any objective evidence of a disease. Cf. *symptom*.

sign stimulus See under *stimulus*.

silk toxicity A lethal hyperaminoacidemia (q.v.) in the silkworm, caused by silk retention. The inability to emit silk is related to structural and functional lesions in the silk glands, caused by endocrine disturbances, genetic factors, or infectious agents.

simian bone disease See *avitaminosis D*.

simian malaria See *malaria*.

simian virus (SV) Any of a group of viruses that infect nonhuman primates. Extensive use of subhuman primates for biomedical studies, commencing with the poliovirus vaccine program, has led to the discovery of a large number of latent or low-virulence viruses mainly in the adenovirus, picornavirus, myxovirus, and papovavirus groups. Their significance lies in the great effort expended in characterizing their chemical, physical, immunological, and biological properties, and in the impact that the knowledge gained thereby has had in extending the understanding of virology and viral oncology. The accompanying table lists the more completely characterized entities collectively called simian viruses.[2, 39, 114] See *classification*, under *virus*.

single pair mating See *breeding system*.

sipunculoid Any member of the minor phylum Sipunculoidea, related to the annelids. The bodies of this small group are slender, gourd-shaped, highly contractile, and nonsegmented, with short hollow tentacles about the mouth. The digestive tract is complete, the coelom large and containing blood with free cells. The sexes are separate, and all forms are marine. Symmetry is bilateral and there are three germ layers. Some of the more common members include *Dendrostoma* (the sausage worm), *Endrostomum* (the peanut worm), *Sipunculus*, and *Phascolosoma*.

Skinner box An enclosure with floors and

Simian Viruses

Classification	Designation	Comment
Picornaviruses; known also as ECMO (enteric cytopathogenic monkey orphans) or enteroviruses	SV2, SV6, SV16, SV18, SV19, SV25, SV29, SV35	Commonly isolated from feces or tissues (kidney)
Myxoviruses	SV5, SV41	Classified with parainfluenza viruses; have been recovered from children with respiratory disease, hence also known as CA or croup associated simian viruses. Isolated from monkey kidney.
Adenoviruses	SV15, SV17	Commonly isolated from feces and tissues (kidney); SV17 causes experimental rhinitis of patas monkeys.
Papovaviruses	SV40	Isolated from monkey kidney. Causes tumors when inoculated into newborn hamsters; but not children receiving SV40 contaminated poliovirus vaccine. Cell changes in culture depend on species; no CPE in rhesus or cynomologous kidney cells, vacuolation in green monkey kidney cells (and also patas monkey kidney cells, and transformation in certain cell lines, e.g., human kidney) without production of infectious virus.

walls from which an animal under study cannot escape. The box is provided with objects which can be manipulated and devices which automatically deliver a reinforcing stimulus in response to a selected operant behavior, such as the pressing of a bar, the pulling of a string, or the pushing of a panel.

skin window A thin cover glass placed over a gently scarified area of skin, an experimental device designed by Rebuck. Leukocytes which migrate from the capillaries and become attached to the glass surface can be stained and observed. This method is useful for studying the dynamics of inflammation and response to infectious agents, toxic materials, and other irritants. Cf. *granuloma pouch.*

Skrjabinema ovis A nematode (pinworm) of sheep.[21]

SLE Systemic lupus erythematosus.

slow virus A term first used by Sigurdsson to describe the cause of viral diseases manifested by extremely long preclinical phase and slow progression once symptoms appear, even though most of these viruses replicate rapidly in the host. Those first studied were maedi, visna, and scrapie (q.v.) of sheep. Later findings have shown that slow viruses possess a narrow host range, usually with intraspecific genetic predilection, that they are probably transmitted both vertically and horizontally, and that there are immunologic responses by the host which are unable to halt progression of the disease. Other slow viruses are the viruses of rubella and kuru of man, lactic dehydrogenase virus and lymphocytic choriomeningitis virus of the mouse, the virus of equine infectious anemia, and the viruses of Aleutian disease and infectious encephalopathy of mink.[14, 44] See *CHINA virus.*

slug See *mollusk.*

smallpox (variola) An acute viral infection of man characterized by vomiting, lumbar pains, a skin eruption that is first papular, then vesicular, and finally pustular, and by fever marked by a distinct remission, beginning with the eruption and ending when the eruption becomes pustular. See *cowpox.*

snail See *mollusk.*

snake A limbless reptile, many species of which are poisonous.

    poisonous s., any snake that secretes substances capable of producing a deleterious effect on the blood (hematoxins) or nervous system (neurotoxins), which are injected into the body of the victim by their bite. See table on page 190.

snuffles See *enzootic pasteurellosis,* under *pasteurellosis.*

Soboliphyme baturini A nematode of the family Soboliphymidae, found in the intestine of the cat, sable, and fox in Siberia, and also in the wolverine in North America.[21]

Society for Cryobiology Suite 308, 11125 Rockville Pike, Rockville, Md. 20853.

Society for Experimental Biology and Medicine 630 W. 168th Street, New York, N.Y. 10032.

Society for Investigative Dermatology, Inc. Stanford University, Palo Alto, Calif. 94305.

Society for the Study of Evolution University of Kansas, Lawrence, Kans. 66044.

Society of Experimental Psychologists, Inc. Department of Psychology, University of Illinois, Urbana, Ill.

Society of General Physiologists Department of Biophysics, The Johns Hopkins University, Baltimore, Md.

Society of Nematologists Department of Entomology, University of Florida, Gainesville, Fla. 32601.

Society of Protozoologists Howard University, Washington, D.C.

Society of Systematic Zoology Division of Entomology and Acarology, University of California, Berkeley, Calif. 94720.

The Society of the Sigma XI 155 Whitney Avenue, New Haven, Conn. 06510.

Society of Technical Writers and Publishers, Inc. 1010 Vermont Avenue, N.W., Suite 421, Washington, D.C. 20005.

Society of Toxicology, Inc. Mellon Institute, 4400 5th Avenue, Pittsburgh, Pa. 15213.

sockeye salmon virus A host-specific virus causing severe disease of hatchery-reared fingerling sockeye salmon, *Oncorhyncus nerka.* The fresh-water form of the salmon (*Kokanee*) is also susceptible. The disease is characterized by acute onset, dark pigmentation, and a circular swimming pattern as the result of unilateral motor paralysis. The abdomen is swollen, the gills are pale, hemorrhagic areas develop at the fin bases, and many of the survivors have residual spinal deformities. Internal lesions include pale spleen; green bile; focal necrosis of the swim bladder, smooth muscle, and liver; and deposition of ceroid in liver and spleen. Extramedullary hematopoiesis may be seen in visceral adipose tissue and is reflected in blood smears. Inclusion bodies have not been observed, but the virus has been passed in vivo.[114]

solipsism The belief that the world exists only in the mind of the individual, or that it consists solely of the individual himself and his own experience.

solochrome cyanin R An acid dye of the hydroxy-triphenylmethane group. Solubility at 15° C.: water 7 per cent, absolute alcohol 5 per cent, and glycerol 3 per cent. It is a pseudoamphoteric dye capable of reacting with cationic or amphoteric anionic dyes to give differential coloring.[57]

Solo man An extinct subspecies of man known from fossil remains found near the Solo River in Java; currently known as *Homo erectus soloensis.*

soluble RNA See *ribonucleic acid.*

somatic cell A body cell of an organism containing diploid chromosomes; any cell other than a germ cell.

IMPORTANT POISONOUS SNAKES OF THE WORLD*

FAMILY AND TYPE OF FANGS	COMMON NAME	TYPE OF VENOM	DISTRIBUTION	REMARKS
Colubridae; rear, immovable, grooved	Colubrids	Mostly mild	Warm parts of both hemispheres	Over 1000 species, the few poisonous ones not dangerous
Example:	Boomslang	Hemorrhagin	South Africa	Arboreal, timid
Elapidae; front, immovable, grooved	Elapids	Predominantly neurotoxin	Mostly in Old World	Over 150 species, very poisonous
Examples:	Cobras	Mostly neurotoxin	Africa, India, Asia, Philippines, Celebes	Spitting cobra in Africa aims at eyes
	Kraits	Strong neurotoxin	India, S.E. Asia, Indonesia	Sluggish, often buried in dust
	Mambas	Neurotoxin	Tropical W. Africa	Arboreal
	Blacksnake	Neurotoxin	Australia	Large snake, wet terrain
	Copperhead	Neurotoxin	Australia, Tasmania, Solomons	Damp environment
	Brown snake	Neurotoxin	Australia, New Guinea	Slender
	Tiger snake	Strong neurotoxin	Australia	Dry environment; aggressive; very dangerous
	Death adder	Neurotoxin	Australia, New Guinea	Sandy terrain
	Coral snakes	Neurotoxin	United States, tropical America	About 26 species, 2 in Southern U.S.A.
Hydrophidae; front, immovable, hollow	Sea snakes	Some mild; others very toxic	Tropical, Indian and Pacific Oceans	Gentle, Rudder-like tail. Over 50 species
Viperidae; front, movable, hollow	True vipers	Predominantly hematoxin	Entirely in Old World	About 50 species
Examples:	European viper	Hematoxin	Europe (rare), N. Africa, Near East	Dry rocky country
	Russell's viper	Hematoxin	S.E. Asia, Java, Sumatra	Mostly open terrain; deadly
	Sand vipers	Hematoxin	N. Sahara	Buried in sand
	Puff adder	Hematoxin	Arabia, Africa	Open terrain; sluggish
	Gaboon viper	Neurotoxin and hematoxin	Tropical W. Africa	Forests; deadly
	Rhinoceros viper	Hematoxin	Tropical Africa	Wet forests
	Habu viper	Neurotoxin	Okinawa	Caves and dry rocky country
Crotalidae; front, movable, hollow	Pit vipers	Predominantly hematoxin	Old and New Worlds; none in Africa	Over 80 species; pit between eye and nostril
Examples:	Rattlesnakes†	Predominantly hematoxin	N., Central and S. America	South American form neurotoxic
	Bushmaster	Hematoxin	Central and S. America	Large. In wet forests
	Fer-de-lance	Hematoxin	Central America, N. South America, few West Indies	Common on plantations
	Palm vipers	Hematoxin (?)	S. Mexico, Central and South America	Arboreal; small, greenish. Bite face
	Copperhead	Hematoxin	United States	Dry stony terrain
	Water moccasin	Hematoxin	Southeast U.S.A. to Texas	Swamps
	Asiatic pit vipers	Hematoxin	Southeast Asia, Formosa	Most arboreal

*From G. W. Hunter, W. W. Frye, and J. C. Swartzwelder: A Manual of Tropical Medicine. W. B. Saunders Co., Philadelphia.
†All rattlesnakes are poisonous.

somatic mutation A mutation occurring in a somatic cell. It is thought that many such mutations occur but that the mutated cells do not survive, and thus abnormal cell populations are prevented from multiplying. Some believe that neoplasms originate as somatic mutations. Other processes of the body, such as the graying of hair and the formation of abnormal pigmented plaques in old age, are thought by some to be related to somatic mutation.

Somogyi unit That amount of amylase that will destroy 1.5 mg. of starch in 8 minutes at 37° C. The normal range of the value in blood serum is considered by some to be between 80 and 200 units per 100 ml.

sore hocks (of the rabbit) A form of decubitus resulting from bruising or chafing of the plantar aspect of the metatarsus from treading on hard floors, seen most frequently in caged domestic rabbits. An elevated tender lesion approximately 2 cm. in diameter, with a scaly hyperkeratotic crust or scab, occurs in certain individual rabbits and is difficult to prevent or cure under laboratory conditions.

sotto disease See *bacillary paralysis,* under *paralysis.*

sound Mechanical radiant energy, the motion of particles of the material medium through which it travels (air, water, or solids) being along the line of transmission (longitudinal); such energy, of frequency between 20 and 20,000 cycles per second, provides the stimulus for the subjective sensation of hearing.

South Carolina Academy of Sciences Savannah River Laboratory, Aiken, S.C. 29801.

South Dakota Academy of Science South Dakota State University, Brookings, S.D.

Southern California Academy of Sciences Los Angeles County Museum of Natural History, 900 W. Exposition Boulevard, Los Angeles, Calif. 90007.

soy bean The bean of the leguminous plant, *Soja hispida* (*Glycine soja*), or Chinese bean. It contains little starch and is rich in albuminoids, and from it is prepared a meal which is used in making bread for diabetics. It also furnishes an enzyme, urease (q.v.).

sparsomycin   An antibiotic produced by a species of *Streptomyces*, which inhibits both gram-positive and gram-negative bacteria and has weak antifungal activity. It is markedly toxic to certain cells in tissue culture and may have value as an antitumor agent. The mechanism of its activity is not well characterized, but it appears to function as an inhibitor of protein synthesis.[36, 49]

species-specific   See under *behavior* and *response.*

spectrophobia   Morbid dread of mirrors or of seeing one's face in a mirror.

spectrophotometer   1. An apparatus for measuring the light sense by means of a spectrum. 2. An apparatus for estimating the quantity of coloring matter in solution by the quantity of light absorbed (as indicated by the spectrum) in passing through the solution.

spectropolarimeter   A combined spectroscope and polariscope for determining optical rotation.

spectrum   A charted band of wavelengths of electromagnetic vibrations obtained by refraction and diffraction. See *invisible s.* and *visible s.* By extension, a measurable range of activity, such as the range of bacteria affected by an antibiotic (antibacterial s.) or the complete range of manifestations of a disease.

   absorption s., one afforded by light which has passed through various gaseous media, each gas absorbing those rays of which its own spectrum is composed.

   chemical s., that part of the spectrum which includes the ultraviolet or actinic rays.

   chromatic s., that portion of the range of wavelengths of electromagnetic vibrations (from 7700 to 3900 Å) which gives rise to the sensation of color (red to violet) to the normally perceptive eye; coincident with the visible spectrum.

   color s., chromatic s.

   diffraction s., a spectrum formed by the passage of light through a diffraction grating.

   gaseous s., one which is afforded by an incandescent gas.

   invisible s., that made up of vibrations of wavelengths less than 3900 Å (ultraviolet rays, grenz rays, x-rays, and gamma rays) and between 7700 and 120,000 Å (infrared).

   ocular s., after-image.

   prismatic s., one produced by the passage of light through a prism.

   solar s., that portion of the range of wavelengths of electromagnetic vibrations emanating from the sun, including the visible (chromatic, or color) spectrum and small portions of the infrared and ultraviolet radiations at either extreme.

   thermal s., that portion of the range of wavelengths of electromagnetic vibrations (>7700 Å) containing the infrared or heat rays.

   toxin s., a diagrammatic representation of the neutralizing power of an antitoxin.

   visible s., that portion of the range of wavelengths of electromagnetic vibrations (from 7700 to 3900 Å) which is capable of stimulating specialized sense organs and is perceptible as light.

   x-ray s., the spectrum of a heterogeneous beam of roentgen rays produced by a suitable grating, generally a crystal.

spermist   A believer in the theory of preformation, which held that the spermatozoon contains a complete miniature individual. See *homunculus.*

SPF   Abbreviation for specific-pathogen free, a term applied to gnotobiotic animals reared for use in laboratory experiments, and known to be free of specific pathogenic microorganisms.[86] See *gnotobiote* and *axenic.*

sphenisciform birds   Members of the avian order Sphenisciformes, comprising a single family, the Spheniscidae, which includes all species of penguins. Penguins are flightless sea birds of the southern hemisphere, well adapted for aquatic life, and unique among birds in having a dense and uniform covering of feathers over the entire body without apteria. Penguins are favorite zoo birds, and a few species are important in research (see table).

SPECIES OF PENGUINS IMPORTANT
IN RESEARCH

SPECIES	COMMON NAME	HABITAT
Aptenodytes forsteri	Emperor penguin	Antarctic
A. patagonica	King penguin	Antarctic
Pygoscelis adeliae	Adelie penguin	Antarctic
Spheniscus demersus	Blackfooted penguin	South Africa
S. humboldti	Humboldt penguin	Peru

spherocytosis   A form of familial hemolytic anemia characterized by spherical rather than biconcave erythrocytes. This condition is also seen in the deer mouse, *Peromyscus moniculatus,* in which the pathophysiology of this autosomal recessive trait appears to be the same as that in the human disease.

spheroplast   Any of the osmotically sensitive bacterial forms derived from gram-negative and some gram-positive bacteria. They are similar to protoplasts but differ in that they retain cell wall structures and have the ability to revert to classical bacteria.[36]

sphingolipidosis   A general designation applied to a disease characterized by abnormal storage of sphingolipids, such as Gaucher's disease, Niemann-Pick disease, Pfaundler-Hurler disease, and Tay-Sachs disease. See *inborn errors of metabolism,* under *metabolism.*

spider monkey   Any member of the genus *Ateles* or *Brachyteles.* See *primate.*

spiradenoma   Adenoma of the sweat glands.

spiramycin   See *macrolide.*

Spirocerca   A genus of nematodes of the

superfamily Filaroidea. The most common species is *Spirocerca lupi*, a parasite of the dog in southern United States, although it has been reported from many parts of the world. The adult worms are frequently found in granulomatous nodules in the walls of the esophagus, aorta, stomach, and other organs. They frequently cause enlargements of the terminal portion of the esophagus and may produce obstruction because of this. Of particular interest to experimental biologists is the fact that they apparently can lead to the formation of tumors, including osteosarcoma and fibrosarcoma, in the wall of the esophagus. It has not been established whether the parasite is the direct cause of these neoplasms, but their close association with them appears to be most significant.[142]

spirochete A spiral-shaped bacterium; a general term given any microorganisms of the order Spirochaetales. See also *spirochetosis*.

spirochetosis (rabbit syphilis; vent disease) A spirochetal disease caused by *Treponema cuniculi*, an agent specific to rabbits of the species *Oryctolagus*. The organism has not been successfully cultivated or subjected to passage in other species. It is a venereal disease characterized by ulcerated areas about the skin of the vulva of females and perineum of males. *T. cuniculi* is similar in morphology and staining reactions to *T. pallidum* but antigenically distinct. It is also transmitted in the same fashion, by coitus. Secondary lesions in the form of excoriations or papules may be seen about the external nares or conjunctivae. Spirochetes are generally abundantly present in all lesions and may be demonstrated by darkfield microscopy or silver impregnation stains (e.g., Warthin-Starry, Levaditi, or Fontana stain). Microscopic lesions include ulceration, edema, hyperkeratosis with deep epithelial pegs, and cellular infiltrations by all types of inflammatory cells that concentrate about necrotic areas.

Immunity is not often conferred by healed infections. Treatment with 50,000 units of penicillin per day is effective, and recovered animals may be retained for breeding. Lues and other syphilitic sequelae of *T. pallidum* infections in man have not been observed in *T. cuniculi* infections of the rabbit.

splayleg See *joint dysplasia*, under *dysplasia*.

spondylitis Spondyloarthritis.

spondyloarthritis Arthritis of the vertebrae.

spontaneous behavior See under *behavior*.

spontaneous recovery In behavioral science, a term applied to the reappearance of a response which had been extinguished, and had not been elicited over a considerable period of time, at a strength greater than that observed at the termination of the extinction procedure.

spore The reproductive element of one of the lower organisms, such as a protozoon or a cryptogamic plant. Exospores or conidio-

spores are asexual spores arising from the end of the hypha by budding. Large ones are called macroconidia; small ones, microconidia. Endospores or gonidospores are formed in the interior of special spore cases called sporangia. Endospores that are free and provided with locomotive flagellae are zoospores, their cases being termed zoosporangia. An ascospore is a variety of endospore contained in a special spore case called an ascus. Basidiospores are spores formed at the ends of club-shaped structures called basidia. Zygospores are formed by a conjugation between two special hyphae. Chlamydospores are asexual resting spores, with thick walls, produced by enlargement of special cells. *Oospores* are spores formed by fertilization in a manner similar to true seeds.

asexual s., a spore produced by division within the walls of a mother cell.

bacterial s's., inactive resting or resistant forms produced within the body of a bacterium.

black s's of Ross, degenerated and pigmented malarial oocysts in the body of a mosquito.

swarm s's, spores made up of numerous active motile individuals.

washed s's, spores of bacteria that have been freed of their toxin by washing.

sporogony Sexual reproduction of the malaria parasite, which occurs in the stomach and body of the mosquito.[109]

sporotrichosis A disease of man and ano-men caused by *Sporotrichum schenckii*, which appears as a single-celled, budding, yeastlike fungus in exudate or tissues. This disease is characterized by a subacute or chronic granulomatous lesion of the skin, the skin lymphatics, and occasionally the internal organs.

Sporozoa A class of parasites which reproduce by spores that contain from one to many sporozoites. It includes Gregarinidia (*Lankesteria* and *Schizocystis*), Coccidia (*Selenococcidium*, *Eimeria*, *Aggregata*, *Schellaskia*, *Hepatozoon*, and *Haemogregarina*), Haemosporidia (*Plasmodium*, *Haemoproteus*, and *Leucocytozoon*), Sarcosporidia (*Sarcocystis*), Myxosporidia, and Microsporidia. The last three groups are mainly parasites of invertebrates and lower vertebrates.[109, 159]

sporozoite A spore formed after fertilization; any one of the sickle-shaped nucleated germs formed by division of the protoplasm of the spore of a sporozoan organism. In malaria, the form that develops in the salivary glands of the mosquito and is transmitted to man.

spring disease A disease of the cutworm *Euxoa segetum*, caused by *Pseudomonas septica*.

squab See *columbiform birds*.

squamous cell carcinoma G8755 A tumor arising spontaneously in the forestomach of a 22-month-old strain of C3H$_f$/He mice in the laboratories of Heston at the National

Cancer Institute in 1949. Subcutaneous transplants grow successfully without regression in 100 per cent of C3H$_f$/He hosts, killing the host in about 60 days.[150]

squid   See *mollusk*.

squirrel   A small to medium-sized rodent of the family Sciuridae, which contains about 50 genera and is widely distributed throughout the world. It has strong hind legs and a well developed tail, which may serve as a balancing organ in tree-dwelling types. The most common squirrels of the forested regions are the gray squirrel (*Sciurus carolinensis*) and the fox squirrel (*S. niger*). Both species have adapted to urban living.

squirrel monkey   A small monkey, *Saimiri sciureus*, weighing 600 to 1100 gm., native to the northern portion of South America. Other than the *Rhesus*, it is the most commonly used primate in experimental laboratories, over 30,000 being imported into the United States each year. They are widely utilized for neurophysiological, neuroanatomical, and behavioral studies, and their propensity toward development of coronary atherosclerosis provides a valuable model for studies of human arteriosclerosis.[23, 122]

SSO disease   An acronym from *sea side organism*. An infection of the connective tissues of the American oyster, *Crassostrea virginica*, found in spring and early summer along the middle Atlantic coast of the United States. The infection, caused by the haplosporidian *Minchinia costalis*, leads to tissue disruption and leukocytic infiltration.

staining   The artificial coloration of a substance, such as the introduction or application of material to facilitate examination of tissues, microorganisms, or other cells under the microscope. See individual stains.

   bipolar s., staining at the two poles only, or staining differently at the two poles.

   differential s., staining with a substance for which different bacteria or different elements of bacteria or specimens being stained show varying affinities, resulting in their differentiation.

   fluorescent s., the coloration of tissues with a fluorescent dye.

   intravital s., vital s.

   multiple s., staining with several different dyes to facilitate identification of different tissue elements.

   negative s., staining of the background and not the organism, to facilitate the microscopical study of bacteria; particularly applied to the phosphotungstic acid staining of tissues for electron microscopy.

   polar s., staining in which the ends of the rod stain deeply while the central portion is nearly or quite unstained, as in *Pasteurella*.

   postvital s., staining that occurs after death of a tissue which has been previously stained by vital methods.

   supravital s., staining of living tissue removed from the body.

   vital s. (intravital staining), staining of a tissue by a dye which is introduced into a living organism and which, by virtue of elective attraction to certain tissues, will stain those tissues.

Stansly leukemia virus   A reticulum cell leukemia virus isolated from Erlich ascites tumors carried in BALB/c mice. It was subject to passage by transplantation of tissues or inoculation of cell-free extracts, leukemia developing from the latter form after a latent period of six to eight months. The agent differed from the Friend virus in having lymphoid elements in the solid tumors. The lymphosarcoma was carried by transplantation, but after the tenth passage it changed back to a reticulum cell sarcoma.[114]

staphylomycin   See *streptogramin*.

starfish   See *echinoderm*.

statocyst   An organ of balance consisting of a sac lined with sensory cells and containing a solid chalky particle (the statolith).

statolith   See *statocyst*.

steapsin   The lipase of the pancreatic juice.

stereo-   A combining form meaning solid, having three dimensions, or firmly established.

stereoisomerism   A type of isomerism in which two or more compounds possess the same molecular and structural formulas but different spatial or configurational formulas, the spatial relationships of the atoms being different, but not the linkages.

stereotyping   In behavioral science, a term used to designate a situation in which a set of successive instances of a response do not vary in their topographic character.

sterilization   1. The complete destruction of microorganisms by heat (wet steam under pressure at 120° C. for 15 minutes, or dry heat at 360 to 380° C. for 3 hours), or by bactericidal chemical compounds. 2. Any procedure by which an individual is made incapable of reproduction, such as castration, vasectomy, or salpingectomy.

   chemical s., sterilization accomplished by means of a chemical substance.

   eugenic s., the process of rendering a person incapable of reproduction because the offspring would probably be undesirable types.

   fractional s., intermittent s., destruction of microorganisms by successive application of the procedure at intervals, to allow spores to develop into adult forms, which are more easily destroyed.

   mechanical s., the eradication of microorganisms by passing the fluid through a bacteria-proof filter.

sterol   A monohydroxy alcohol of high molecular weight; one of a class of compounds widely distributed in nature, which, because their solubilities are similar to those of fats, have been classified with the lipids. Cholesterol is the best known member of the group.

stetho-   A combining form denoting relationship to the chest.

stethoscope   An instrument of various form, size, and material for performing auscultation. By means of this instrument the respiratory, cardiac, pleural, arterial, venous, uterine, fetal, intestinal, and other sounds are conveyed to the ear of the observer.

stimulus   1. Any agent, act, or influence that produces functional or trophic reaction in a receptor or in an irritable tissue. 2. In behavioral science, a physical event impinging on the receptors of an animal and capable of exciting those receptors to induce a response.

aversive s., a stimulus which, when applied following the occurrence of a response, decreases the strength of that response on later occurrences.

conditioned s. (CS), in classical conditioning, a stimulus which through conditioning acquires the capability of eliciting a response not evoked before conditioning was initiated.

conditioned s., reinforcing, see *reinforcing s.*

consummatory s., the stimulus for a consummatory act (q.v.).

discriminative s., a stimulus the response to which is reinforced only when the specific stimulus is present and which eventually results in the response occurring at a higher rate or in greater magnitude in the presence of that stimulus than in its absence.

drive s., the stimulus, usually internal, which is thought to be determined by a given drive state.

eliciting s., the stimulus evoking a reflex act or the conditioned stimulus of a classical conditioned response.

reinforcing s., a stimulus the occurrence of which under specified conditions alters some aspect of the response of the experimental animal as determined by measurement of this response on subsequent trials.

reinforcing s., negative, a stimulus which, when administered following the occurrence of a response, reduces or diminishes the magnitude of the response, and which, when terminated following a response, increases the strength of that response. See also *punishment* and *aversive s.*

reinforcing s., primary, any stimulus that is effective as a reinforcing stimulus for all members of a strain or of a species at the beginning of an experiment.

reinforcing s., secondary (conditioned), a stimulus which is ineffective as a reinforcing stimulus until it has been presented with a reinforcing stimulus one or more times, and which then acts as a reinforcing stimulus when presented by itself.

sign s., the particular physical attributes or behavior of one animal that induces stimulation or release of a particular response in another animal of the same species. The response is referred to as a *social response.*

sign s., supernormal, a term used to designate certain sign stimuli that have proven quantitatively to have greater effect in re-

sponse strength than the normal sign stimulus (e.g., an oversized artificial egg presented to the oyster catcher causes it to respond with more vigorous brooding activity than does its own egg).

trace s., a hypothetical state that persists for a short time after the termination of a stimulus and which has the property of a stimulus in controlling response.

stimulus generalization   The condition in which a response conditioned to one stimulus can be elicited by or will occur in the presence of another stimulus.

stimulus-response correlation (SR, or S-R, correlation)   The observation that a particular response is dependent for its occurrence upon the administration of a specific stimulus.

stimulus threshold   The quantitative value of a stimulus that will elicit some defined constant response at a fixed strength of less than maximal value. See *response threshold.*

stolon   A stalk-like structure.

stoma   1. Any minute pore, orifice, or opening on a free surface; specifically, one of the openings (stigma or pseudostoma) between epithelial cells of a lymph space, forming a means of communication between adjacent lymph channels. 2. The opening established in the abdominal wall in colostomy, cecostomy, ileostomy, etc.; also the opening between two portions of a structure, as the intestine or blood vessels, in an anastomosis.

stomatitis   Inflammation of the oral mucosa, due to local or systemic factors, which may involve the buccal and labial mucosa, palate, tongue, floor of the mouth, and the gingivae.

contagious s. (cryoicthyozoose virus disease), a viral disease of aquarium fish, especially *Geophagus braziliensis.* Signs of infection include lethargy, skin ulcers, hemorrhages at the fin bases, pale gills, and peculiar swimming patterns. The digestive system is filled with mucus, and the gallbladder is reddish with yellow contents (as contrasted to the normal dark green). Healthy fish introduced into a tank with diseased fish may die after an incubation period as short as 24 hours. Microscopically, the key lesion is stomatitis with eosinophilic and reticulated cytoplasmic inclusions in oral mucosal cells. Transmission occurs only in water temperatures below 12 to 14° C., hence the descriptive synonym.[114]

papular s. (proliferative s.), a common viral disease of calves characterized by wartlike eruptions on the tongue, lips, palate, and buccal mucosa.

vesicular s. (sore mouth of cattle and horses; mal de jerbe), a viral disease of horses, cattle, swine, and occasionally man. Fluid-filled vesicles appear in the tongue and oral mucosa which closely resemble the lesions of foot-and-mouth disease. VS should be differentiated from foot-and-mouth disease by animal inoculation. Vesicular stomatitis follows a benign course and does not show secondary lesions on other parts of the body.

-stomy   A word termination denoting the surgical creation of an artificial opening into a hollow organ (colostomy, tracheostomy) or a new opening between two such structures (gastroenterostomy, pyeloureterostomy).

stone brood   A disease of larval and adult bees, caused by the fungi *Aspergillus flavus* and, less frequently, *A. fumigatus.* Diseased larvae usually die in the sealed stage, before pupation. See *aspergillosis.*

stork   See *ciconiiform birds.*

strain cross   See *breeding system.*

Streptobacillus moniliformis   A species of gram-negative, extremely pleomorphic organisms which form long filaments with swellings up to five times their width, and chains of bacilli and cocci. L forms are also produced. It is highly pathogenic for mice, and in man produces rat-bite (Haverhill) fever.

Streptococcus   A genus of gram-positive, spherical organisms that characteristically develop into chains. Members of this group are classified on the basis of hemolysis (alpha, beta, and gamma streptococci), the presence of group antigens in the cell wall (see Lancefield classification), and the presence of "M" and "T" proteins in the cell wall. Hemolytic strains produce a large number of extracellular enzymes and toxins.[16, 36] See table.

DISEASES CAUSED BY STREPTOCOCCI

AGENT	HOST	DISEASE
S. pyogenes	Man, occasionally the cow	Septic sore throat, scarlet fever, erysipelas, endocarditis, nephritis, rheumatic heart disease (?)
S. agalactiiae	Cow	Mastitis
S. dysgalactiae	Cow	Mastitis
S. uberis	Cow	Mastitis
S. equi	Horse	Strangles
S. genitalium	Mare	Metritis, cervicitis
S. zoopidemicus, or S. gallinarum	Chicken	Septicemia

streptogramin   A group of antibiotics produced by species of *Streptomyces* which includes the original streptogramin, as well as staphylomycin, ostreogrycin, synergistin, mikamycin, pristinamycin, and vernamycin. They are divided into groups A and B, which are markedly synergistic in their activities. The agents in group A are active against gram-positive cocci, while those in group B are mainly active against gram-positive bacilli. The activity of the group is based on inhibition of protein synthesis at the ribosomal level.[36, 49]

streptokinase   An enzyme produced by streptococci that catalyzes the conversion of plasminogen to plasmin.

    s.-streptodornase, a mixture of enzymes elaborated by hemolytic streptococci; used as a proteolytic and fibrinolytic agent.

streptomycin   An antibiotic produced by species of *Streptomyces* which possesses a broad range of activity against gram-positive and gram-negative bacteria and against mycobacteria. Its mechanism of action is complex but appears to be directed against protein synthesis.[49]

streptonigrin   A broad-spectrum antibiotic produced by a species of *Streptomyces* which acts by inhibition of DNA synthesis.[36, 49]

stress   The sum of all nonspecific biological phenomena elicited by adverse external influences including damage and defense. See *general adaptation syndrome.*

stridulation   The production of noise by rubbing parts of the body together.

strigiform birds   Any member of the avian order Strigiformes, which comprises two families. All members are known under the substantive name of owls. They are divergent from the falconiform birds in having no crop and long ceca with club-shaped ends.

Strongyloides   A genus of nematodes which parasitize man and animals. They enter the body through the skin, go through the blood stream to the lungs, where they undergo further development, then invade the surrounding tissues, and enter the intestinal tract. *S. stercoralis* occurs in man; certain species in rhesus and cynomolgus monkeys, *S. papillosus* in sheep, and *S. ransomi* in pigs.[21]

Strongylus   A genus of nematodes which are the most common parasites of the cecum and colon of the family Equidae. There are several species, including *S. vulgaris, S. edentatus,* and *S. equinus.* The larvae of strongyles migrate widely throughout the mesentery and surrounding tissues and frequently give rise to endarteritis in the major branches of the aorta, particularly the mesenteric and celiac branches. These lesions frequently result in thrombosis and the formation of aneurysms, which may lead to partial occlusion of the vessels and weakness in the hind limbs or recurrent anoxic spasms of the large intestine.[21]

structural gene   See *gene.*

structure unit   The smallest building unit of the capsid of a virus. Clumps of structure units are known as capsomeres.

struthioniform birds   Members of the avian order Struthioniformes, huge flightless birds with unkeeled sternum and powerful legs with two toes, typified by the ostriches.

sub-   A prefix signifying under, near, almost, or moderately.

subacute sclerosing panencephalitis (SSPE)   See *Dawson's encephalitis,* under *encephalitis.*

submetacentric   Denoting a chromosome with an off-center centromere.

substrain   See *inbred strain.*

succinic dehydrogenase   An enzyme of the Krebs cycle that converts succinate to fumarate, requiring Fe^{++} and flavin as co-factors.

sudan III   A non-ionic dis-azo dye. Solubility at 15° C.: water nil, absolute alcohol 0.25 per cent, and insoluble in glycerol; used to differentiate old from fresh blood in spinal fluids and to stain lipids in tissues.[57, 153]

Sudan black B A non-ionic dye of the disazo group. Solubility at 15° C.: water nil, absolute alcohol 0.25 per cent, and glycerol 0.05 per cent. It is used with pyronin for staining tubercle organisms, with safranin for fat in bacteria, and with eosin-methylene blue for lipid granules in leukocytes.[57]

Sudan blue A non-ionic dye of the anthraquinone group. Solubility at 15° C.: water nil, absolute alcohol 1.4 per cent, and glycerol 2.5 per cent.[57]

Sudan violet A non-ionic anthraquinone dye. Solubility at 15° C.: water nil, absolute alcohol 3.2 per cent, and glycerol 12 per cent. It is used to stain the nucleus of the malarial parasites.[57]

suggillation A bruise or ecchymosis.

sulfo- A prefix used in naming chemical compounds, indicating the presence of divalent sulfur or of the group SO_2OH.

summer sleep See *estivation*.

sun yellow G An acid dye. Solubility at 15° C.: water 1 per cent, insoluble in absolute alcohol, and glycerol 3 per cent. It is used as a decolorizer.[57]

super- A prefix signifying above, or implying excess.

superfemale A female organism whose cells contain more than the ordinary number of sex-determining (X) chromosomes. See also *chromosomal aberration*.

superstition In behavioral science, a condition resulting from lack of care in specifying the response which is reinforced in experiments (e.g., if a reinforcing stimulus such as food is randomly delivered to an animal irrespective of his behavior, he may develop response patterns [superstitions] which are repeated but which are not part of the experimental behavior being reinforced).

suppression See *conditioned suppression*.

supra- A prefix signifying above or over.

supravital Denoting the staining of tissues in the living state.

SV Simian virus.

swan See *anseriform birds*.

swayback 1. Abnormal downward curvature of the spinal column in the dorsal region in horses. 2. A congenital demyelinating disease of lambs, characterized by incoordination, tremor, blindness, and paralysis which is caused by deficiency of copper in the diet of pregnant ewes, resulting in incomplete embryological development of the central nervous system of the offspring.

sweet clover poisoning See *dicoumarol*.

swimmer's itch (cercarial dermatitis) An itching dermatitis caused by penetration into the skin of larval forms (cercaria) of schistosomes. It occurs in bathers in waters infested with these organisms.

swine See specific diseases of swine, and see *miniature swine*.

swine erysipelas See *erysipelas*.

swine fever Hog cholera.

swine influenza (hog flu) An acute respiratory infection caused by the combined action of a myxovirus of the influenza A group and *Hemophilus suis*. The disease usually appears suddenly and begins with fever, anorexia, and extreme weakness. The agent may persist in masked form for several years, during which it passes through a most unusual cycle. It is carried from infected swine by the larvae of the lungworm *Metastrongylus apri*. Shope showed that the larvae are harbored by the earthworm, which may transmit the infective lungworm larvae, still containing influenza virus, back to swine. The swine influenza virus resembles the human strain in its ability to grow in amniotic and allantoic cavities of embryonated hen's eggs.[76, 142]

sykes monkey Any member of *Cercopithecus mitis*. See *primate*.

symbiont (symbiote) An organism living in symbiosis; usually the smaller member of a symbiotic pair of dissimilar size (also called *microsymbiont*), and frequently, such microorganisms associated in a regular mutualistic manner with insects and other invertebrates.[159]

symbiosis The living together or close association of two dissimilar organisms, each of the organisms being known as a symbiont. The association may be beneficial to both (mutualism), beneficial to one without effect on the other (commensalism), beneficial to one and detrimental to the other (parasitism), detrimental to one without effect on the other (amensalism), or detrimental to both (synnecrosis).[159]

symbiote Symbiont.

symbolophobia A morbid fear that one's acts may contain some symbolic meaning.

symptom Any functional evidence of disease or of a patient's condition; a change in a patient's condition indicative of some bodily or mental state. *Symptom* should be used in reference to the evaluation of subjective feelings about disease; thus it is usually less appropriate when referring to a disease in anomen, for which the word *sign*, the manifestation of disease as interpreted by the observer, is more correct. Used in plant pathology as synonymous with lesion (q.v.).

syn- A prefix signifying union or association.

syndactyly The most common congenital anomaly of the hand, marked by persistence of the webbing between adjacent digits, so that they are more or less completely attached; generally considered an inherited condition, the anomaly may also occur in the foot.

syndesmo- A combining form denoting relationship to connective tissue, or particularly to the ligaments.

syndesmoma A neoplasm or tumor composed of connective tissue.

syndrome A set of symptoms which occur together; the sum of signs of any morbid state; a symptom complex.

synergistin See *streptogramin.*

Syngamus A genus of nematodes of the family Syngamidae, superfamily Strongyloidia, that are parasitic for vertebrates, especially birds.[21]

S. laryngeus, a species parasitizing the cow (cattle gapeworm), cat, and man, as well as birds.

S. trachea, a species that parasitizes the trachea of the chicken, turkey, pheasant, and other birds. Infection may occur either directly or indirectly, with the earthworm serving as intermediate host.

syngeneic Isogeneic.

synthetase Ligase.

Syphacia obvelata A common nematode (pinworm) of laboratory rats which has also been found in man. The life cycle of this parasite resembles that of *Enterobius*[21.] See also *helminth parasites,* under *rat.*

syphilis See *spirochetosis.*

syringo- A combining form denoting relationship to a tube or a fistula.

syringoma Adenoma of the sweat glands.

systemic lupus erythematosus (SLE) See under *lupus.*

T

Tabanidae A family of large flies of the order Diptera. The males feed on plants, whereas the females are blood-sucking and serve as intermediate hosts in protozoan infections. *Chrysops* and *Tabanus* are two important genera.

tabes Any wasting of the body; progressive atrophy of the body or a part of it.

tachy- A combining form meaning swift or rapid.

tachyauxesis See *heterauxesis.*

tachytelic See *evolutionary rate.*

Taenia A genus of cestodes of the family Taeniidae that parasitize man and other vertebrates. The most important species are *T. solium* (the pork tapeworm), the most common large tapeworm of man; *T. pisiformis,* the tapeworm of the dog, cat, rabbit, and hare; and *T. taeniaeformis,* the tapeworm of the cat and rat. See also *cestodiasis.*

Talfan disease See *baby pig encephalomyelitis* under encephalomyelitis.

tamarin A small South American monkey of the genus *Saguinus,* family Callithricidae, sometimes called a marmoset (q.v.). It reacts to injection of serum from human hepatitis victims in a manner which indicates that it may be susceptible to hepatitis virus. The tamarin is susceptible to Rous sarcoma virus, which produces in it a metastasizing tumor. It is also useful for study of twin births.[85] See *primate.*

tandem schedule See *schedules of reinforcement,* under *reinforcement.*

T antigen A foreign antigenic determinant found within cells that have been transformed by oncogenic viruses such as adenoviruses, SV 40, and polyoma virus. These antigens are present in the nucleus of nearly all transformed cells and usually are detected by complement fixation or fluorescent antibody procedures. They are specific for the virus that caused the transformation and are immunologically identical in all transformed cells.

tapeworm A parasitic intestinal cestode worm having a flattened, tapelike form, and composed of separate joints. The ova of tapeworms are taken into the alimentary canal of the intermediate host, whence they make their way into the tissues, where they form small cystlike masses, called scolices (see *hydatid disease*). When the flesh of the intermediate host is eaten, the scolices develop within the alimentary canal of the new host into the adult tapeworm, which consists of a head, neck, and a various number of segments, called proglottids, each of which is hermaphroditic and produces ova. See table accompanying *cestode.*

tarantula A venomous spider. See *arachnid.*

tarsier A member of genus *Tarsius.* See *primate.*

tarsus In tetrapods, the ankle; in some arthropods, the end of the limb.

teleonomy The doctrine that the existence of a structure or a function in an organism implies that it has had evolutionary survival value. Also used to refer to the development or presence of cellular structures as being the result of a design for a specific purpose.

teleost Any member of the typical bony fishes of the chordate class Osteichthyes, subclass Neopterygii, i.e., the modern fishes.

telo- A combining form denoting relationship to an end.

telocentric Denoting a chromosome with a terminally located centromere.

telophase The last of the four stages of mitosis (q.v.).

telson The last segment of the abdomen of an arthropod, modified in scorpions as a powerful sting. Absent in adult insects.

Tennessee Academy of Science University of Tennessee, Martin, Tenn. 38237.

tera- A combining form used in naming units of measurement to indicate a quantity one trillion (10^{12}) times the unit specified by the root with which it is combined.

teras A fetal monster.

terato- A combining form denoting relationship to a monster.

teratoblastoma A neoplasm containing embryonic elements and differing from a teratoma in that its tissue does not represent all the germinal layers.

teratogen A substance that causes abnormal development of the embryo.

teratology That branch of pathology that deals with abnormal development and congenital malformations.

teratoma A true neoplasm made up of a number of different types of tissue, none of which is native to the area in which it occurs.

teratoma E6496 A spontaneous tumor observed at necropsy in the ovary of a C3HeB substrain inbred mouse in the laboratory of E. Fekete at the Jackson Memorial Laboratory in 1951. It contains elements of all three primary germ layers and transplants of it grow progressively in nearly 100 per cent of C3He, C3H, C3H$_f$ and C3H × C57B1 hybrid hosts. Subcutaneous transplants are palpable in seven to nine days and kill the host in six to seven weeks without metastasis.[150]

teratophobia 1. Morbid fear or aversion to monsters. 2. Morbid dread of giving birth to a monster.

terminal ileitis of hamsters See under *ileitis*.

tertian malaria See *malaria*.

Tertiary Denoting the period of the Cenozoic Era extending from about 63 million to one million years ago. See *geologic time divisions*.

Teschen disease See *porcine encephalomyelitis*, under *encephalomyelitis*.

tetracycline A group of antibiotics referred to as broad-spectrum antibiotics because they are able to inhibit the growth of a wide range of microorganisms, including many gram-positive and gram-negative bacteria, rickettsiae, mycoplasma, and certain protozoa. The tetracyclines are active against a number of metabolic processes, including respiration, enzyme formation, cell wall synthesis, and chelation of metallic ions, but most evidence indicates that their primary activity is inhibition of protein biosynthesis at the level of the ribosome by interference with formation of the complex between ribosome, messenger RNA, and aminoacyl-s-RNA.[36, 49]

Tetrahymena A genus of ciliate protozoa used frequently in genetic studies.

tetrapod A four-legged vertebrate.

The Texas Academy of Science, Inc. Department of Statistics, Southern Methodist University, Dallas, Tex. 75222.

Theiler's mouse encephalomyelitis See under *encephalomyelitis*.

Thelazia rhodesii (oriental eyeworm) A genus of nematodes of the family Thalaziidae. *T. rhodesii* is found in the tear ducts and between the eyes and the lids of cattle; the intermediate host is the fly, *Musca*. Other members of this group are *T. californiensis* found in the dog in California, *T. erschowi* in the pig, *T. leesei* in the camel, *T. lacrymalis* in the horse, and *T. callipaeda* in the dog, rabbit, and man.

theory 1. The doctrine or the principles underlying an art as distinguished from the practice of that particular art. 2. A formulated hypothesis or opinion not based upon actual knowledge. 3. A generic term for the empirical and theoretical study of behavior in experimental psychology.

cognitive t., in behavioral science, the tendency to stress latent learning and place learning in experiments, and perception and cognition in theory.

contiguity t., that which considers the occurrence of the responses in the presence of a stimulus as a necessary and sufficient condition for learning.

continuity t., that which states that the animal's response is determined by the total number of responses reinforced in the presence of, or shortly after, the positive discriminative stimulus.

drive-reduction t., a theory of learning which asserts that there must be a reinforcing stimulus and that it must be contiguous in time with a response in order for sufficient conditions to exist for learning. Also that the reinforcing stimulus must reduce some drive or need if learning is to occur.

Hullian t., a generic term for the drive-reduction theory of learning or a reference to the entire empirical and theoretical statements put forward by Hull and his school.

noncontinuity t., a theory of discrimination learning which asserts that the animal's behavior is not dependent upon the total number of responses reinforced in the presence of, or shortly after, the positive discriminative stimulus, but rather upon the expectancy of stimuli which may not be contiguous with the response.

reinforcement t., a term used to refer to the work of stimulus response theorists, who stress the operation of reinforcement in their experiments.

stimulus-response t. (S-R t.), a term almost synonymous with reinforcement theory, which presents all descriptions of behavior in terms of stimulus and response.

thermobiosis Ability to live in a high temperature.

thermochroic Reflecting some of the heat rays and absorbing or transmitting others.

thermophilic Growing best at or having a fondness for high temperatures; said of bacteria which grow best at temperatures between 50° and 60° C. Cf. *mesophilic* and *psychrophilic*.

thiaminase An enzyme, especially common in fish, which destroys thiamine and can cause vitamin deficiency in animals which consume large amounts of fish containing the enzyme, as the fox (see *Chastek's paralysis*), mink, and cat.[142]

thiamine pyrophosphate See *cocarboxylase*.

thin layer chromatography See *chromatography*.

thio- A prefix signifying the presence of sulfur.

thioflavin T A stain used in fluorescent microscopy to demonstrate amyloid in tissue sections.[153]

6-thioguanine A purine analog used as an immunosuppressant and antitumor drug.

thionine A basic dye of the thiazine group. Solubility at 15° C.: water 1 per cent, absolute alcohol 1 per cent, and glycerol 5 per cent. It is used with orange G for staining infected plant tissues and with 25 per cent buffered methanol to stain chondroitin sulfates; also used to stain mucins of epithelial and connective tissue.[57, 153]

thionine blue A basic dye of the thiazine group. Solubility at 15° C.: water 4.5 per cent, absolute alcohol 1.8 per cent, and glycerol 3 per cent.

thiouracil A thiourea derivative, 2-mercapto-4-pyrimidone, which affects adversely the synthesis of the thyroid hormone.

thoracopagus A double fetal monster consisting of two nearly complete individuals joined at or near the sternal region, so that the two components are face to face.

threat See under *behavior.*

threshold 1. That value at which a stimulus just produces a sensation, is just appreciable, or comes just within the limits of perception. See also under *response* and *stimulus.* Called also *Schwelle.* 2. That concentration of a substance in the blood above which it is excreted by the kidneys and below which it is retained.

-thrix A word termination denoting a resemblance or a relationship to hair.

thrombin (thrombin; fibrin ferment) The enzyme derived from prothrombin which converts fibrinogen to fibrin. Also, a pharmaceutical preparation (*topical t.*), which is a sterile protein substance prepared from prothrombin of bovine origin through interaction with added thromboplastin in the presence of calcium.

thrombo- A combining form denoting relationship to a clot, or thrombus.

thrombocytopathy A general term applied to a qualitative disorder of the blood platelets; sometimes used to designate specifically a qualitative abnormality due mainly to deficiency of platelet factor 3, causing defective generation of intrinsic thromboplastin.

thrombocytopenia Decrease in the number of blood platelets.

thrombolysis The phenomenon by which preformed thrombi are lysed by a complex series of events, the most important of which involves the local action of plasmin confined within the substance of the thrombus.

thromboplastin A coagulation factor essential to the production of thrombin and proper hemostasis.

thrombus A plug or clot in a blood vessel or in one of the cavities of the heart, formed by coagulation of the blood, and remaining at the point of its formation. Cf. *embolus.*

thwarting See *frustration.*

thymectomy Removal of the thymus.

thymus A bilobed lymphoepithethial organ situated in the anterior superior portion of the thorax and ventral and lateral to the trachea in the neck. The epithelial portion is derived from the third and fourth pharyngeal pouches, around which lymphocytes develop early in embryonic life. These are the first lymphocytes to be found in the body, and it is believed that colonization from this organ forms lymphoid follicles in the rest of the body. The thymus is thus very important in the development of immunological competence, especially cellular or transplantation immunity. It is thought by some that the formation of abnormal clones of immunologically competent cells in the thymus may be responsible for certain kinds of auto-antibodies, as in systemic lupus erythematosus, NZB mouse disease, and myasthenia gravis.[48, 93] See also *central lymphoid tissue* and *bursa of Fabricius.*

tick A blood-sucking arachnid parasite of the superfamily Ixodoidea.

tiger snake See table accompanying *snake.*

tinamiform birds Members of the avian order Tinamiformes, largely ground-dwelling birds with little power to fly, typified by the tinamou.

Tissue Culture Association Department of Microbiology, University of Michigan, Ann Arbor, Mich. 48104.

titan yellow An acid dye of the thiazole group. Solubility at 15° C.: water 1.5 per cent, absolute alcohol 1 per cent, and glycerol 3 per cent. It is used to stain magnesium in plant tissues.[57]

titi A member of genus *Callicebus.* See *primate.*

TL antigen Thymus leukemia antigen. In the mouse, the Tla locus determines the presence (Tla[a]) or absence (Tla[b]) in the normal thymus of the alloantigen called the thymus leukemia antigen. It is present in the thymus of inbred strains A and C58, absent in the thymus of strains C57BL/6, C3H/An, BALB/c, and AKR. The antigen is found in no other normal tissue, but it is found in a proportion of the leukemias of probably all mouse strains. Heterozygote Tla[a]/Tla[b] mice are intermediate between the two homozygotes in the quantity of antigen present in the thymus.[51]

T-maze A T-shaped path or runway with the starting box at the base of the T and the goal boxes at each end of the cross piece. Discriminative stimuli are sometimes placed in the opposite arms of the T.

    multiple T-m., a series of T-shaped runways with a starting box at the base of the first T and a goal box at the end of one of the arms of the last of the series.

tobacco mosaic virus (TMV) A plant virus producing lesions on the leaves of tobacco plants. The virus is rod shaped, with a core of RNA surrounded by 21,000 protein subunits of molecular weight about 17,000 each. TMV was the virus first obtained in crystalline form (Stanley) and has been an important biological model in studying the function of nucleic acids in heredity.

toco- A combining form denoting relationship to childbirth, or labor.

tocophobia Abnormal dread of childbirth.

tolerance In immunology, the inability to react against an antigen, an immunological state that occurs when an excess of antigen reaches normal or primed immunologically competent cells without the action of the reticuloendothelial system. As a result the recipient responds toward the antigen as though it were self-protein.[93]

toluidine blue A basic dye of the thiazine group. Solubility at 15° C.: water 3.25 per cent, absolute alcohol 1.75 per cent, and glycerol 10 per cent. It is used to demonstrate amyloid metachromasia; as a counterstain in the substrate film method for deoxyribonuclease; for staining cartilage matrix, chondroitin sulfates, the mucin of connective and epithelial tissue; and with acid fuchsin and aurantia as a differential stain for mitochondria and starch grains in plant cells.[57, 153]

tom Mature male domestic turkey (*Meleagris gallopavo*).

topography In behavioral science, the physically measurable dimensions of a response. The term pattern of response is also used.

topophobia A morbid dread of particular places.

torpor A body state in which the temperature and the heart, respiratory, and metabolic rates are reduced, but not as drastically as in deep hibernation, as in the "carnivorean lethargy" of *Ursus* (bears). Cf. *hibernation*.

tortoiseshell cat Calico cat.

touffe See under *flacherie*.

TO virus See *Theiler's mouse encephalomyelitis*, under *encephalomyelitis*.

Toxascaris leonina A nematode of the family Ascaridae that parasitizes the small intestine of the dog, cat, lion, tiger, and other carnivorous animals. The larvae do not migrate through the viscera as do *Ascaris* and *Toxocara*, but burrow into the crypts of Lieberkuhn, submucosa, and muscular layer. After several days, the larvae return to the lumen of the small intestine and grow to maturity.[21]

toxemia of pregnancy In anomen, a condition of acute onset occurring in near-term pregnant or postparturient animals. Species exhibiting a recognized syndrome include the dog, cow, sheep, guinea pig, and rabbit. In these species, the characteristic biochemical derangement appears to be in the Krebs cycle metabolism of glucose precursors or storage forms such that the animal suffers severe hypoglycemia and is forced into an accelerated phase of fat metabolism to provide 2-carbon fragments for entry into the oxidative cycle. It is believed that a poor plane of nutrition potentiates a genetic predisposition to the toxemia.

In the guinea pig and rabbit, the genetic and biochemical parameters have been explored in detail. The characteristic gross lesions include a swollen yellow liver and enlarged brownish adrenal glands. Microscopically, one sees fatty infiltration of the liver and degeneration of cells in the zona fasciculata of the adrenal gland. Intravenous glucose administration reverses the clinical signs.[119, 142, 144]

toxin A substance produced by plants (phytotoxin), animals (zootoxin), or bacteria (endotoxin and exotoxin) which may produce severe damage to tissues or cells. Endotoxins (q.v.) or pyrogens are produced when bacterial cells break down and release their protoplasm. Exotoxins (q.v.) or true toxins are secreted by bacterial cells and usually exhibit high specificity and antigenicity. Toxins may be further classified by their affinity for certain cells: neurotoxins (nerve cells), hemolytic toxins (erythrocytes), and leukocidins (leukocytes).[16, 36]

Toxocara A genus of nematode worms.

T. canis, a species of intestinal parasites of the dog. They exhibit two phases of infection depending on the age and species of the host. The tissue phase occurs in the adult dog and in children and rodents. The larvae migrate through the arterial system to muscles, kidneys, and the central nervous system, where they remain. See *visceral larva migrans*. The intestinal phase occurs in pups. The larvae go through the venous circulation to the lungs. After they reach the bronchi and trachea they are coughed up, swallowed, and develop into maturity in the small intestine. The life cycle is similar to that of *Ascaris lumbricoides*. Prenatal infection of puppies by transplacental migration of larvae is very common.[21]

T. cati, a species which parasitizes the cat. Infection may occur in man causing a syndrome known as visceral larva migrans (q.v.). Prenatal infection is not known to occur.[21]

toxoid A bacterial exotoxin which has lost its toxicity from treatment such as heat or formalinization, but which retains antigenicity and can be used to immunize animals against the corresponding toxin.

Toxoplasma See *toxoplasmosis*.

toxoplasmosis Disease of vertebrate animals noted for its wide host range, caused by a genus of parasites with the single species *Toxoplasma gondii*, although the nomenclature often includes species named after the species from which the organism is isolated, e.g., *Toxoplasma cuniculi*. In the rabbit, the disease is comparatively infrequent in the United States, but is much more common in Europe. It may occur sporadically in individuals or as an epizootic, with mortality up to 30 per cent in some rabbit colonies. In the rabbit the disease may be acute, chronic, or clinically silent. In the acute form, lesions include swelling and necrosis of mesenteric lymph nodes and spleen, and multiple miliary foci of necrosis in the liver, kidney, and lungs. The organism is seen in these lesions intracellularly in pseudocysts in the proliferative form of the disease, and extracellularly as individual organisms in the necrotizing form. The organism is small and crescent-shaped, measuring 2 to 4μ by 4 to 7μ. Granuloma formation in all the above-mentioned organs, but especially in the spleen and brain, characterizes the proliferative form of the disease, and these may be the only organs involved in the chronic form. Presumably this is because, as humoral antibody is elaborated by survivors of the acute and necrotizing phase, the organisms require intracellular shielding; hence a reticuloendotheliosis or latent central nervous system infection results. Diagnosis is established by demonstration of the organisms in microscopic sections and by serologic assay for specific antibody, using the Sabin-Feldman dye test. No method of treatment or control is advocated. See also *nosematosis* for differential diagnosis.[142]

TPN Triphosphopyridine nucleotide, the former name for nicotinamide adenine dinucleotide phosphate (NADP).

tragus (pl. *tragi*) A fleshy protuberance anterior to the external ear of a mammal

train In behavioral science, to subject an animal to experimental procedures until one or more of its responses become conditioned.

training See *discrimination training.*

transaminase An enzyme that catalyzes the reversible transfer of an amino group from an α-amino acid to an α-keto acid, usually α-ketoglutaric acid. Most, if not all, transaminases require pyridoxal-5-phosphate.[90, 118]

    glutamic-oxalacetic t. (GOT), an enzyme normally present in serum and in various body tissues, especially the heart and liver; it is released into the serum as the result of tissue injury, hence the concentration in the serum may be increased in myocardial infarction or acute damage to hepatic cells.

    glutamic-pyruvic t. (GPT), an enzyme normally present in serum and body tissues, especially in the liver; it is released into the serum as a result of tissue injury, hence the concentration in the serum may be increased in patients with acute damage to hepatic cells.

    tyrosine t., an enzyme concerned with catabolism of tyrosine and the physiological regulation of gluconeogenesis, found in the liver, kidney, brain, and other tissues. An increase in the liver enzyme can be rapidly induced by numerous hormones (insulin, glucagon, glucocorticoids, etc.) on injection into intact animals, or on perfusion of the isolated liver. Increased activity results from increased synthesis of the apoenzyme. The enzyme has a striking 24-hour cycle of variation, with the ascending phase correlated to the intake of protein. Rapid transient increases can also be induced by stress, such as cold, laparotomy, etc.

transamination The reversible transfer of an amino acid to what is originally an α-keto acid, forming a new amino acid and keto acid, without the appearance of ammonia in the free state.

transcription The formation of messenger RNA against a DNA template.

transduction The transfer of new genetic material to a bacterial genome, through the intermediate action of a bacteriophage.[32, 64]

transfaunation Transfer of symbiotic fauna (usually mutualistic protozoa) from one host to another. See also *mutualism, defaunate, infaunate,* and *refaunation.*

transfer The phenomenon in which over several trials a set of responses originally given to one set of stimuli, are given to other sets of stimuli. See *stimulus generalization* and *insight.*

transferase An enzyme that catalyzes the transfer, from one molecule to another, of a chemical group that does not exist in free state during the transfer.[90, 118]

transfer factor An immunological mechanism by which reacting cells release substances that can transfer hypersensitivity to normal individuals or may initiate inflammatory reactions.

transferrin (siderophilin) Serum β-globulin that binds and transports iron. Several hereditary variants have been distinguished.

transfer RNA (soluble RNA) A low molecular weight RNA existing in 20 species, each designed to transfer a specific amino acid to ribosomal particles and deposit it there to be formed into a polypeptide chain.[32, 90]

transformation 1. A phenomenon originally observed in pneumococci wherein one strain of organism can be changed into another. This was shown to be a result of the entry of DNA from one cell into the genome of another. Subsequently similar transfers of genetic activity from one cell to another were found to occur in virus-infected bacteria (transduction) and in mammalian cells in culture (polykaryon formation). The same phenomenon probably occurs in vivo and, if so, is of great biological significance. The original experiments with DNA and bacteria by Griffith and by Avery, McCleod, and McCarty comprised one of the most important modern steps leading to the current concepts of genome function.[32, 36, 59] 2. More recently, the term has been applied to cellular transformation in which cell cultures are induced to lose contact inhibition (q.v.) and undergo neoplastic change.

transketolase An enzyme present in the hexose-monophosphate shunt that catalyzes the conversion of D-erythrose-4-phosphate to glycolaldehyde, and the conversion of D-ribose-5-phosphate to D-sedo-heptulose-7-phosphate, and D-xyulose-5-phosphate to D-glyceraldehyde-3-phosphate, using thiamine pyrophosphate and Mg^{++} as co-factors.

translation The formation of protein in ribosomes by ribosomal RNA as directed by specific messenger RNA.

translocation In genetics, the transfer of a

segment of one chromosome to a nonhomologous chromosome.

reciprocal t., the mutual exchange of fragments between two nonhomologous chromosomes.

transmissible gastroenteritis A viral disease of swine that is highly fatal to pigs less than 10 days old.[16]

transmissible venereal tumor (canine) See *venereal tumor.*

transovarian transmission A mode of transovum transmission (q.v.) in which the passage of microorganisms from mother to egg is known to occur within the ovary. First demonstrated in Texas cattle fever in 1893 by Smith and Kilborne.

transovum transmission The transmission of microorganisms from one generation to the next by way of the egg. Transovarian transmission is a special case of transovum transmission.

transphosphorylase An enzyme that catalyzes the transfer of a phosphate group. See *kinase.*

transplantation The grafting of tissues taken from the same body or from another. See *xenograft, allograft,* and *isograft.*

transstadial transmission The transmission of microorganisms from one stage in the life cycle of the host to the next, throughout part or all of the host's life cycle.

transvestism (cross-dressing; eonism) A sexual deviation characterized by overwhelming desire to assume the attire, and be accepted as a member of the opposite sex.

tree shrew See *primate.*

trematode Any member of the class Trematoda, commonly referred to as flukes, which are parasitic in man and other animals. See table, and see individual genera.

Treponema A genus of slender spiral microorganisms which belongs to the family Treponemataceae, order Spirochaetales, comprising species pathogenic and saprophytic in man and other animals.

DISEASES CAUSED BY *Treponema*

SPECIES	HOST	DISEASE
T. pallidum	Man	Syphilis
T. pertenue	Man	Yaws
T. carateum	Man	Pinta (caraate)
T. cuniculi	Rabbit	Syphilis
T. genitalis	Man	None
T. macrodentium	(Saprophytic)	None
T. microdentium	(Saprophytic)	None

trial A single experimentally manipulated occasion on which an instance of a specific response is elicited.

trial and error Denoting a form of learning; see under *learning.* Also, *vicarious trial and error,* the back and forth movement of the head of an animal at a choice point in a T-maze. See *intention movement.*

Triassic Denoting that portion of the Mesozoic Period extending from 225 to 180 million years ago. See *geologic time divisions.*

Triatoma A genus of the family Reduviidae (assassin bugs), important as a vector of *Trypanosoma cruzi.*

Trichinella spiralis A nematode of the family Trichinellidae which may infest the muscle of man, hog, rodents, and other carnivorous animals. The infestation is acquired by eating contaminated meat. The free larvae circulate through the arteries and capillary beds, then encyst in the diaphragm and other muscles and produce the disease known as trichinosis. Immunity has been obtained through the injection of larval secretions and excretions into mice. See *helminth parasites,* under *rat.*

trichinosis A disease caused by the muscle parasite *Trichinella spiralis,* and acquired by eating contaminated meat. This disease is particularly common in swine and rats. Rat-infested pig farms are a potential source of trichinosis in man and therefore comprise a very important public health hazard. It is marked in its early stages by diarrhea, nausea, colic, and fever, and later by stiffness, pain, swelling of the muscles, fever, sweating, and insomnia.

trichloroethylamine An alkylating agent used as an oncolytic drug.

trichloroethylene poisoning A condition characterized by thrombocytopenia, granulocytopenia, and hypoplastic anemia, which occurs in cattle fed soy bean oil meal extracted with trichloroethylene. The mechanism is unknown.

tricho- A prefix denoting relationship to hair.

trichoepithelioma An epithelial tumor that frequently calcifies and involves the hair follicle.

trichomonad A parasite of the genus *Trichomonas.*

Trichomonas A genus of parasitic flagellate protozoa that cause disease in birds and animals, including man. See *trichomoniasis.*

T. muris, see *protozoan parasites,* under *rat.*

trichomoniasis Infestation with *Trichomonas.*

avian t., the most important trichomonad of birds is *Trichomonas gallinae* (syn: *T. columbae, T. halli, T. diversa, T. hepaticum*). This organism, which inhabits the upper digestive tract, appears to act as a primary pathogen, especially in columbiform, passerine, falconiform, and gallinaceous birds. In falcons the disease has been called frounce, and in pigeons canker, but in all affected species the infection is manifested by focal necrosis of the mucosa of the crop, esophagus, buccal cavity, and occasionally the liver. The affected areas become ulcerated or thrown up into hard, caseous, yellow masses which tend to become contiguous and extend in furrows along the epithelium. Diagnosis is established by demonstration of the trichomonads in smears of the lesion. It may be treated with the use of 2-amino-5-nitrothiazole (Enheptin) in the drinking wa-

(Text continued on page 207.)

TREMATODE	PRINCIPAL HOSTS	HABITAT	MAIN CHARACTERISTICS	DISEASE CAUSED
Schistosomatoidea				
Schistosoma mansoni	Man	Blood	Male and female paired, male 6.4–9.9 mm. long, female 7.2–14 mm. long, conspicuous tuberculations on male, 6–9 testes, eggs 114–175 μ by 45–68 μ	Schistosomiasis mansoni
S. japonicum	Man, dogs, cats, rats, mice, cattle, pigs, horses	Blood	Male and female paired, male 12–20 mm. long, female 26 mm. long, cuticle spinous on males, seven testes, eggs 70–100 μ by 50–65 μ	Schistosomiasis japonicum
S. haematobium	Man, monkeys	Blood	Male and female paired, male 10–15 mm. long, female 20 mm. long, cuticular tuberculations on males, four to five testes, eggs 122–170 μ by 40–70 μ	Schistosomiasis haematobium
Schistosomatium douthitti	Muskrats, (skin of man)	Blood	Anterior 2/5 of male body is flattened, 14–18 testes	Schistosome dermatitis in man and dogs
Fascioloidea				
Fasciola hepatica	Man, sheep, cattle	Bile ducts	20–30 mm. long, 13 mm. wide, cone shaped process at anterior end, eggs 130–150 μ by 63–90 μ	Fascioliasis (liver rot)
F. gigantica	Horses, cattle	Bile ducts	Similar to F. hepatica only larger	Fascioliasis gigantica
Fascioloides magna	Cattle, horses, sheep	Liver	Larger than F. hepatica, often over 200–300 mm. long, eggs 109–168 μ by 75–100 μ	Fascioloidiasis
Fasciolopsis buski	Man, pigs	Duodenum, jejunum	Broadly ovate, 30–75 mm. long, 8–20 mm. wide, highly dendritic testes, eggs 130–140 μ by 80–85 μ	Fasciolopsiasis
Plagiorchioidea				
Dicrocoelium dendriticum	Sheep, cattle, goats, horses, pigs, rabbits, dogs, man	Liver, bile ducts	Slender, lancet shaped, 5–12 mm. long, 1 mm. wide, extremities pointed, eggs 38–45 μ by 22–30 μ	Dicrocoeliasis
Opisthorchioidea				
Opisthorchis felineus	Cats, rarely man	Biliary and pancreatic ducts	Lancet shaped, rounded posteriorly, 7–12 mm. long, 2–3 mm. wide, intestinal caeca along entire length of body, eggs 30 μ by 11 μ	Opisthorchiasis
Opisthorchis (=Clonorchis) sinensis	Man, dogs, cats	Bile ducts	10–25 mm. long, 3–5 mm. wide, deeply lobed testes, eggs 27.5–35 μ by 11.7–19.5 μ	Clonorchiasis(?)
Metorchis conjunctus	Dogs, cats, foxes, man	Gallbladder, bile ducts	1–6.6 mm. long, 590 μ to 2.6 mm. wide, linguiform, testes slightly lobed, cirrus absent, eggs 22–32 μ by 11–8 μ	Experimental hosts killed in heavy infections
Parametorchis complexus	Cats	Bile ducts	3–10 mm. long, 1.5–2 mm. wide, uterus rosette shaped and located in anterior half of body	Cirrhosis of liver(?)
Amphimerus pseudofelineus	Cats, coyotes	Bile ducts	12–22 mm. long, 1–2.5 mm. wide, uterus with only ascending limb, eggs 25–35 μ by 12–15 μ	Cirrhosis of liver(?)

*From T. C. Cheng: The Biology of Animal Parasites. W. B. Saunders Co., Philadelphia, 1964.

(Table continues)

203

TREMATODE	PRINCIPAL HOSTS	HABITAT	MAIN CHARACTERISTICS	DISEASE CAUSED
Opisthorchioidea (*Cont'd*)				
Paramonostomum parvum	Ducks	Intestine	Ovoid, 250–500 μ long, 200–350 μ wide	Nonpathogenic
Notocotylus imbricatus	Water fowls	Caecum	2–4 mm. long, no acetabulum	Nonpathogenic
Heterophyoidea				
Heterophyes heterophyes	Man, cats, dogs, foxes	Small intestine	Elongate, pyriform, 1–1.7 mm. long, 0.3–0.4 mm. wide, small oral sucker	Heterophyiasis
Metagonimus yokogawai	Man, dogs	Small intestine	Similar to *H. heterophyes* but with acetabulum deflected to right of midline	Metagonimiasis
Apophallus venustus	Cats, dogs, raccoons	Small intestine	950 μ to 1.4 mm. long; 250–550 μ wide; no cirrus or cirrus sac; few eggs, 26–32 μ by 18–22 μ	Nonpathogenic
Cryptocotyle lingua	Usually in fish-eating birds, also found in dogs and cats	Small intestine	902 μ to 1.6 mm. long, 430–470 μ wide, conspicuous genital pore at anterior margin of acetabulum, anterior portion of body often attenuated, eggs 32–48 μ by 18–22 μ	Nonpathogenic
Phagicola longa	Dogs, cats, foxes, wolves	Small intestine	500 μ to 1 mm. long, 300–400 μ wide, oral sucker surrounded by double row of 16 spines, eggs 18 μ by 9 μ	Nonpathogenic(?)
Euryhelmis monorchis	Minks	Small intestine	410 μ long, 610 μ wide, only one testis, eggs 29 μ by 14 μ	Nonpathogenic
Strigeata				
Alaria americana	Dogs	Small intestine	4–5 mm. long, posterior portion of body cylindrical, crescentric projection on each side of oral sucker, testes bilobed, eggs 106–134 μ by 64–80 μ	Nonpathogenic
A. arisaemoides	Dogs, foxes	Small intestine	7–10 mm. long, small projections on each side of oral sucker, body constricted, eggs 140 μ by 90 μ	Nonpathogenic
A. michiganensis	Dogs	Small intestine	1.8–1.91 mm. long, right testis bilobed, genital atrium more than twice the size of suckers, eggs 80–140 μ by 76–80 μ	Nonpathogenic
A. canis	Dogs	Small intestine	2.8–4.2 mm. long, small projections on each side of oral sucker, anterior testis lobed, posterior testis horseshoe shaped, eggs 107–133 μ by 70–99 μ	Nonpathogenic
Strigea falconis	Turkeys	Intestinal	Body divided, vitellaria extend into both portions, eggs 110–125 μ by 75–80 μ	Nonpathogenic
Cotylurus flabelliformis	Ducks, chickens	Small intestine	Body divided, 560–850 μ long, 200 μ wide, eggs 100–112 μ by 68–76 μ	Nonpathogenic(?)
Postharmostomum gallinum	Chickens	Caecum	Elongate body, 3.5–7.5 mm. long, 1–2 mm. wide, vitellaria well developed along lateral margins of body	Irritation in heavy infections

Strigeata (Cont'd)

Sphaeridiotrema globulus	Ducks, swans	Small intestine	Body subspherical; 500-850 μ long; uterus short, in front of acetabulum, containing four to five eggs; eggs 90-105 μ by 60-75 μ	Ulcerative enteritis
Ribeiroia ondatrae	Chickens, fish-eating birds, muskrats	Proventriculus	1.6-3 mm. long; testes at posterior end of body, ovary anterior to testes; eggs 82-90 μ by 45-48 μ	Proventriculitis
Echinostomatoidea				
Clinostomum attenuatum	Chickens	Trachea	5.7 mm. long, 1.5 mm. wide; dorsal body surface convex, ventral surface concave, oral sucker surrounded by collar	Nonpathogenic
Euparyphium melis	Mink	Stomach, small intestine	Lancet shaped; 3.8-10.5 mm. long; 650 μ to 2.1 mm. wide; collar of 27 spines; eggs large, 117-130 μ by 72-84 μ	Nonpathogenic(?)
Echinoparyphium recurvatum	Chickens, turkeys, usually in water birds	Small intestine	700 μ-4.5 mm. long, 500-600 μ wide; collar of 45 spines around oral sucker, four larger corner spines, others arranged in two rows	Severe inflammation of small intestine
Echinostoma ilocanum	Man, rats, dogs	Small intestine	2.5-6.5 mm. long, 1-1.35 mm. wide, circumoral disc with 49-51 spines, eggs 83-116 μ by 58-69 μ	Colic, diarrhea
E. revolutum	Chickens, (usually also in water birds)	Caecum, rectum	10-22 mm. long, 2-3 mm. wide, collar of 37 spines, five grouped together as corner spines, eggs 90-126 μ by 59-71 μ	Hemorrhagic diarrhea in heavy infections
Himasthla muehlensi	Man	Intestine	11-17.7 mm. long, 0.41-0.67 mm. wide, body thin, elongate, collar of 32 spines, two on each side, remaining 28 arranged in horseshoe pattern, eggs 114-149 μ by 62-85 μ	Unknown
Hypoderaeum conoideum	Ducks, chickens, pigeons	Small intestine	6-12 mm. long, 1.3-2 mm. wide, collar of 47-53 spines in two rows, eggs 95-108 μ by 61-68 μ	Nonpathogenic
Troglotrematoidea				
Paragonimus westermani	Man, cats	Encapsulated in lungs	Plump, ovoid, 7.5-12 mm. long, 4-6 mm. wide, scalelike spines, deeply lobed testes, no cirrus pouch or cirrus, ovary lobed, eggs 80-118 μ by 48-60 μ	Paragonimiasis
P. kellicotti	Man, dogs, cats, sheep, goats, rats, lions	Encapsulated in lungs	Plump, ovoid, 9-16 mm. long, 4-8 mm. wide, similar to *P. westermani*, eggs 78-96 μ by 48-60 μ	Kellicotti paragonimiasis
Nanophyetus (=Troglotrema) salmincola	Dogs, foxes, bobcats, coyotes, cats, raccoons, man	Intestine	Pyriform, 0.8-1.1 mm. long, 0.3-0.5 mm. wide, uterus simple with few eggs, vitellaria profuse, eggs 60-80 μ by 34-50 μ	Salmon poisoning
Sellacotyle mustelae	Mink, foxes	Intestine	335 μ long, 190 μ wide, pyriform, eggs 60 μ by 54 μ	Slight enteritis
Collyriclum faba	Chickens, turkeys	Encysted in skin	Each cyst with two worms unequal in size 4-5 mm. long, 3.5-4.5 mm. wide, eggs 19-21 μ by 9-11 μ	Emaciation and anemia resulting in death

(Table continues)

205

TREMATODE	PRINCIPAL HOSTS	HABITAT	MAIN CHARACTERISTICS	DISEASE CAUSED
Paramphistomatoidea *Watsonius watsoni*	Man	Intestine	Pear shaped, 8–10 mm. long, 4–5 mm. wide, thick body, acetabulum near posterior end, eggs 122–130 μ by 75–80 μ	Severe diarrhea
Gastrodiscoides hominis	Man	Caecum	Pyriform, 5–10 mm. long, 4–6 mm. wide, prominent genital cone, large acetabulum covering posterior half of body, eggs 150–152 μ by 60–72 μ	Mucous diarrhea
Paramphistomum microbothrioides (*Cotylophoron cotylophorum*)	Cow	Rumen	3–11 mm. long, 1–3 mm. wide, conical convex dorsally, concave ventrally, acetabulum at posterior end, testes large and lobate, eggs 132 μ by 68 μ	Paramphistomiasis
P. cervi	Cow, moose, deer	Rumen	Similar to *P. microbothrioides*	Nonpathogenic (?)
Zygocotyle lunata	Chickens, (usually also in water birds)	Caecum, small intestine	3–9 mm. long, 1.5–3 mm. wide, testes lobed, acetabulum at posterior end, ovary behind posterior testis, eggs 130–150 μ by 72–90 μ	Nonpathogenic
Cyathocotylioidea *Mesotephanus appendiculatum*	Dogs, cats	Small intestine	900 μ to 1.75 mm. long, 400–600 μ wide, large adhesive organ behind acetabulum, genital pore posterior, uterus short with four to five eggs, eggs 117 μ by 63–68 μ	Nonpathogenic (?)
Cyclocoelioidea *Typhlocoelum cymbium*	Ducks, geese	Trachea, bronchi and air sacs	6–12 mm. long, 3–6 mm. wide, caeca form complete ring, eggs 122–154 μ by 63–81 μ	Suffocation in heavy infections

206

(Text continued from page 202.)

ter. Although numerous other trichomonads, especially in the lower digestive tract, have been described in birds, none appear to be significant as agents of disease.[11, 112]

trichopathophobia   Morbid anxiety with regard to the hair, its growth, disease, etc.

Trichophyton   A genus of the imperfect keratinophilic fungi, the dermatophytes, which exhibit pigmented colonies with a granular to powdery, or a cottony to velvety appearance. Characteristic microconidia and macroconidia may be used as a guide in the identification of the various members of this group. See table.

Trichosomoides crassicauda   See *helminth parasites*, under *rat*.

trichostrongylosis   Infestation with nematodes of the family Trichostrongyloidea, common parasites of cattle and sheep. The disease may occur as multiple infections, with several species simultaneously parasitizing the host and resulting in severe anemia, cachexia, diarrhea, and sometimes death, particularly in young animals. Some of the commonest of this group of parasites are *Haemonchus contortus* (the common stomach worm), *Osertagia* (the brown stomach worm), and *Trichostrongylus axei* (the hairlike stomach worm).

Trichostrongylus   A genus of nematodes of the family Trichostrongylidae, superfamily Strongyloidea. *T. axei* is the hairlike stomach worm of cattle, sheep, and horses. Other members of the genus are *T. ransomi*, *T. affinis*, and *T. calcaratus*, which are found in rabbits; *T. colubriformis* and *T. capricola*, in the stomach and small intestine of ruminants; *T. delicatus*, in squirrels; and *T. tenuis* in birds.[21, 109]

tricothecin   An antibiotic produced by *Trichothecium roseum*, which is active against fungi, including *Actinomyces*, *Coccidioides*, and *Blastomyces*. Its mechanism of action is not known, but its toxicity precludes therapeutic use.[49]

Trichuris   (*Trichocephalus;* whipworm)   A genus of nematodes of the family Trichuridae which parasitizes many species. *T. trichiura* is the whipworm of man. Other members of the genus are *T. felis*, found in the cecum and colon of the cat; *T. discolor*, in the cow; *T. leporis*, in the rabbit; *T. muris*, in the rat; *T. suis*, in the pig; *T. vulpis*, in the dog; and *T. ovis* in the cow and sheep.[21]

Diseases Caused by *Trichophyton*

Agent	Host	Disease
T. verrucosum, *T. violaceum*	Cattle	Ringworm of cattle
T. equinum	Horse	Ringworm of horses
T. rubrum	Dog, cow, man	Dermatomycosis
T. mentagrophytes	Mouse, rat, dog, cat, rabbit, chinchilla, guinea pig	Dermatomycosis
T. schoenleini	Dog, cat, mice, man	Dermatomycosis
T. gallinae	Chicken, turkey	Favus of fowl

trinactin   See *nonactin*.

triose isomerase   An enzyme of the Embden-Meyerhof pathway that catalyzes the conversion of dihydroxyacetone phosphate to D-glyceraldehyde-3-phosphate.

triphenylmethane   See *rosaniline*.

triplet   A sequence of three nucleotides in RNA which codes for a specific amino acid. See *codon*.

trisomy   Abnormal additional chromosome of one type in an otherwise diploid cell; seen in Down's syndrome and Klinefelter's syndrome. See *chromosomal aberration*.

Troglotrema   See *Nanophyetus*.

trogoniform birds   Members of the avian order Trogoniformes, composed of a single family, the Trogonidae, which includes the trogons and quetzal, the latter a resplendent American species sacred to the Mayans and Aztecs.

-trophic, -trophin   Word termination denoting relationship to nutrition.

trophoblastoma   Chorioepithelioma.

trophology   The science of nutrition.

trophozoite   A motile protozoan stage that multiplies and maintains the colony in the host. In the malaria parasite, the state of schizogony.

-tropic   A word termination denoting turning toward, changing, or tending to turn or change.

tropism   A growth response in a nonmotile organism, elicited by an external stimulus. Such response may be either positive (toward) or negative (away from the stimulus). By extension, used as a word termination affixed to a stem denoting the nature of the stimulus (phototropism) or the material or entity for which an organism or substance shows a special affinity (neurotropism).

true vipers   See table accompanying *snake*.

trypan blue   An acid dis-azo dye. Solubility at 15° C.: water 1 per cent, absolute alcohol 0.2 per cent, and glycerol 7 per cent. It is used for staining fungi and as a vital stain for calcifying bone and dentine.[37, 57, 153]

Trypanosoma   A genus of heteroxenous hemoflagellates of the family Trypanosomatidae, order Protomastigida, all species of which are parasitic. During its life cycle, the individual trypanosome passes through four stages: the leishmanial, leptomonad, crithidial, and trypanosomal. The first three forms occur in the vector, and the last in the definitive host. The trypanosome stage is found in blood, lymph, and cerebrospinal fluid of man and anomen as an extracellular parasite. It has a very wide host range, being found in the blood of pigs, cattle, sheep, antelope, fish, birds, and reptiles. The life cycle is complex and cannot be adequately discussed here. The trypanosome stage measures 15 to 20μ and the crithridial stage 15μ in length. Each has a flagellum and undulating membrane and multiplies by longitudinal fission.[21, 109, 142, 159] See table on page 208.

T. duttoni, see *protozoan parasites*, under *rat*.

T. lewisi, see *protozoan parasites*, under *rat*.

DISEASES CAUSED BY TRYPANOSOMES [21, 142, 159]

AGENT	VECTOR	RESERVOIR HOST	HOST	DISEASE
T. brucei	Tsetse fly (Glossina)	Dog	Horse, mule, dog	Nagana
T. gambiense, T. rhodesiense	Glossina palpalis	– – –	Man	Trypanosomiasis
T. congolense	Tsetse fly	Wild animals	Cow, horse, sheep, goat, camel, dog	Nagana
T. simiae	Tsetse fly	– – –	Pig, camel, monkey	– – –
T. vivax, T. uniforme	Tsetse fly	Antelope	Cow	– – –
T. evansi	Tabanidae (horse fly)	Water buffalo	Horse, camel, elephant, dog	Surra
T. equinum	Tabanus, Stomoxys	Capybara, native cattle	Horse	Mal de caderas
T. hippicum	Tabanus, Desmonus rotundus (Sat)	Cow, native burro	Horse, mule	Murrina or derrengadera
T. venezuelense	(?)	Capybara	Horse, dog	Surra, murrina
T. equiperdum	Tabanidae, Stomoxys	– – –	Horse	Pourine or maladie du coit
T. cruzi	Triatoma Panstrongylus	– – –	Man	Chagas' disease
T. ariari	Reduviidae (Rhodnius prolixus)	– – –	Man	Trypanosomiasis

trypanosome 1. Any member of the genus *Trypanosoma*. 2. One of the forms achieved in the life cycle of various members of the family Trypanosomatidae.

trypansomiasis Infestation with members of the genus *Trypanosoma*. See table.

trypsin One of the proteolytic enzymes of pancreatic secretion.

trypsinogen The crystallizable zymogen occurring in the pancreas from which trypsin is formed when it comes in contact with enterokinase.

tryptophan An essential amino acid, the precursor of serotonin and nicotinamide. It is essential for optimal growth in infants and for nitrogen equilibrium in adults.

tryptophanase An enzyme that catalyzes the cleavage of tryptophan into indole, pyruvic acid, and ammonia.

tsetse fly A member of the genus *Glossina*, which transmits sleeping sickness.

tsutsugamushi Scrub typhus.

tubercle In pathology, the nodular granulomatous lesion most frequently associated with tuberculosis, but also seen in other chronic inflammations, as in bacterial and mycotic infections. Cf. *granuloma*.

tuberculin A sterile liquid containing the growth products of, or specific substances extracted from, the tubercle bacillus. The original form (old tuberculin), prepared by boiling, filtering, and concentrating a bouillon culture of tubercle bacilli, was put forth as a cure for tuberculosis by Koch in 1890 (Koch's lymph). In various forms, tuberculin is presently used in the diagnosis of tuberculosis, especially in children and cattle, and also in the treatment of tuberculosis. The tuberculin test, as commonly applied, consists in the injection of tuberculin under or into the skin: the injection has no effect in nontuberculous subjects, but causes inflammation at the site of the injection in tuberculous subjects. [36, 142]

tuberculosis An infectious disease caused by an acid-fast bacillus, *Mycobacterium tuberculosis*, and characterized by the formation of tuberculous granulomata. It remains one of the world's most devastating diseases, and is especially serious in man, cattle, swine, birds, and subhuman primates. The three principal types are human, bovine, and avian. [16, 36, 136, 142] See table.

tularemia A disease of rodents, resembling plague, which is transmitted by the bites of flies, fleas, ticks, and lice, and may be acquired by man through handling of infected animals. It is caused by *Pasteurella tularensis*. In man the disease is marked by the formation of an ulcer at the site of inoculation, followed by inflammation of the lymph nodes and the development of severe constitutional symptoms such as headache and other pains, chills, and rapid rise of temperature. Called also *deer fly fever, Pahvant Valley plague, rabbit fever, alkali disease*, and *Francis' disease*.

tumor A mass of tissue which grows independently of its surrounding structures and which has no apparent physiological function; see *neoplasm*. Sometimes also used to denote a swelling such as that caused by a bruise or inflammation.

tunicate Any member of the subphylum Tunicata, classified with the lower chordates. Tunicates inhabit the seas, various forms being found in depths from shallow beaches to 3 miles below the surface. Some are free-

PRINCIPAL TYPES OF TUBERCULOSIS

AGENT	HOST	COMMENT
M. tuberculosis (var. hominis)	Man	Most frequently pulmonary but may spread and be manifested in many organs
	Cow	Occasionally contracted from man
	Swine	By contact with garbage or human offal
	Horse	Occasional infection
	Nonhuman primates very susceptible	Important problem in zoos and research laboratories; can infect guinea pig and mouse
M. bovis	Cow	Lesions most prominent in lymph nodes; frequently calcified
	Man	Intestinal tract, lymph nodes, and especially bones; elimination of tuberculosis from bovine population of U.S. has reduced this form in man to very low level. Still a serious problem in many other parts of the world
	Horse	Occasional infections
	Cat	Occasional infections
	Swine	By ingestion of excrement; guinea pig, mouse and rabbit can be infected
M. avian	Birds	Swine and occasionally the cat; guinea pig, rabbit, and mouse can also be infected

living, others sessile. They may be solitary or colonial. The group name refers to the self-secreted "tunic" over the body. There are three classes of tunicates, the Larvacea, the Ascidiacea (ascidians or sea squirts), and the Thaliacea (salpians or chain tunicates, e.g., *Doliolum*). They are widely used in the study of chordate physiology and phylogeny. See also *chordate* and *ascidian*.

turbidity reducing unit The amount of hyaluronidase which is just sufficient to reduce the turbidity produced by 0.2 mg. of hyaluronate to that produced by 0.1 mg. after addition of acidified horse serum.

turkey See *galliform birds*.

Tween 80 Trademark for a sorbitan polyoxyalkalene derivative used as an emulsifier.

tyrocidine An antibiotic produced, together with gramicidin, (q.v.) by *Bacillus brevis*. The original mixture of tyrocidine and gramicidin was referred to by its discoverer, Dubos, as tyrothricin. Tyrocidine is active against many gram-positive and some gram-negative organisms. It is not used systemically because early studies indicated considerable toxicity. Its antibiotic activity is due to its cationic detergent effect on cell membranes causing leakage of vital metabolites.[36, 49]

Tyzzer's disease A disease originally described in Japanese waltzing mice by Tyzzer, but the agent, *Bacillus piliformis*, is now known to have a host range that includes the mouse, rat, rabbit, gerbil, dog, subhuman primate, and man. Clinical signs include diarrhea, loss of weight, and high mortality in early stages of disease outbreaks, although it may be asymptomatic in certain individuals. Gross lesions include target-shaped necrotic foci on the surface of the liver, enteritis of the terminal ileum and cecum, and mesenteric lymphadenitis. The organisms lie in palisades or clusters within hepatocytes or epithelial cells at the periphery of the necrotic lesions. The intracellular location of the organism may account for the inability to culture the organism on artificial media. Nothing is known of the immunology of infection with *B. piliformis;* control measures consist in destruction of affected colonies or repopulation with gnotobiotic derivation.[27]

U

uakari A member of the genus *Cacajao*. See *primate*.

UDP Uridine diphosphate.

ultra- A prefix denoting excess, or beyond.

ultracentrifugation A method used for the characterization of viruses, immunoglobulins, or other molecules by means of an extremely high rate of rotation, and based on the sedimentation rates of molecules in a centrifugal field. The measurement of the sedimentation rate can be taken by photographic devices which record the state of sedimentation at various intervals of time.[32, 64] See also *density gradient*, under *centrifugation*.

ultracentrifuge A centrifuge with a very high rate of rotation capable of sedimenting viruses and macromolecules such as proteins, nucleic acids, and polysaccharides. See *centrifugation.*

ultramicrotome   An instrument designed for cutting sections in preparation for electron microscopy.

ultrasonic   Pertaining to mechanical radiant energy having a frequency beyond the upper limit of perception by the human ear, that is, beyond about 20,000 cycles per second.

ultrastructure   The structure of biological materials as seen under the electron microscope.

ultraviolet   That portion of the electromagnetic spectrum just beyond the visible, with wavelengths from 1800 to 3900 Å.

ultraviolet absorption   A measurement of the relative amount of ultraviolet light transmitted or absorbed by a substance in solution. Absorption of specific frequencies can be plotted on a curve and used as a qualitative and quantitative estimate of materials under study.

Uncinaria stenocephala   A species of hookworms which infect the dog, cat, fox, and other carnivores.[21]

unit membrane   A trilaminar cell membrane varying in thickness from 80 to 100 Å and consisting of two electron-dense lines of protein each about 30 Å in thickness and separated from each other by an intermediate light region of lipid of about the same thickness. It occurs in most types of cells as plasma membrane and is also seen in internal structures such as endoplasmic reticulum. This similarity in structure does not imply that there is not great diversity in composition and function of the lipoprotein constituents.[38]

Universities Associated for Research and Education in Pathology, Inc.   9650 Rockville Pike, Bethesda, Md. 20014.

urea   A white, crystallizable substance, the diamide of carbonic acid, $NH_2CO \cdot NH_2$, from the urine, blood, and lymph. It is the chief nitrogenous constituent of the urine, and is the final product of the decomposition of proteins in the body, being the form under which the nitrogen of the body is given off. It is believed to be formed in the liver out of amino acids and other compounds of ammonia.

urease   A colorless, crystalline globulin that was first extracted by Takeuchi from the soy bean. It is also found in mucous urine passed during inflammation of the bladder. It is formed by various microorganisms, and is capable of causing the change of urea into carbon dioxide and ammonia, and of hippuric acid into benzoic acid and glycocoll.

uricase   An enzyme found in most mammals except man, which catalyzes the complicated transformation of uric acid into allantoin.

uricoxidase   An enzyme that oxidizes uric acid.

uridine diphosphate glucose pyrophosphorylase   An enzyme concerned with glycogenesis that catalyzes the conversion of D-glucose-1-phosphate to D-glucose-6-phosphate, utilizing uridine triphosphate (UTP) as a co-factor.

uridine diphosphate glucose transglucosylase (glycogen synthetase)   An enzyme concerned with glycogenesis that catalyzes the conversion of glycogen to uridine diphosphoglucose.

urodeum   See *cloaca.*

urokinase   A substance found in the urine of mammals, including man, and of other vertebrates, which activates the fibrinolytic system, acting enzymatically by splitting plasminogen.

uropod   An appendage found on the segment immediately anterior to the telson in some crustaceans.

Utah Academy of Sciences, Arts and Letters   Brigham Young University, Provo, Utah.

uviosensitive   Sensitive to ultraviolet rays.

V

vaccination   The injection of vaccine for the purpose of inducing immunity. Coined originally to apply to the injection of smallpox vaccine, the term has come to mean any immunizing procedure in which vaccine is injected. The original observation by Jenner that milkmaids exposed to cowpox were immune to smallpox was subsequently confirmed and led to the adoption of vaccination as one of the strongest measures available for control of diseases.[36, 136]

vaccine   A suspension of attenuated or killed microorganisms (bacteria, virus, or rickettsiae), administered for the prevention, amelioration, or treatment of infectious diseases.

   attenuated v., a vaccine containing living viruses which have been passed through abnormal hosts or cell cultures until they have lost their virulence but are still antigenic and useful in producing immunity against this specific disease without risk of infection to the host, as vaccines of yellow fever, canine distemper, rabies, and poliomyelitis.

   autogenous v., a vaccine prepared from microorganisms that have been freshly isolated from the lesion of the patient who is to be treated with it.

   BCG v. (bacille Calmette Guérin), a preparation for the prophylactic inoculation of young infants against tuberculosis. It consists of living cultures of bovine tubercle bacilli that have been grown over a period of many years on glycerinated ox bile so that their virulence is greatly reduced. Originally given by mouth, the preparation is now administered subcutaneously. The research leading up to the production of BCG vaccine has remained a classical example of the tremendous profit reaped by the cooperation of scientists in human and animal medicine: Calmette, a physician, and Guérin, a veterinarian, based their cooperative studies on background gained in working with bovine tuberculosis.

measles virus v., a preparation derived from the causative virus of rubeola grown in monkey kidney or chick embryo tissue, and inactivated or attenuated; used to produce immunity to naturally occurring rubeola.

polyvalent v., a vaccine prepared from more than one strain or species of organism.

Sabin's oral polio v., an orally administered vaccine consisting of the three types of live, attenuated polioviruses grown in monkey kidney tissue culture.

Salk v., a vaccine containing three types of poliomyelitis virus which, although inactivated with formalin, still retain the capacity to produce resistance against the natural disease.

vaccinia (cowpox) A viral disease of cattle. Communicated to man, usually by vaccination, it confers a greater or less degree of immunity against smallpox. See *vaccination*.

vacuolating virus A simian virus of the papovavirus group that causes vacuolation in cultured kidney cells of the green monkey.

vacuum activity The occurrence of a fixed action pattern apparently in the absence of its usual releaser or sign stimulus.

vaginal plug A fibrinous coagulum formed from the secretions of the seminal vesicles and prostate glands of the male in many species, including rodents and primates. The secretions are part of the coital ejaculate from the male and usually fill the vagina from the vulva to the cervix. They usually persist from 16 to 36 hours and are useful as indicators of mating.[51]

valinomycin An antibiotic produced by a species of *Streptomyces* possessing activity against mycobacteria, fungi, and some gram-positive organisms. It increases the permeability of mitochondrial membranes and interferes with oxidative metabolism.[49]

valvular fibrosis (verrucous endocardiosis) Thickening of the cusps of the mitral and tricuspid valves of unknown cause, it is common in old dogs.[142] See *endocarditis*.

vancomycin An antibiotic isolated from a species of *Streptomyces* which has a strongly bactericidal action against gram-positive organisms, particularly *Staphylococcus*, by interference with mucopeptide manufacture in the bacterial cell wall.[36, 49]

varicella Chickenpox.

variola Smallpox.

vector A carrier, especially an animal (usually an arthropod) that transfers an infectious agent from one host to another. See table on page 212 for examples of some of the most important vectors and the disease agents which they transmit.

vehicle Denoting the transmission of an infection by means other than physical or direct contact.

venereal tumor (canine condyloma; canine histiocytoma; infectious sarcoma; infectious lymphosarcoma; Sticker's sarcoma; transmissible sarcoma; venereal lymphosarcoma) An undifferentiated neoplasm of the dog usually acquired in nature by coitus. The canine venereal tumor appears to have a world-wide distribution and is the earliest known transmissible tumor. The first successful experimental transplantation was performed by M. A. Novinsky, a Russian veterinary student, in 1876. In 1934, Stubbs and Furth found that subcutaneous inoculations of tumor emulsions were successful in 72 per cent of dog hosts and that all of the tumors, with one exception, regressed spontaneously. Recovered dogs were immune to repeated tumor inoculations. Early lesions on the glans penis or vaginal mucosa occur as small reddish nodules, but as they mature they may assume a cauliflower-like appearance, with necrosis and hemorrhage.[150]

venom A poison, especially a toxic substance normally secreted by a serpent, insect, or other animal.

cobra v., see *snake v.* and *cobra factor*.

Russell's viper v., the venom of the Russell viper, which acts in vitro as an intrinsic thromboplastin and is useful in defining deficiencies of blood coagulation factor X.

snake v., the poisonous secretion of snakes, containing hemotoxins, hemagglutinins, neurotoxins, leukotoxins, and endotheliotoxins. The venoms of various species have been used as hemostatics.

spider v., the venom of a poisonous spider such as *Latrodectus, Atrax, Ctenus,* and *Lycosa*.

vent disease (of rabbits) See *spirochetosis*.

vernamycin See *streptogramin*.

verruca 1. An epidermal tumor of viral origin; called also *wart*. 2. One of the wartlike elevations developing on the endocardium in various types of endocarditis.

v. necrogenica, a verrucous growth, occurring usually about the knuckles, or elsewhere on the hands, of those who dissect cadavers or perform autopsies. A form of cutaneous tuberculosis, it is usually a single, hyperkeratotic dull red lesion which persists harmlessly and indefinitely, with little growth. Called also *anatomical, dissection,* or *postmortem tubercle,* or *anatomical, necrogenic, postmortem,* or *prosector's wart*.

v. vulgaris, a designation once given the common viral epidermal tumor of the skin.

vervet (green monkey) A member of the species *Cercopithecus aethiops*. See *primate* and *Marburg virus*.

vesicular exanthema (VE) A viral disease of swine which produces vesicles on the

RELATIONSHIP OF VECTOR GROUP TO PARASITE GROUP*

VECTOR GROUP	Protozoa	Bacteria	Spirochetes	Rickettsiae	Viruses
Triatomin bugs	*Trypanosoma cruzi, T. rangeli,* etc.				
Lice			*Borrelia recurrentis*	Epidemic typhus Trench fever Murine haemobarto- nellosis	
Fleas	*Trypanosoma lewisi, T. duttoni,* etc.	*Pasteurella pestis*		Endemic (murine) typhus Canine haemobarto- nellosis	
Mosquitoes	*Plasmodium* spp.				Encephalitides Dengue Yellow fever Rift Valley fever
Midges (*Culicoides*)	*Haemoproteus Leucocystozoon Hepatocystis*				Blue tongue
Sandflies (*Phlebotomus*)	*Leishmania*	*Bartonella bacilliformis*			Pappataci fever (sandfly fever)
Blackflies (*Simulium*)	*Leucocytozoon*				
Tabanid flies (*Tabanus, Chrysops,* etc.)	*Trypanosoma evansi*	*Pasteurella tularensis*		Anaplasmosis	
Tsetse flies (*Glossina*)	*Trypanosoma brucei, T. gambiense, T. rhodesiense, T. con- golense, T. vivax,* etc.				
Hippoboscid flies	*Haemoproteus*				
Ixodid ticks	*Babesia Theileria*	*Pasteurella tula rensis*		Q fever Rocky Mountain spotted fever Boutonneuse fever Siberian tick typhus Anaplasmosis	Colorado tick fever Omsk hemorrhagic fever Russian spring-summer encephalitis
Argasid ticks	*Aegyptianella*		*Borrelia* spp.		
Mites other than ticks	*Hepatozoon Lankesterella*			Rickettsialpox Scrub typhus	

*From D. Weinman and M. Ristic: Infectious Blood Diseases of Man and Animals. Vol. I. Academic Press, New York, 1968.

snout, lips, tongue, footpads, and skin be- tween the claws. The foot lesions usually cause lameness, which may be complicated by secondary bacterial infection. Animal in- oculation is used to differentiate this disease from foot-and-mouth disease and vesicular stomatitis.[16]

vesicular stomatitis   See under *stomatitis*.

Vibrio   A genus of polymorphic, highly mo- tile, gram-negative rods which may appear as curved rods arranged singly or united into spiral forms.[16, 36] Many are pathogenic (see table).

Victoria blue B   A basic triarylmethane dye. Solubility at 15° C.: water 4.3 per cent, abso- lute alcohol 8.25 per cent, and glycerol 12.5 per cent.

Victoria blue 4R   A basic triphenylmethane dye. Solubility at 15° C.: water 3 per cent, absolute alcohol 20 per cent, and glycerol 20 per cent. It is used to stain elementary virus bodies.[57]

Victoria green G   An acid tris-azo dye. Solu- bility at 15° C.: water 1.85 per cent, absolute alcohol 1.85 per cent, and glycerol 5 per cent.

villoma   A villous tumor, chiefly of the rec- tum.

vinblastine   An alkaloid extracted from *Vinca rosea* which inhibits mitosis and is used as a neoplastic depressant; $C_{46}H_{58}N_4O_9$.

vincristine   An alkaloid extracted from *Vinca rosea* which inhibits mitosis and is used as a neoplastic depressant; $C_{46}H_{56}N_4O_{10}$.

vinegar eel   A free-living ovoviviparous nematode, *Turbatrix aceti,* commonly found in old vinegar. Adults, which are about 2 mm. in length, feed on bacteria.

viomycin   An antibiotic produced by a species of *Streptomyces* which is active

Diseases Caused by *Vibrio*

Species	Host	Disease
V. comma	Man	Asiatic cholera
V. fetus	Cattle, ewe	Abortion
V. jejuni	Cattle, calf	Black scours or winter dysentery
V. coli	Swine	Diarrhea
Other species	Fowl	Avian vibrionic hepatitis

against mycobacteria. Its mechanism is not understood.[49]

viper A snake of the genus *Vipera;* see table accompanying *snake.*

   pit v., any of a group of venomous snakes having a depression or pit between the nostril and the eye. They include the rattlesnake, copperhead, water moccasin, and fer-de-lance. See table accompanying *snake.*

   Russell's v., the daboia, a venomous snake of Southeastern Asia. See table accompanying *snake,* and see under *venom.*

Viperidae See table accompanying *snake.*

viral diarrhea of cattle (mucosal disease) A viral disease of cattle which closely resembles infectious bovine rhinotracheitis, shipping fever, and rinderpest. Viral diarrhea has a mild clinical course and mortality seldom exceeds 5 per cent. Affected animals manifest a high temperature, leukopenia, depression, anorexia, excessive salivation, and dehydration.[16]

viral enteritis of mink See under *enteritis.*

viral hemorrhagic septicemia See *Egtved virus.*

Virginia Academy of Science P.O. Box 9211, Richmond, Va. 23227.

virion The mature and potentially infectious virus particle.

virology That branch of microbiology which is concerned with viruses and viral diseases.

virucidal Capable of neutralizing or destroying viruses.

virulence The degree of ability of a microorganism to cause disease as indicated by case fatality rates and/or its ability to invade the tissues of the host. It is measured experimentally by the median lethal dose (LD_{50}) or median effective dose (ED_{50}). By extension, the competence of any infectious agent to produce pathologic effects. Cf. *pathogenicity.*

virus A group of ultramicroscopic infectious agents which can replicate only within living cells. For a comparison of viruses and other microscopic forms, see *microorganism.*

   v. III (herpesvirus cuniculi) A herpesvirus isolated from rabbit tissues by Rivers at The Rockefeller Institute in the 1920's. Experimental infections have been used to produce cardiac lesions in laboratory rabbits, but the agent is not associated with any known spontaneous disease of the rabbit, nor has it been reported since.

   classification of v's, with full recognition that no completely satisfactory taxonomic system has yet been devised, an adaptation of the system presented by Fenner[39] has been selected for emphasis (see table). This classification is based on certain physical, chemical, and biological properties. There may be some conflict when terms are compared to those used by epidemiologists, e.g., arbovirus is not used in Fenner's classification although it is an important category in epidemiological studies. Fenner uses encephalovirus instead.[2, 39, 64, 114] See also main entries for description of each group.

   Adenovirus: A group of nonenveloped icosahedral deoxyriboviruses that multiply in the nucleus of infected cells to produce crystalline arrays of virions. Most adenoviruses

Animal Viruses and Their Basic Properties[*]

Virus Group	Nucleic Acid			Virion			Nucleocapsid	
	Type	Config-uration	Molecular Weight[†] (×10⁶)	Shape	Size (Å)	En-velope	Symmetry	No. of Capsomers or Diameter of Helix
Papovavirus	DNA	DS[‡]	3–5	Spherical	300–500	−	Icosahedral	72
Adenovirus	DNA	DS	20–25	Spherical	800–900	−	Icosahedral	252
Adenovirus-associated viruses	DNA	DS	3.6	Spherical	200	−	Icosahedral	(?)
Herpesvirus	DNA	DS	54–92	Roughly spherical	1000–1500	+	Icosahedral	162
Poxvirus	DNA	DS	160–200	Brick-shaped	3000 x 2000 x 1000	−	Complex	−
Parvovirus	DNA	SS[‡]	1.8	Spherical	200	−	Icosahedral	32
Picornavirus	RNA	SS	about 2	Spherical	200–300	−	Icosahedral	60 (?)
Encephalovirus	RNA	SS	2–3	Spherical	500	+	Cubical (?)	(?)
Myxovirus	RNA	SS	about 3	Roughly spherical	800–900	+	Helical	80–90 Å
Paramyxovirus	RNA	SS	7.5	Picomorphic	800–1200	+	Helical	170–180 Å
Rhabdovirus	RNA	SS	6	Bullet-shaped	1750 x 700	+	Helical	50 Å
Leukovirus	RNA	SS	10–12	Roughly spherical	1000–1200	+	Complex	(?)
Reovirus	RNA	DS	10	Spherical	600–900	−	Icosahedral	180 or 270

[*]From F. Fenner: The Biology of Animal Viruses. Academic Press, New York, 1968.
[†]Extreme figures within group shown.
[‡]DS = double-stranded, SS = single-stranded.

The Adenoviruses*

Subgroup	Recognized Serotypes	Adenovirus Group Antigen
Human	28	+
Simian	12	+
Bovine	2	+
Canine (canine hepatitis virus)	(?)	+
Murine	(?)	+
Avian	(?)	−

*From F. Fenner: The Biology of Animal Viruses, Academic Press, New York, 1968.

are associated with respiratory infections, and many are characterized by prolonged latency. Some strains of adenoviruses are oncogenic (see *oncogenic virus*). See table.

Encephalovirus: A group of spherical enveloped riboviruses containing single-stranded RNA which multiply in the cytoplasm and mature by budding from cytoplasmic membranes. Chemical and physical data for their classifications are rather meager See table, and see also *arbovirus*, under A.

Herpesvirus: A group of deoxyriboviruses enclosed within an envelope which is acquired as the virus matures either at the nuclear membrane or the cytoplasmic membrane (see table). Other viruses probably in this group are those of pachecos disease of parrots, fatal disease of owls, inclusion disease of owls, feline rhinotracheitis, malignant catarrhal fever of cattle, renal carcinoma of leopard frogs, salivary gland infection of mice and guinea pigs, and inclusion body rhinitis of pigs. See table.

Leukovirus: A group of enveloped riboviruses which mature by budding from cytoplasmic membranes. This group is divided into two subgroups, avian and murine. See tables.

Myxovirus: A group of spherical riboviruses enclosed within an envelope derived from modified cytoplasmic membranes.

The Encephaloviruses*

Group A: Grow well in cultured cells, show extensive serological cross-reactivity; all are mosquito-borne viruses.

Equine encephalitis—Western, Eastern, and Venezuelan; Semliki Forest; Chikungunya; Sindbis; and 11 to 13 other named viruses.

Group B: More difficult to grow in cultured cells, show extensive serological cross-reactivity; some are mosquito-borne and some are tickborne viruses.

Yellow fever, St. Louis encephalitis, Japanese encephalitis, dengue (4 serotypes), West Nile, Murray Valley encephalitis, Russian tickborne encephalitis, and 23 other named viruses.

*From F. Fenner: The Biology of Animal Viruses. Academic Press, New York, 1968.

Some viruses of this group have been placed in a second group, referred to as paramyxovirus, because of nucleic acid content. The viruses of influenza type A of man, swine, horse, duck, and fowl share type-specific nucleoprotein antigen; this group includes the fowl plague virus. The viruses of influenza types B and C have distinctive nucleoprotein antigens; they are recovered only from man.[39]

Papovavirus; A group of small nonenveloped icosahedral deoxyriboviruses that replicate in the nucleus. There are two subgroups, which have capsids of different sizes containing different amounts of DNA. They are typified by papilloma and polyoma viruses. The papilloma subgroup includes the viruses of rabbit papilloma, rabbit oral papilloma, human papilloma (wart), canine papilloma, and bovine papilloma. The polyoma subgroup includes the virus of mouse polyoma, simian virus 40, "K" virus, and rabbit vacuolating virus.[39]

Paramyxovirus: A group similar to the myxoviruses but separated because of the differing RNA content. Of this group, the viruses of mumps, Newcastle disease, and

The Herpesviruses*

Virus	Comment
Herpes simplex	Serologically related by cross-neutralization tests
B viruses	Serologically related by gel-diffusion tests
Pseudorabies Infectious bovine rhinotracheitis Equine abortion (equine herpes type 1), rhinopneumonitis	Serologically related by complement-fixation tests
Varicella-zoster	The diseases of varicella and herpes zoster are different manifestations of infection by one virus
Infectious laryngotracheitis	Probably other related viruses in birds
Cytomegaloviruses	Several related viruses, each highly host-specific
Canine herpes	A fatal infection in puppies
Herpesvirus T	A fatal infection in the owl monkey and marmoset
Virus III of rabbits	A latent infection

*Adapted from F. Fenner: The Biology of Animal Viruses. Academic Press, 1968.

The Leukoviruses: Avian Subgroup[*]

DESIGNATION OF VIRUS	ABBREVIATIONS OF VIRUS TYPES ARRANGED IN SUBGROUPS		
	A	B	C
Rous-associated viruses			
Isolated from the Bryan high-titer strain	RAV-1 RAV-3	RAV-2	– – –
Isolated from the Bryan standard strain	RAV-4 RAV-5	– – –	– – –
Fujinami-associated virus	FAV-1	– – –	– – –
Avian myeloblastosis virus strain BAI-A	AMV-1	AMV-2	– – –
Resistance-inducing factors (field strains of avian leukosis found in congenitally infected chick embryos)	RIF-1	RIF-2	– – –
Strain RPL-12 avian leukosis virus	RPL-12	– – –	– – –
Schmidt-Ruppin strain of Rous sarcoma virus	SR-RSV-1	SR-RSV-2	– – –
Harris strain of Rous sarcoma virus	– – –	HA-RSV	– – –
Mill Hill strain of Rous sarcoma virus	MH-RSV	– – –	– – –
Carr-Zilber strain of Rous sarcoma virus	– – –	– – –	CZ-RSV
Prague strain of Rous sarcoma virus	– – –	– – –	PR-RSV

[*]From F. Fenner: The Biology of Animal Viruses. Academic Press, New York, 1968.

The Leukoviruses: Murine Subgroup[*][†]

VIRUS (NAMED AFTER INVESTIGATOR)	HOST SENSITIVITY	NEOPLASTIC CELL (TYPE)	COMMENT
Gross	Mice, rats	Lymphoid	Possibly the "natural" form of the murine leukovirus
Rauscher	Mice, rats	Lymphoid (with erythrocytopoiesis)	⎫ Show serological cross reactivity
Friend	Mice, rats	Reticulum cell with erythroblastosis	⎬
Moloney	Mice, rats, hamsters	Lymphoid	⎭
		Rhabdomyosarcoma (Moloney) Sarcoma (Harvey)	⎫ Obtained by passage of high titer Moloney virus ⎭
Bittner	Mice	Mammary carcinoma	Incidence of tumors greatly affected by genetic and hormonal factors

[*]From F. Fenner: The Biology of Animal Viruses. Academic Press, New York, 1968.
[†]A leukovirus has recently been isolated from feline leukemia.

parainfluenza 1, 2, 3, and 4 contain neuraminidase; the simian myxovirus (SV5) is related to parainfluenza 2 virus; and the viruses of measles, distemper, and rinderpest are serologically related, but lack neuraminidase.[39]

Parvovirus: A group of small deoxyriboviruses found mainly in rodents; they are unique among animal viruses in that they contain a small single-stranded molecule of DNA. Sometimes referred to as *picodnaviruses.* See table.

The Parvoviruses[*]

SEROTYPE (MOORE, 1962)	DESIGNATION	ORIGIN	REFERENCE
1	H-1 (T)	H-Ep No. 1 tumor growing in conditioned rats	Chandra and Toolan (1961)
2	H-3 (T)	H-Ep No. 3 tumor growing in conditioned rats	Moore (1962)
2	RV	Rat neoplasms	Kilham and Oliver (1959)
2	X-14	Mammary tissue of X-irradiated rats	Payne et al., (1964)
(?)	Minute mouse	Contaminant of stock of mouse adenovirus	Crawford (1966)

[*]From F. Fenner: The Biology of Animal Viruses. Academic Press, New York, 1968.
[†]Poxviruses of mammals not yet allocated to subgroups.

Picornavirus: A large group of vertebrate viruses which are small, nonenveloped, and icosahedral in shape. Most infections with picornaviruses are inapparent, but some, such as foot-and-mouth disease and poliomyelitis, are important. This group is divided into subgroups: the enteroviruses include poliovirus (3 serotypes), coxsackievirus (A 24 serotypes; B-6 serotypes), and echovirus (30 serotypes); the cardioviruses include EMC (encephalomyocarditis) virus, mengovirus, and ME (Maus Elberfeld) virus; the rhinovirus has about 80 serotypes; and the virus of foot-and-mouth disease contains many serotypes.[39]

Poxvirus: The largest and most complex viruses of vertebrates. They differ from all other viruses in that they consist of a brick-shaped DNA-containing core surrounded by a complex series of membranes. See table.

Reovirus: A group of nonenveloped riboviruses that are distinctive in that they contain double-stranded RNA. They multiply and mature in the cytoplasm and cause infections in many animals, but their pathogenic significance is unknown. The viruses of bluetongue and African horse sickness may be in this group.

Rhabdovirus: A group of enveloped riboviruses that are characteristically bullet-shaped. They were previously included in the arbovirus group, and are still considered to be in that group from an epidemiological standpoint. In this group are the viruses of vesicular stomatitis and possibly rabies.

Unclassified viruses: There are, in addition, viruses about which insufficient information is available to put them in specific categories. Some of these, which may be of great importance in the diseases of man and anomen, are the viruses of lymphocytic choriomeningitis, mouse hepatitis, rubella, scrapie, visna, Aleutian mink disease, African swine fever, and equine anemia, and the lactic dehydrogenase virus.

oncogenic v., see under *O.*

replication of v's, the mechanisms by which viruses multiply within host cells are of intense interest to experimental biologists. Each virus contains only one kind of nucleic acid, either DNA or RNA, covered by a protein coat. Attachment, penetration, and subsequent replication of viruses depend to a variable extent upon enzymes furnished by the host cell. The nucleic acid of different viruses may be synthesized in either the nucleus or the cytoplasm; all viral proteins are synthesized on cellular polyribosomes in the cytoplasm, although they may be polymerized to form virus subunits or virus particles in the nucleus or in the cytoplasm in different cases (see table).

THE POXVIRUSES*

VACCINIA	MYXOMA	ORF	SHEEPPOX	BIRDPOX	OTHERS†
Vaccinia	California myxoma	Orf	Sheeppox	Fowlpox	Swinepox
Cowpox	Brazilian myxoma	Bovine papular	Goatpox	Canarypox	Molluscum
Ectromelia	Rabbit fibroma	stomatitis	Lumpy skin	Pigeonpox	contagiosum
Rabbitpox	Squirrel fibroma	Pseudo-cowpox	disease	Turkeypox	Yaba monkey
Monkeypox	Hare fibroma	(milker's nodes)	(Neethling		tumor virus
Variola			strain)		
Alastrim					

*From F. Fenner: The Biology of Animal Viruses. Academic Press, New York, 1968.
†Poxviruses of mammals not yet allocated to subgroups.

CELLULAR SITES OF VIRAL REPLICATION, ASSEMBLY, AND MATURATION

GROUP	REPLICATION OF NUCLEIC ACID	ASSEMBLY OF PROTEIN ANTIGENS	MATURATION OF VIRUS
Poxvirus	Cytoplasm	Cytoplasm	Cytoplasm
Herpesvirus	Nucleus	Nucleus	By acquiring envelope from nuclear membrane
Adenovirus	Nucleus	Nucleus	Nucleus
Papovavirus	Nucleus	Nucleus	Nucleus
Picornavirus	Cytoplasm	Cytoplasm	Cytoplasm
Encephalovirus (arbovirus)	Cytoplasm	Cytoplasm	Bud from plasma membrane or into vacuoles
Myxovirus	Nucleus (?)	Nucleoprotein core in nucleus, other antigens in cytoplasm	As envelope is acquired by budding from plasma membrane
Paramyxovirus	Cytoplasm (?)	Cytoplasm	Bud from plasma membrane
Leukovirus	Cytoplasm	Cytoplasm	Bud from plasma membrane or into cytoplasmic vacuoles. Some maturation after release
Reovirus	Cytoplasm	Cytoplasm	Virions associated with spindle apparatus
Rhabdovirus	Cytoplasm	Cytoplasm	Bud from plasma membrane or into vacuoles

*From F. Fenner: The Biology of Animal Viruses. Academic Press, New York, 1968.

Details elucidated with poliovirus, an RNA virus, and vaccinia virus, a DNA virus, are as follows. The single-stranded RNA of poliovirus serves as messenger RNA for making viral proteins, including RNA polymerase, from cellular precursors. Vaccinia virus contains double-stranded DNA and an RNA polymerase to transcribe this information. It has recently been shown that some viruses possess RNA-dependent DNA polymerase, which may be of fundamental significance in oncogenesis, as well as casting doubt on some of the currently held dogma concerning protein synthesis.

Many different virus-specified enzymes and other proteins are synthesized during the growth cycle. See accompanying two tables.

visceral larva migrans The migration of larvae, especially those of nematodes, through the tissues. Ascarid larvae may wander to many sites such as the brain, kidney, eye, etc. *Toxocara canis* and *T. cati* (q.v.) have been found in the eye, brain, and visceral organs of children and therefore constitute a health hazard.[142] See also *cerebrospinal nematodiasis*, under *nematodiasis*.

visceropallium The visceral mass covered with the mantle on the dorsal aspect of a mollusk.

visna A disease of the central nervous system of sheep characterized by meningitis, perivascular cuffing, and demyelination. It is caused by a virus closely related to the virus of maedi and was one of the first agents described as a slow virus.

vital stain A dye used to stain living cells, as Janus green, trypan blue, etc.

vitellarium A gland that forms yolk.

viviparous Giving birth to live young.

vole A small rodent of the family Muridae which is closely related to the rat and mouse. Common forms are the water rat (*Microtus amphibius*), which is large, diurnal, and aquatic, and the short-tailed field mouse (*M. agrestis*), which is small and damages gardens and crops. Voles differ from rats and mice in their small eyes, blunt snout, stout body, small ears, and short limbs and tail. See also *vole bacillus*.

vole bacillus An acid-fast agent, *Mycobacterium muris*, typical of the mycobacteria, isolated from small rodents in England, including the vole, *Microtus agrestis*, the bank vole, *Clethrionomys glareolus*, the wood mouse, *Apodemus sylvaticus*, and the shrew, *Sorex araneus*. Both natural and experimental infections exhibit gross and histologic lesions typical of those caused by *Mycobacterium tuberculosis*. The vole bacillus is serologically similar to human and bovine (but not avian) tuberculosis bacilli, and it induces cross-hypersensitivity to tuberculin produced by either of these *Mycobacterium* species. The vole bacillus has been used in anomen as an efficacious vaccine organism, analogous to BCG.[92]

MAJOR FEATURES OF THE REPLICATION OF DEOXYRIBOVIRUSES OF FOUR GROUPS*

	POXVIRUS	HERPESVIRUS	ADENOVIRUS	PAPOVAVIRUS
Model virus(es)	Vaccinia	Herpes simplex and pseudorabies	Adenoviruses, types 2 and 5	Polyoma and SV40
Number of cistrons	~400	~120	~50	6–8
Effects on host-cell macromolecular syntheses				
DNA	Inhibited early	Inhibited early	Inhibited late (after 24 hours)	Stimulated early
RNA	Inhibited early	Inhibited early	Inhibited late (after 24 hours)	No effect
Protein	Inhibited early	Inhibited early	Inhibited late (after 24 hours)	No effect
Site of synthesis of viral				
DNA	Cytoplasm	Nucleus	Nucleus	Nucleus
Protein	Cytoplasm	Cytoplasm	Cytoplasm	Not determined
Site of assembly of capsid	Cytoplasm	Nucleus	Nucleus	Nucleus
Site of maturation of virion	Cytoplasm	Crossing nuclear membrane	Nucleus	Nucleus
Viral release	Slight, late	Slight, late	Slight, late	Slight, late
Times of appearance				
New virions	5–14 hours	5–10 hours	13–28 hours	Begins at 24 hours
Viral DNA	1.5–7 hours	2–8 hours	6–24 hours	Begins at 12–14 hours
Early proteins	1–6 hours	1–6 hours	Begins at 3–4 hours	Begins at 8–9 hours
Structural proteins	A few begin at 2 hours, most begin at 6 hours	2.5–10 hours	10–28 hours	Begins at 14 hours

*From F. Fenner: The Biology of Animal Viruses. Academic Press, New York, 1968.

MAJOR FEATURES OF THE REPLICATION OF RIBOVIRUSES OF THE SEVEN MAJOR GROUPS*

	PICORNAVIRUS	ENCEPHALOVIRUS	MYXOVIRUS	PARAMYXOVIRUS	LEUKOVIRUS	RHABDOVIRUS	REOVIRUS
Model virus	Poliovirus	Several group A viruses	Influenza type A	Newcastle disease virus	Avian leukosis virus	Vesicular stomatitis virus	Reovirus
Estimated number of cistrons	~10	~10	~15	~35	~50	~30	~25
Effects on host cell macromolecular syntheses							
DNA	Late inhibition	Late inhibition	?	Late inhibition	Nil	Late inhibition	Late inhibition
RNA	Early inhibition	Late inhibition	?	Late inhibition	Nil	Inhibition by 4 hours	Late inhibition
Protein	Early inhibition	Late inhibition	?	Late inhibition	Nil	Late inhibition	Late inhibition
Site of synthesis of viral RNA	In virus-synthesizing bodies in cytoplasm	Cytoplasm	Nucleus	Cytoplasm	Probably nucleus	Cytoplasm	Cytoplasm
Proteins	In virus-synthesizing bodies in cytoplasm	Cytoplasm	?, probably all in cytoplasm	Cytoplasm	?, probably all in cytoplasm	Cytoplasm	Cytoplasm
Site of assembly of nucleocapsid	In virus-synthesizing bodies in cytoplasm	Cytoplasm	Nucleus	Cytoplasm	Probably nucleus	Cytoplasm	Cytoplasm
Maturation and release by budding							
Into cytoplasmic vacuoles	−, release by cell lysis	+, late in growth cycle; release by cell lysis	−	+, with some strains of virus; release by cell lysis	Rarely	−	−, late release by cell destruction
From cytoplasmic membrane	−, release by cell lysis	+	+, inhibited by anti-neuraminidase	+	+	+	−, late release by cell destruction
Dependence of replication on DNA							
Synthesis	−	−	−	−	+, early requirement only	−	−
Function	−	−	+, early requirement only	−	+, continual requirement	−	−
Does the viral RNA act as its own messenger RNA?	Yes	Probably	Unknown	Unknown, possibly minus strands smaller than viral RNA act as mRNA	Unknown	Unknown	No

*From F. Fenner: The Biology of Animal Viruses. Academic Press, New York, 1968.

W

Waldtracht disease Poisoning of adult honeybees foraging on honeydew from conifers, usually spruce. The poisoned bees first show agitation, then become incapable of flight, crawl rapidly in front of the hive, and die.

walleye sarcoma virus A virus causing skin sarcomas in walleye pikes (*Stizostedion vitreum*) with characteristic cytoplasmic inclusion bodies.[114]

warfarin An anticoagulant, 3-(α-acetonylbenzyl)-4-hydroxycoumarin, which was developed as a result of investigations of sweet clover poisoning. See *dicoumarol*.

warm-up A rapid increase in strength of response which occurs over the first few occasions in which reinforcement is provided.

wart An epidermal tumor of viral origin. See *verruca*.

wart hog disease African swine fever.

Washington Academy of Sciences 1530 P Street, N.W., Washington, D.C. 20005.

wassersucht Watery disintegration.

water moccasin See table accompanying *snake*.

watery disintegration (wassersucht) A lethal viral disease of cockchafer grubs (*Melolontha*). The diseased larva appears transparent, especially in the abdomen, following atrophy and disintegration of its fat-body. As the disease progresses, the muscles as well as other tissues become atrophic. The virus particles are isometric, 60 to 70 mμ in diameter, and are found in the cytoplasm of fat-body cells. There are some similarities between this disease and Heidenreich's disease (q.v.).

wattles (lappets) Lobulated erythematous, apterygous skin appendages of sexual significance situated in pendulous folds ventral to the larynx in birds, especially galliform birds.

wavelength The distance between the top of one wave and the identical phase of the succeeding one. See table for the wavelengths of the more common colors.

W chromosome A sex chromosome in species in which the female is heterogametic (WZ), and the male homogametic (ZZ), as in *Bombyx mori*, the silkworm.

Wellcomia A genus of nematodes (pinworms) found in rodents.[21]

West Virginia Academy of Science West Virginia University, Morgantown, W. Va. 26506.

wet-tail Terminal ileitis of hamsters; see under *ileitis*.

whale See *cetacean*.

white blood cell count See *hemogram*.

white graft rejection The violent, Arthus-

WAVELENGTHS OF THE MORE COMMON COLORS

Wavelength (mμ)	Color	Complementary Color
400–430	Violet	Greenish yellow
430–490	Blue	Yellowish orange
490–510	Blue-green	Red
510–530	Green	Purple
530–560	Yellowish green	Violet
560–590	Yellow	Blue
590–610	Orange	Greenish blue
610–750	Red	Blue-green

like reaction of the recipient in rejecting an allograft transplanted during the course of a first- or second-set rejection.

white head An abnormality in the development of honeybees, characterized by lack of brown pigment in the cuticle of the head and of the first pair of logs. Absence of oxygen has been considered a factor responsible for the lack of pigmentation in "whiteheaded" or "Linthal" bees. As the result of an imperfect pupal molt, both prothoracic tracheae of these abnormal bees are obstructed and, consequently, the oxygen flow to the prothorax and head is arrested. The head does not develop normally and death usually occurs at the end of the pupal period.

white muscardine See under *muscardine*.

Wildlife Disease Association P.O. Box 886, Ames, Iowa 50010.

wild rat pneumonia See under *pneumonia*.

Wilms' tumor Embryonal carcinosarcoma of the kidney.

wilt disease Nucleopolyhedrosis (q.v.) of gypsy-moth caterpillars, *Porthetria dispar*, and lepidopteran larvae; not the preferred term.

Wipfelkrankheit Nucleopolyhedrosis (q.v.) of the larva of the nun moth, *Lymantria monacha*. The tendency of diseased caterpillars to produce to the tops (Wipfeln) of trees caused the malady to be known in Germany by the name "Wipfelkrankheit" or "Wipfelsucht."

WMI virus See *lactic dehydrogenase virus*.

wombat See *marsupial*.

woolly monkey A member of the genus *Lagothrix*. See *primate*.

woolsorter's disease A form of pulmonary anthrax attacking those who handle wool.

work decrement A decrease in response magnitude which appears to be a function of the increased number of occurrences of the response. See *fatigue*.

World Wildlife Fund 910 17th Street, N.W., Suite 728, Washington, D.C. 20006.

X

xanthelasma (xanthelasma palpebrarum) A form of xanthoma affecting the eyelids and characterized by soft yellowish spots or plaques.

xanthinoxidase An enzyme that oxidizes xanthine and hypoxanthine into uric acid.

xanthism An abnormal amount of yellow-orange pigmentation in birds resulting either from melanocarotenoid schizochromism or from carotenism, depending on etiology. See also *schizochromism*.[112]

xantho- A combining form meaning yellow.

xanthochroia Yellowish discoloration caused by changes in the pigmentary layer of the skin.

xanthogranuloma A tumor having the histological characteristics of both granuloma and xanthoma.

xanthoma A condition characterized by the presence of small, flat plaques of a yellow color in the skin, due to deposits of lipids. Microscopically the lesions show light cells with foamy protoplasm (foam cells, or xanthoma cells).

xanthomatosis An accumulation of an excess of lipids in the body due to disturbance of lipid metabolism and marked by the formation of fatty tumors in various parts of the body and sometimes by profound effects on bodily health.

xanthomycin A mixture of three antibiotics, xanthomycin A, B, and C, produced by a species of *Streptomyces,* active against the gram-positive bacteria and highly toxic against mammalian cells in culture. Its mode of action is interference with DNA metabolism.[36, 49]

xanthosarcoma (xanthomyeloma) Giant cell sarcoma of tendon sheaths and aponeuroses containing xanthoma cells and regarded as a phase of xanthomatosis.

X chromosome See *chromosome* and see *late-replicating X chromosome,* under *chromosome.*

xeno- A combining form meaning strange, or denoting relationship to foreign material.

xenodiagnosis Diagnosis by means of finding, in the feces of clean laboratory-bred bugs fed on the patient, the infective forms of the organism causing the disease; used in the early stages of Chagas' disease.

xenogeneic Originating in a different, or foreign, species.

xenograft A graft of tissue in which donor and recipient are of different species. Formerly called *heterograft.*

xenoma A symbiotic complex formed by hypertrophic host cells and intracellular parasites, such as certain microsporidians.

xenophobia Dread of strangers.

Xenopsylla cheopis A species of rat flea. See *arthropod parasites,* under *rat.*

x-ray See *roentgen ray.*

XYZ factor See *Brown-Pearce tumor.*

Y

Yaba virus A poxvirus originally isolated from an epizootic of superficial tumors of the limbs and head of rhesus monkeys and a baboon at Yaba, Nigeria. The tumor is a histiocytoma containing cytoplasmic inclusion bodies which grows for about eight weeks and then regresses in both natural and experimental cases. The agent causes similar tumors in man. The inconstant susceptibility among simian species is now known to result from acquired immunity in many African species. Yaba virus is antigenically unrelated to monkey poxvirus.[3, 114]

Yaba-like poxvirus Poxlike disease.

Y chromosome See *chromosome.*

Yoshida tumor (Yoshida ascites tumor; Yoshida ascites sarcoma; reticulum cell-line sarcoma of Yoshida; Yoshida sarcoma) An undifferentiated tumor induced in an albino rat fed with *o*-aminoazotoluol and painted with potassium arsenite in the laboratory of T. Yoshida in Nagasaki, Japan, in 1943. Yoshida established two lines of tumors by serial passage from the original rat: a solid tumor line and an ascites line. Later it was found that a solid tumor could give rise to an ascites variant, and conversely that solid variants could be selected from the ascites line. The tumor grows progressively in Wistar and Marshall inbred rats. The ascites variant induces an early inflammatory infiltrate of polymorphonuclear leukocytes and lymphocytes, but within 48 to 72 hours it becomes essentially a pure culture of ascites tumor cells.[150]

young rabbit enteritis See *mucoid enteritis,* under *enteritis.*

Z

Z chromosome A sex chromosome found in species in which the female is heterogametic (ZW) and the male homogametic (ZZ).

zeiosis Bubbling or blebbing activity, giving the appearance of boiling in slow motion, observed just before mitosis at the periphery of cells cultured in artificial media.

zoo- A combining form denoting relationship to an animal.

zoology The biology of animals; the sum of what is known regarding animals.

zoonosis An infection or infestation shared in nature by man and anomen.[66, 136, 156] See table, Addendum II.

zoophile 1. Zoophilic. 2. An antivivisectionist.

zoophilic Preferring animals to man; said of certain mosquitoes. Cf. *anthropophilic.*

zoophilic dermatophytes See *dermatomycosis.*

zoophilism 1. Fondness for animals; opposition to vivisection. 2. The state of being zoophilic.

erotic z., sexual pleasure experienced in the fondling of animals.

zoophobia Abnormal dread of animals.

zygo- A combining form meaning yoked or joined, or denoting relationship to a junction.

zygodactylous Having two toes directed backwards and two directed forwards, as in psittacine birds.

zygote The cell produced when the male and female gametes unite.

zygotene See *meiosis.*

zymo- A combining form denoting relationship to an enzyme, or to fermentation.

zymosan A mixture of lipids, polysaccharides, proteins, and ash, of variable concentration, derived from the cell walls or the entire cell of yeast, commonly *Saccharomyces cerevisiae.*

zymurgy The art of brewing, distilling, and winemaking; the branch of chemistry that deals with the commercial application of fermentation.

ADDENDUM I—TABLE OF ANIMAL MODELS

(See *animal model* in text for references.)

HUMAN DISEASE	ANIMAL SPECIES	ANIMAL COUNTERPART OR COMMENT
	CARDIOVASCULAR SYSTEM	
Milroy's disease	Dog, pig	Hereditary lymphedema
Hypertension	Mouse, rat, rabbit, primates	– – –
Pulmonary hypertension	Cow	High altitude disease
Atherosclerosis	Pigeon, swine, dog, primates, many other species	Pigeon and swine probably show lesions most similar to those of human coronary atherosclerosis
Arteriosclerosis	Cow, cat, rabbit, mouse, dog, steelhead trout, iguana	– – –
Polyarteritis	Sheep, cow, rat (breeder rats), horse, mink	Aleutian mink disease; viral in the horse
Aneurysm	Turkey, hamster, horse, cow, primates	Lathyritic in the turkey; parasitic in the horse
Endocardial fibroelastosis	Cat, dog, cow	– – –
Aortic arch syndrome	Dog, cow, pig	– – –
Aortic medial necrosis	Komodo dragon	– – –
Aortic stenosis	Dog	– – –
Anomaly of Fallot	Cow, dog, pig	Many congenital cardiac anomalies in many species
Ectopic heart	Dog, cow	– – –
Myocardial infarction	Dog, horse, primates	– – –
Wolff-Parkinson-White syndrome (paroxysmal tachycardia)	Horse, cow	– – –
	HEMATOPOIETIC SYSTEM AND BLOOD	
Chédiak-Higashi syndrome	Mink, cow	Hereditary recessive giant lysosomes
Erythroblastosis fetalis	Horse, dog, pig	Isohemolytic disease
Hemophilia (several factors)	Dog, pig, horse	– – –
Cyclic neutropenia	Dog	– – –
Polycythemia vera	Cow, deer, dog	– – –
Porphyria	Cow, pig, cat	Recessive inheritance in the cow and pig; dominant in the cat
Anemia (many types)	Many species	See also *classification*, under *anemia*
Congenital erythrocytic porphyria	Short-horned cattle, Holstein-Friesian cattle, swine, fox, squirrel, cat	Recessive in all species except the cat, in which it is dominant
Pelger-Huët anomaly	Cow, dog, rabbit	– – –
Niemann-Pick disease	Mouse	– – –
Lipid storage disease	Budgerigar	– – –
Leukemia	Chicken, cow, cat, dog	– – –
Sickling of erythrocytes	Deer	Different molecular process than in man
Hereditary spherocytosis	Deermouse	– – –
Elliptocytosis	Guanaco	– – –
Thrombotic thrombocytopenia	Horse	– – –
Idiopathic thrombocytopenic purpura	Dog	– – –
di Guglielmo's disease	Bird, dog	Caused by virus in fowl
	GASTROINTESTINAL SYSTEM	
Achalasia	Dog	– – –
Achlorhydria	Dog	– – –
Esophageal dilatation	Mouse	– – –
Esophageal stenosis and dilatation	Dog, cat	Persistent right aortic arch
Regional ileitis	Pig, dog	Similar but not identical to Crohn's disease
Streptococcal uveitis	Horse	– – –
Cleft palate	Horse, dog	– – –
Gingival hyperplasia (familial)	Dog	– – –
Papillomatosis (oral)	Dog	– – –
Ulcer (gastric)	Cow, pig, rat	– – –
Hypoamylasemia	Rabbit	– – –
Mucus hypersecretion	Rabbit	– – –
Malabsorption syndrome (nontropical sprue)	Dog	– – –

223

Human Disease	Animal Species	Animal Counterpart or Comment

GASTROINTESTINAL SYSTEM (*Continued*)

Ulcerative colitis	Dog	Granulomatous colitis of the boxer dog
Chronic enteritis	Cow	Johne's disease
Milk allergy	Rabbit	– – –
Hemorrhagic colitis	Rabbit, pig	– – –
Megacolon	Mouse, dog	– – –
Pancreatitis	Dog	Common idiopathic disease
Emphysema (intestinal)	Pig	– – –
Pyloric stenosis	Dog	– – –

THE LIVER

Viral hepatitis	Primates, dog, turkey, duck, rat	Possible transmission of human hepatitis in the marmoset
Transfusion hepatitis	Horse	– – –
Idiopathic hepatitis	Red rattlesnake	– – –
Aflatoxicosis	Sheep, dog	Facial eczema of sheep in New Zealand, hepatitis X in the dog
Cholelithiasis	Rabbit, dog, cat, weakfish, deer, mouse	– – –
Cirrhosis	Cow, horse, sheep, dog, cat, alligator	Many causes: toxins, flukes, post-necrosis, unknown
Crigler-Najjar syndrome	Rat	Nonhemolytic hyperbilirubinemia
Hepatocellular melanosis	Howler monkey, sheep	Pigmentary liver disease in monkeys, environmental hepatic lipofuscinosis in sheep
Hepatorenal syndrome	Dog	– – –
Hepatic coma	Horse	Poisoning from *Amsinckia* (tarweed)
Nutritional hepatic necrosis	Cow, pig	Probably vitamin B and selenium deficiency
Hepatoma	Trout	Dietary, possibly aflatoxin
Hepatic lipidosis and fibrosis	Sheep	Lupinosis
Hepatic megalocytosis	Rat	Pyrrolizidine plant alkaloids
Veno-occlusive disease	Cow	Pyrrolizidine plant alkaloids

MUSCULOSKELETAL SYSTEM

Achondroplasia	Dog, cow, chicken, mouse, rabbit	There are several types of dwarfism involving achondroplasia. Some are intentionally maintained in breed selection, as in Dachshund dogs; others have been discovered accidentally
Arthropathy (hemophilic)	Dog	– – –
Acetabular dysplasia	Dog	Extensively studied in German Shepard
Fibrous osteodystrophy	Primates, dog, cat, horse, goat	– – –
Hyperostosis (polyostotic)	Budgerigar	– – –
Hypertrophic pulmonary osteoarthropathy	Dog, horse, lion	Usually associated with pulmonary tumors
Intervertebral disc protrusion	Dog	Very common in dogs with long backs, as the dachshund
Osgood-Schlatter disease	Dog	– – –
Osteochondritis dissecans	Mouse, dog	– – –
Osteogenesis imperfecti	Dog, cat, sheep	– – –
Legg-Perthes disease	Dog, cow	– – –
Muscular dystrophy	Dog, cow, chicken, mouse, hamster, turkey, rat, sheep, duckling	Some disorders are hereditary in nature; others appear to be of nutritional origin
Myoclonia congenita	Pig	Possibly resulting from transplacental viral infection
Harelip	Dog, cow, mouse, pig	– – –
Osteoarthritis	Many species	
Myoglobinuric nephrosis	Horse	Similar to crush syndrome of man
Myotonia congenita	Goat, horse	– – –
Rheumatoid arthritis	Pig, rat, mouse	None of the animal diseases is an exact counterpart, but there are similarities to the disease in man; agents such as *Erysipelothrix* and *Mycoplasma* are involved

TABLE OF ANIMAL MODELS (*Continued*)

Human Disease	Animal Species	Animal Counterpart or Comment

MUSCULOSKELETAL SYSTEM (*Continued*)

Rickets	Tortoise, crocodile, toad	– – –
Osteopetrosis	Rabbit, chicken	– – –
Osteomalacia	Spanish terrapin, carp	– – –
Osteoporosis	Spanish terrapin, toad, dog, birds	– – –

NERVOUS SYSTEM

Cerebellar hypoplasia	Cat, dog, cow, hamster, ferret, rat, mink	Established as neonatal or transplacental viral infection in the cat; see *cerebellar ataxia*
Amaurotic familial idiocy	Dog, pig	– – –
Cerebral palsy	Rhesus monkey	– – –
Demyelinating disease	Primates, sheep, dog, mink	– – –
Epilepsy	Dog, cow, primates, rabbit, gerbil	– – –
Familial metachromatic leukodystrophy	Mink, dog, pig, cow	– – –
Hydrocephalus	Cow, mink, dog, pig, horse, mouse	– – –
Pachymeningitis (ossifying)	Dog	– – –
Kuru	Chimpanzee	Experimental transmission

REPRODUCTIVE SYSTEM

Prolonged gestation	Cow	
Persistent corpus luteum	Mouse, cow	– – –
Twinning	Marmoset, cow, armadillo	Regularly dizygotic with fused placenta (marmoset); frequently dizygotic with blood chimerism (cow); multiple monozygotic (armadillo)
Siamese twins	Trout, terrapin, slow worm	– – –
Cryptorchidism	Pig, horse	– – –
Uterine cystic hyperplasia	Dog, mouse	Frequently accompanied by pseudocyesis in the dog
Prostatic hyperplasia	Dog	Neoplasia rare
Pseudocyesis	Dog, rat	– – –
Sex chromosome anomalies	Cat, mouse, cow, swine, mink, marmoset	– – –
Ectopic pregnancy	Dog, cat, rabbit, mouse	– – –
Viral embryopathy	Hamster, pig, sheep	The hamster provides a particularly sensitive model for assay of teratogenic materials; in the pig, associated with hog cholera vaccination of the mother; in sheep, associated with blue tongue virus vaccination of the mother.
Hermaphroditism	Terrapin, tortoise, lizard, pig, dog, cat, sheep, goat	– – –
Indeterminate sex	Grass frog, toad, newt	– – –
Cystic ovary	Cow, primates, dog, pig, cat	– – –
Hydrops amnii	Cow	– – –

RESPIRATORY SYSTEM

Acute pulmonary emphysema	Cow	– – –
Chronic pulmonary emphysema	Horse, dog	– – –
Adenomatosis (pulmonary)	Sheep, cow, guinea pig, chinchilla	– – –
Giant cell interstitial pneumonia	Dog, primates	Hecht's pneumonia
Pulmonary tumors	Mouse	– – –
Anthracosis	Dog	– – –
Bronchiectasis	Dog, cat	– – –
Bronchiolitis obliterans	Cow	– – –
Farmer's lung	Cow	– – –
Silo-filler's disease	Cow	– – –
Hyaline membrane disease	Cow, horse, rat, guinea pig	– – –

HUMAN DISEASE	ANIMAL SPECIES	ANIMAL COUNTERPART OR COMMENT
THE SKIN		
Acanthosis nigricans	Dog (Dachshund)	– – –
Albinism	Mouse, rabbit, guinea pig, cow, axolotl, frog, newt, all fishes, python	– – –
Allergy	Dog	– – –
Melanism	Asp, viper, lizard	– – –
Alopecia	Mouse, swine, guinea pig, cow	– – –
Angioneurotic edema	Cow, horse, dog	– – –
Baldness (male pattern)	Stumptail, macaque	– – –
Ehlers-Danlos syndrome	Dog	– – –
Eczema	Dog	– – –
Hyperkeratosis	Mouse, cow	Lack of sebaceous glands (mouse); poisoning with chlorinated hydrocarbon (cow)
Ichthyosis	Mouse, cow	– – –
Hypotrichosis	Cow	– – –
Xanthomatosis	Chicken	– – –
Pityriasis	Pig	– – –
Apocrine tumor	Pig	– – –
Calcinosis cutis	Dog	– – –
Contact dermatitis	Dog, guinea pig	– – –
Atopic dermatitis	Dog	– – –
Seborrheic dermatitis	Dog	– – –
Dermatofibroma	Dog	– – –
Epidermal inclusion cyst	Dog	– – –
Granuloma pyogenicum	Cow, cat	– – –
Suppurative hidradenitis	Dog	– – –
Impetigo	Dog	– – –
Mastocytoma	Dog, cat	Similar to urticaria pigmentosa
Sebaceous retention cyst	Dog	– – –
Molluscum contagiosum	Chimpanzee	– – –
Mycetoma	Dog	– – –
Neurofibroma	Dog, horse, cow	– – –
Trichoepithelioma	Dog	– – –
Vitiligo	Horse	– – –
Trichostasis spinulosa	Dog, rat	– – –
Herpes	Primates	– – –
Subcutaneous tissue deficiency	Pig	– – –
Epitheliogenesis imperfecta	Cow, horse, pig	– – –
URINARY SYSTEM		
Hereditary hydronephrosis	Rat, mouse	– – –
Hydronephrosis	Dog, cow, sheep, pig, goat	– – –
Polycystic kidney	Rat, cat, pig, goldfish, carp	– – –
Renal aplasia	Mouse, cat	– – –
Glomerulonephritis	Dog, mouse, mink, sheep	Lupus-like in the dog and mouse; infectious in the mink
Pyelonephritis	Dog, cat, cow, rat, pig	Most commonly *Corynebacterium* or *Escherichia coli*
Urolithiasis	Dog, cat, sheep, horse, mink, cow, frog, striped marlin, leech	– – –
Diabetic glomerulosclerosis	Mouse, dog	– – –
Nephrosis (hemoglobinuria)	Horse	Crush syndrome, hemaglobinuria
Nephrocalcinosis	Mouse, rainbow trout	– – –
Renal hemosiderosis	Goat	– – –
THE EYE		
Glaucoma	Rabbit, dog, rat	– – –
Cataract	Dog, cow, mouse, rat, trout	– – –
Lens rupture	Mouse	– – –
Hereditary heterochromia	Cow	– – –
Aniridia	Horse	– – –
Scleral ectasia	Dog	– – –
Retinal degeneration	Mouse, dog	– – –
Congenital retinal dysplasia	Dog	– – –
Retinitis pigmentosa	Dog, mouse	– – –
Diabetic microaneurysms	Dog	– – –
Microphthalmia	Pig, mouse	– – –

HUMAN DISEASE	ANIMAL SPECIES	ANIMAL COUNTERPART OR COMMENT

THE EYE (*Continued*)

Entropion	Dog, sheep	– – –
Corneal opacity (hereditary)	Cow	– – –
Horner's syndrome	Cat, dog	– – –

THE EAR

Deafness (hereditary)	Mink, dog, cat, mouse	– – –
Cochlear degeneration	Mouse	– – –
Defective semicircular canals	Mouse	Partial deafness, ataxia
Hypoplasia of organ of Corti	Dog	– – –

IMMUNOLOGIC, IMMUNOPROLIFERATIVE, AND CONNECTIVE TISSUE DISEASES

Amyloidosis	Mouse, cow, horse, dog, mink, primates, badger, boa constrictor	Thymectomized mice and rabbits
Anaphylaxis	Dog, guinea pig, cow	– – –
Lupus erythematosus	Dog, mouse	– – –
Hay fever	Dog, cow	– – –
Plasmacytosis	Mink	– – –
Serum sickness	Dog, horse, rabbit	– – –
Chronic thyroiditis	Dog	– – –
Myeloma	Horse, cow, pig, dog, cat, mouse, mink	Variant of Aleutian mink disease
Urticaria (hives)	Dog	– – –
Atopic dermatitis	Dog	– – –
Myeloma	Horse, cow, pig, cat, mouse, mink, dog	Aleutian disease in the mink; IgG and IgM gammopathies in the dog
Complement defects	Mouse, rabbit	Various fractions
Graft-vs.-host reaction	Mouse	– – –
Cortical renal necrosis	Rabbit, pig, calf	Generalized Shwartzman phenomenon
Leukemia	Chicken, mouse, cat	Variety of transmissible agents
Arteritis	Horse	Viral arteritis
Aging immunologic deficiency	Mouse	– – –
Immunologic tolerance	Calf, marmoset, dog	Blood chimerism of dizygotic twins (calf, marmoset); irradiation blood chimera (dog)

NEOPLASMS

(Tumors are so common and widespread in many species that only a few, considered unusual or especially significant, are listed below. For complete tabulation, see references. See also *transmissible tumors, leukemia,* and *oncogenic viruses.*)

Dermal papilloma	Sand lizard, green turtle, musk turtle	– – –
Papilloma of gallbladder	Green turtle	– – –
Thyroid adenoma	Turtle	– – –
Pulmonary fibroadenoma	Horsfield's tortoise	– – –
Cardiac rhabdomyoma	Black terrapin	– – –
Benign hepatoma	Massurana, toad, frog	– – –
Bile duct adenoma	Black cobra	– – –
Chondroma	Monitor lizard, newt	– – –
Rhabdomyoma	Pine snake	– – –
Osteoma	Green lizard, crocodile	– – –
Epithelioma	Great tegu, puff-faced water snake, sand lizard, Gila monster, Ceylon terrapin, alpine newt	– – –
Carcinoma of parotid	Black-pointed tegu	– – –
Carcinoma of thyroid	Ceylon terrapin	– – –
Carcinoma of stomach	Side-necked turtle	– – –
Adenocarcinoma of stomach	Bull snake, giant tortoise	– – –
Carcinoma of pancreas	Pine snake, rattle snake, water moccasins, black racers	– – –
Adenocarcinoma of bile duct	Water snake	– – –
Adenocarcinoma of kidney	Grass snake, leopard frog, edible frog, toad	– – –
Nephroblastoma	Toad	– – –
Adenocarcinoma of colon	Bull snake	– – –
Sarcoma of stomach	Water moccasin	– – –

TABLE OF ANIMAL MODELS (*Continued*)

HUMAN DISEASE	ANIMAL SPECIES	ANIMAL COUNTERPART OR COMMENT
	NEOPLASMS (Continued)	
Lymphosarcoma	Egyptian cobra, hognose snake, river jack	– – –
Malignant melanoma	Reticulated python, pine snake, axolotl, toad, fruit fly	– – –
Osteogenic sarcoma	Rufous-beaked snake, meadow frog	– – –
Lipoma	Toad	– – –
Myxofibrochondroma	Brown-throated frog	– – –
Pulmonary carcinoma	Natterjack	– – –
Cutaneous adenoma	Meadow frog	– – –
Cutaneous adenocarcinoma	Crested newt, bullfrog, frog	– – –
Ovarian carcinoma	Edible frog	– – –
Fibroma	Giant salamander, frog	– – –
Fibrosarcoma	Frog	– – –
Neurogenic sarcoma	Bullfrog	– – –
Myxosarcoma	Green frog	– – –
Lymphosarcoma	Newt, frog, toad (*Xenopus laevis*)	– – –
Myogenic tumor	Earthworm (*Lumbricus terrestris*)	X-irradiation
Sarcoma-like tumor	Annelid (*Nereis diversicolor*)	*Bacillus tumefaciens*
Sarcoma of midgut	Roach, Leucophaea	Severance of recurrent nerve

METABOLIC AND ENDOCRINE DISEASES

HUMAN DISEASE	ANIMAL SPECIES	ANIMAL COUNTERPART OR COMMENT
Acromegaly	Dog	– – –
Aminoaciduria	Mouse	– – –
Cystinuria	Dog	– – –
Bialbuminemia	Pig, chicken	– – –
Toxemia of pregnancy	Hamster, sheep, guinea pig, rabbit	Generalized Shwartzman phenomenon in the hamster
Postparturient hypocalcemia	Rabbit, cow	– – –
Phenylketonuria	Mouse	Phenylalanine hydroxylase deficiency
Hypomagnesemia	Cow	Grass tetany
Diabetes mellitus	Dog, sand rat, Chinese hamster, horse, rat, mouse, sculpin	– – –
Diabetes insipidus	Dog, rat, mouse, Chinese hamster	– – –
Polydipsia	Mouse	Adrenal-induced polydipsia
Cushing's disease	Dog	– – –
Goiter	Cow	Congenital goiter
Hypothyroidism	Dog, chicken, cow, brook trout, rat	– – –
Hypoparathyroidism	Dog	– – –
Hyperadrenocorticism	Dog, mouse, steelhead trout	– – –
Thyrotropin deficiency	Mouse	Snell's dwarf
Adenohypophyseal aplasia	Cow, mink	– – –
Adenohypophyseal cysts	Birds	– – –
Hyperparathyroidism	Dog, primates	Common in chronic nephritis
Hyperthyroidism	Dog, cow	– – –
Hyperinsulinism	Dog, mouse	Islet cell tumor
Hypopituitarism	Dog	– – –
Obesity	Mouse, rat	Familial disease
Insulin tolerance	Mouse	Inherited disease
Parturient hypoglycemia (ketosis)	Cow, sheep	Defect in gluconeogenesis
Premature aging	Syrian hamster	Early senility
Dubin-Johnson syndrome	Sheep	– – –
Gilbert's syndrome	Southdown sheep	Hereditary photosensitivity and hyperbilirubinemia
Crigler-Najjar syndrome	Rat	Nonhemolytic hyperbilirubinemia
von Gierke's disease	Dog	– – –
Glycogen storage disease	Duck	– – –
Gout	Birds, dog, alligator, lizard, turtle	– – –
Urate nephropathy	Iguana, gavial, pig	– – –
Caisson disease	Salmonids	– – –
Mucus hypersecretion	Marine worm, *Sipunculus*, rabbit	– – –
Gynecomastia	Dog	– – –
Oxygen toxicity	Frog	– – –
Addison's disease	Dog	– – –
Fröhlich's disease	Dog	– – –

(See *animal model* in text for references.)

INFECTION	AGENT	MODE OF TRANSMISSION	COMMON NONHUMAN VERTEBRATE HOSTS	PREVALENCE IN MAN	SERIOUSNESS OF INFECTION IN MAN
VIRAL INFECTIONS					
Contagious ecthyma	Virus	Contact	Sheep	Sporadic	Mild
Cowpox	Virus	Contact	Cow	Common	Mild
Encephalomyocarditis	Virus	Vehicle	Rodents, swine, primates	Sporadic	Serious
Foot-and-mouth disease	Virus	Contact	Sheep, cow, swine, wild mammals	Sporadic	Mild
Influenza, parainfluenza	Type A influenza virus	Contact	Swine, fowl, horse	Common	Serious
	Type D influenza virus	Contact			
Lymphocytic choriomeningitis	Virus	(?)	Rodents	Sporadic	Serious
Newcastle disease	Virus	Contact	Fowl, wild birds	Sporadic	Mild
Rabies	Virus	Contact	Dog, wild mammals	Sporadic	Fatal
Simian herpes (B virus)	Virus	Contact	Primates	Sporadic	Serious
Vesicular stomatitis	Virus	Contact mechanical vector)	Cattle, horse, swine	Sporadic	Usually mild
Cat-scratch fever	Virus (?)	Contact(?)	Cat	Common	Mild
Herpes simplex	Virus	Contact	– – –	Common	Usually mild
Smallpox	Virus	Contact	– – –	Sporadic, common locally	High mortality
Poliomyelitis	Virus	Vehicle	– – –	Common	Usually mild
Coxsackie infection	Virus	Vehicle	– –	Common	Mild
Salivary gland virus infection	Virus	Contact	Monkeys, rodents	Sporadic	May be serious
Mayaro fever	Group A arbovirus	Mosquito	– – –	Sporadic	Serious
Eastern equine encephalomyelitis	Group A arbovirus	Mosquito	Fowl, wild birds, equines	Sporadic	Serious
Western equine encephalomyelitis	Group A arbovirus	Mosquito	Fowl, wild birds, equines	Sporadic	Serious
Venezuelan equine encephalomyelitis	Group A arbovirus	Mosquito	Fowl, wild birds, equines	Sporadic	Serious
Pixuna	Group A arbovirus	Mosquito	– – –	Sporadic	Serious
Middleburg fever	Group A arbovirus	Mosquito	Sheep	Sporadic	Serious
Wesselsbron fever	Group B arbovirus	Mosquito	Sheep	Sporadic	Serious
Zika fever	Group B arbovirus	Mosquito	– – –	Sporadic	Serious
West Nile fever	Group B arbovirus	Mosquito	Wild birds, horse	Sporadic	Serious
Kyasanur Forest disease	Group B arbovirus	Tick	Monkeys, rodents	Sporadic	Serious
Omsk hemorrhagic fever	Group B arbovirus	Tick	Rodents	Sporadic	Serious
Japanese B encephalitis	Group B arbovirus	Mosquito	Wild birds, swine, horse, cattle	Sporadic	Serious
Murray Valley encephalitis	Group B arbovirus	Mosquito	Wild birds	Sporadic	Serious
St. Louis encephalitis	Group B arbovirus	Mosquito	Fowl, wild birds	Sporadic	Serious
Ilheus fever	Group B arbovirus	Mosquito	Primates, marsupials	Sporadic	Serious
Russian spring-summer encephalitis	Group B arbovirus	Tick	Birds, small mammals	Sporadic	Serious
Diphasic meningoencephalitis	Group B arbovirus	Tick	Cattle, goat, sheep	Sporadic	Serious
Louping ill	Group B arbovirus	Tick	Sheep	Sporadic	Serious
Yellow fever	Group B arbovirus	Mosquito	Primates	Sporadic	Serious
European tick fever	Group B arbovirus	Tick	Cattle, goat, sheep	Sporadic	Serious
Dengue fever	Group B arbovirus	Mosquito	– – –	Sporadic	Serious
Oriboca fever	Group C arbovirus	Mosquito	– – –	Sporadic	Serious
Caraparu fever	Group C arbovirus	Mosquito	– – –	Sporadic	Serious
Apeu fever	Group C arbovirus	Mosquito	– – –	Sporadic	Serious
Murutueu fever	Group C arbovirus	Mosquito	– – –	Sporadic	Serious
Itaqui fever	Group C arbovirus	Insect	– – –	Sporadic	Serious
Oropouche	Simbu virus	Mosquito	– – –	Sporadic	Serious
Quaranfil	Quaranfil virus	Tick	– – –	Sporadic	Serious
Colorado tick fever	Ungrouped virus	Tick	Squirrel, porcupine	Sporadic	Serious
Argentinian hemorrhagic fever	Ungrouped virus	Mite(?)	Rodents	Sporadic	Serious
Crimean hemorrhagic fever	Ungrouped virus	Tick	Horse	Sporadic	Serious
Rift Valley fever	Ungrouped virus	Mosquito	Sheep, goat, cattle	Sporadic	Serious
RICKETTSIAL INFECTIONS					
Boutonneuse fever	*Rickettsia conori*	Tick	Dog, rodents	Sporadic	Serious
Epidemic typhus fever	*R. prowazeki*	Louse (animal ticks)	Sheep, goat	Common	Serious
Murine typhus fever	*R. (typhi) mooseri*	Flea	Rat	Sporadic	Serious
Q fever	*R. (Coxiella) burneti*	Tick	Sheep, cattle, goat, other mammals, fowl	Sporadic	Serious
Rickettsialpox	*R. akari*	Mite	Mouse	Sporadic	Mild
Scrub typhus fever	*R. tsutsugamushi*	Mite	Rodents	Sporadic	Serious
Spotted fever	*R. rickettsii*	Tick	Rabbit, rodents, dog	Sporadic	High mortality

(Table continues)

*Adapted from C. W. Schwabe: Veterinary Medicine and Human Health, 2nd ed. The Williams & Wilkins Co., Baltimore, Md. 21202, U.S.A. © 1969. (See also Hull[66] and Van der Hoeden.[156])

INFECTION	AGENT	MODE OF TRANS-MISSION	COMMON NONHUMAN VERTEBRATE HOSTS	PREVALENCE IN MAN	SERIOUSNESS OF INFECTION IN MAN
		BACTERIAL INFECTIONS			
Anthrax	*Bacillus anthracis*	Contact	Cattle, horse, swine, sheep	Sporadic	High mortality
Brucellosis	*Brucella abortus*	Vehicle, contact	Cattle, sheep	Sporadic	Serious
	B. melitensis	Vehicle, contact	Sheep, goat	Sporadic	Serious
	B. suis	Vehicle, contact	Swine	Sporadic	Serious
Salmonellosis	*Salmonella* spp.	Vehicle	Fowl, rodents, swine, poikilotherms	Common	Serious
Staphylococcosis	*Staphylococcus* spp.	Vehicle, contact	Dog, other anomen	Common	Serious
Streptococcosis	*Streptococcus* spp.	Vehicle, contact	Cattle, dog	Common	Serious
Colibacillosis	*Escherichia* spp.	Vehicle, contact	Cattle, swine	Common	Serious
Erysipeloid	*Erysipelothrix rhusiopathiae*	Contact	Swine, fowl, fish(?)	Sporadic	Serious
Glanders	*Actinobacillus mallei*	Contact	Horse	Sporadic	Serious
Leptospirosis	*Leptospira* spp.	Vehicle, contact	Dog, cattle, rodents	Sporadic	Serious
Listeriosis	*Listeria mono-cytogenes*	(?)	Cattle, sheep, fowl	Sporadic	High mortality
Melioidosis	*Pseudomonas pseudo mallei*	Vehicle, contact	Rodents	Sporadic	Serious
Pasteurellosis	*Pasteurella multocida*	Contact	Cattle, horse, sheep, swine, dog, cat	Sporadic	Serious
Pseudotuberculosis	*P. pseudo-tuberculosis*	Contact	Rodents	Sporadic	Serious
Psittacosis-ornithosis	*Chlamydia*	Contact	Fowl, wild birds	Sporadic	Usually mild, sometimes fatal
Rat-bite fever	*Spirillum minus*	Contact	Rodents	Sporadic	Serious
	Streptobacillus moniliformis	Contact	Rodents	Sporadic	Serious
Tuberculosis	*Mycobacterium bovis*	Vehicle, contact	Cattle	Common	Serious
	M. tuberculosis var. *hominis*	Vehicle, contact	Cattle, dog	Common	Serious
	M. avium	Vehicle, contact	Fowl, swine	Sporadic	Serious
Tularemia	*Pasteurella tularensis*	Contact	Wild animals	Sporadic	Serious
Vibriosis	*Vibrio fetus*	Contact	Cattle	Sporadic	Serious
Tetanus	*Clostridium tetani*	Vehicle	Horse	Common	High mortality
Bacillary dysentery	*Shigella* spp.	Vehicle	Dog	Common	Serious
Diphtheria	*Corynebacterium diphtheriae*	Vehicle	– – –	Common	Usually mild, sometimes serious
Plague	*Pasteurella pestis*	Flea	Rodents	Sporadic	High mortality
Endemic relapsing fever	*Borrelia* spp.	Tick	Rodents, wild animals	Sporadic	Serious
Botulism	*Clostridium botulinum*	Vehicle	Domestic mammals, fish	Sporadic	Highly fatal
		FUNGAL INFECTIONS			
North American blastomycosis	*Blastomyces dermatitidis*	Vehicle	Dog	Sporadic	Serious
Coccidioidomycosis	*Coccidioides immitis*	Vehicle	Rodents, other mammals	Sporadic	Usually mild
Cryptococcosis	*Cryptococcus neoforms*	Vehicle	Cat, other mammals	Sporadic	Serious
Histoplasmosis	*Histoplasma capsulatum*	Vehicle	Dog, rodents, other mammals	Common	Usually mild
Nocardiosis	*Nocardia asteroides*	(?)	Dog, other mammals	Sporadic	Serious
Actinomycosis	*Actinomyces bovis*	(?)	Cattle	Sporadic	Serious
Sporotrichosis	*Sporotrichum schenckii*	(?)	Horse, dog, rodents	Sporadic	Serious
Rhinosporidiosis	*Rhinosporidium seeberi*	(?)	Cattle, horse	Sporadic	Serious
Aspergillosis	*Aspergillus* spp.	Vehicle	Birds, mammals	Sporadic	Serious
Mucormycosis	*Mucor* spp.	(?)	Cattle	Sporadic	Serious
Haplomycosis	*Emmonsia* spp.	(?)	Rodents, carnivores	Rare	(?)
Streptothricosis	*Dermatophilus* spp.	(?)	Insectivores, cattle, horse, goat, sheep, dog	Rare	Mild
Ringworm	*Microsporum* spp.	Contact	Dog, cat	Common	Serious
	Trichophyton spp.	Contact	Cattle, horse	Common	Serious
Candidiasis	*Candida albicans*	Contact	Fowl	Common	Serious

Infection	Agent	Mode of Trans-mission	Common Nonhuman Vertebrate Hosts	Prevalence in Man	Seriousness of Infection in Man
PROTOZOAN INFECTIONS					
Balantidiasis	*Balantidium coli*	Vehicle	Swine	Sporadic	Serious
Amebiasis	*Entamoeba histolytica*	Vehicle	Dog, monkey	Common	Usually mild, sometimes serious
Toxoplasmosis	*Toxoplasma gondii*	(?)	Mammals	Common	Usually mild, sometimes serious
Pneumocystis infection	*Pneumocystis carinii*	(?)	Dog	– – –	– – –
Sarcosporidiosis	*Sarcocystis* spp.	(?)	Cattle, rodents, wild birds	Sporadic	No disease
Giardiasis	*Giardia lambia*	Vehicle	Primates	Sporadic	Sometimes serious
Iodamoeba infection	*Iodamoeba butschlii*	Vehicle	Primates, swine	Sporadic	No disease
Leishmaniasis	*Leishmania donovani*	Sandfly	Dog, rodents	Sporadic	Serious
	L. tropica	Sandfly	Dog, rodents	Common	Serious
	L. braziliensis	Sandfly	Dog, rodents	Sporadic	Serious
Malaria	*Plasmodium malariae*	Mosquito	Apes	Sporadic	Serious
	P. vivax schwetzi	Mosquito	Apes	Sporadic	Serious
	P. cynomolgi bastianellii	Mosquito	Monkeys	(?)	Serious
Trypanosomiasis	*Trypanosoma cruzi*	Reduviid bug	Many mammals	Common	Serious
	T. rhodesiense	Tsetse fly	Bushbuck	Common	Serious
	T. rangeli	Reduviid bug	Dog, other, mammals	Sporadic	No disease
Piroplasmosis	*Babesia* spp.	Tick	Many mammals	Single case	
Coccidiosis	*Isospora* spp.	Vehicle	Dog, cat	Sporadic	Mild
NEMATODE INFECTIONS					
Visceral larva migrans	*Toxocara* spp. and other ascarids	Vehicle	Dog, cat	Sporadic	Serious
Cutaneous larva migrans	*Ancylostoma* spp.	Vehicle	Dog	Common	Serious
Strongyloidiasis	*Strongyloides stercoralis*	Vehicle	Dog, monkeys	Sporadic	Serious
Capillaria hepatica infection	*Capillaria hepatica*	Vehicle	Rodents	Sporadic	Serious
Trichostrongylosis	*Trichostrongylus* spp.	Vehicle	Herbivores	Common	Mild
Oesophagostomiasis	*Oesophagostomum apiostomum*	Vehicle	Primates	Common	Mild
	O. stephanostomum	Vehicle	– – –	Sporadic	Serious
Trichuriasis	*Trichuris trichiura*	Vehicle	Swine, primates	Common	Mild
Ternidens infection	*Ternidens deminutus*	Vehicle	Primates	Sporadic	Serious
Syngamus infection	*Syngamus kingi*	Vehicle	– – –	Rare	– – –
	S. laryngeus	Vehicle	Cattle	Sporadic	Serious
Loaiasis	*Loa loa*	Deer fly	Monkeys	Common	Serious
Dracunculiasis	*Dracunculus medinensis*	Copepod	Dog, other mammals	Common	Serious
Eosinophilic meningoencephalitis	*Angiostrongylus cantonensis*	Slugs, other invertebrates	Rat	Common	Serious
Filariasis	*Brugia malayi*	Mosquito	Cat, primates	Common	Serious
	Dipetalonema perstans	Culicoides	Primates	Common	Mild
	D. streptocerca	Culicoides	Apes	Sporadic	Mild
	Dirofilaria spp.	Mosquito	Dog, other mammals	Sporadic	Serious
	Tetrapetalonema berghei	– – –	– – –	Rare	– – –
Physaloptera infection	*Physaloptera caucasica*	Insects	Monkeys	Common	Mild
Thelaziasis	*Thelazia* spp.	Fly	Cattle, dog, other mammals	Sporadic	Serious
Gnathostomiasis	*Gnathostoma spinigerum*	Cyclops	Cat, dog, other carnivores, poikilotherms	Common	Serious
Kidney worm infection	*Dioctophyma renale*	Annelids	Dog, other mammals, fish	Rare	Serious
Gongylonemiasis	*Gongylonema pulchrum*	Insects	Cattle, sheep	Sporadic	Serious
Trichinosis	*Trichinella spiralis*	Vehicle	Swine, rodents, fox, dog, wild animals	Sporadic Sporadic	Serious Serious

231

INFECTION	AGENT	MODE OF TRANS-MISSION	COMMON NONHUMAN VERTEBRATE HOSTS	PREVALENCE IN MAN	SERIOUSNESS OF INFECTION IN MAN
TREMATODE INFECTIONS					
Clonorchiasis (opisthorchiasis)	*Opisthorchis sinensis*	Snail	Fish-eating mammals	Common	Serious
Paragonimiasis	*Paragonimus westermani*	Snail	Crab-eating mammals	Common	Serious
Schistosomiasis	*Schistosoma*	Snail	Many animals	Common	Serious
	S. mansoni	Snail	Rodents, primates	Common	Serious
	S. haematobium	Snail	Rarely seen	Common	Serious
	S. bovis	Snail	Cattle	Sporadic	Serious
	S. mattheei	Snail	Sheep	Sporadic	Serious
	S. rodhaini	Snail	Rodents, dog	Sporadic	Serious
	S. intercalatum	Snail	– – –	Sporadic	Serious
	S. margrebowiei	Snail	Antelope	Sporadic	Serious
Paramphistomum infection	*Paramphistomum sufrartyfex*	Snail	(?)	Sporadic	
Phaneropsolus infection	*Phaneropsolus bonnei*	Snail	– – –	Rare	– – –
Philophthalmus infection	*Philophthalmus* spp.	Snail	Birds	Rare	Serious
Poikilorchiasis	*Poikilorchis congolensis*	Snail	– – –	Sporadic	Serious
Swimmer's itch	*Ornithobilharzia* spp. and others	Snail	Birds, aquatic mammals	Common	Mild
Echinostomiasis	*Echinostoma* spp.	Snail	Birds, dog, rodents	Common	Mild
Prohemistomiasis	*Prohemistomum vivax*	Snail	Dog, cat, fish, tadpole	Rare	Usually mild
Pseudamphistomiasis	*Pseudamphisto-mum* spp.	Snail	Dog, cat, fox	Rare	Mild
Heterophyiasis	*Heterophyes heterophyes*	Snail	Fish-eating mammals	Common	Usually mild, sometimes serious
Haplorchiasis	*Haplorchis* spp.	Snail	Fish-eating mammals	Sporadic	Sometimes serious
Dicrocoeliasis	*Dicrocoelium dendriticum*	Snail (ant)	Sheep, cattle	Sporadic	Sometimes serious
Metagonimiasis	*Metagonimum yokogawai*	Snail	Fish-eating mammals	Common	Sometimes serious
Himasthla infection	*Himasthla muehlensi*	Snail	Birds(?)	Sporadic	– – –
Metorchiasis	*Metorchis conjunctus*	Snail	Fish-eating mammals	Sporadic	Serious
Nanophyetus infection	*Nanophyetus schikhobalowi*	Snail	Fish-eating mammals	Common	Usually mild
Navigiolum infection	*Navigiolum nigrum*	Snail	– – –	Rare	– – –
Paralecithodendrium infection	*Paralecithodendrium molenkampi*	Snail	– – –	Rare	– – –
Fascioliasis	*Fasciola hepatica*	Snail, vehicle	Cattle, sheep	Common	Serious
	F. gigantica	Snail, vehicle	Sheep, cattle	Sporadic	Serious
Fasciolopsiasis	*Fasciolopsis buski*	Snail, vehicle	Mammals	Common	Serious
Gastrodiscoidiasis	*Gastrodiscoides hominis*	Snail, vehicle	Swine, rodents, monkeys	Common	Serious
CESTODE INFECTIONS					
Diphyllobothriasis	*Diphyllobothrium latum*	Copepod, fish	Dog, other fish-eating mammals	Common	Usually mild, sometimes serious
Sparganosis	*Spirometra* spp. and others	Copepod	Many vertebrates	Sporadic	Serious
Dipylidiasis	*Dipylidium caninum*	Flea	Dog	Sporadic	Mild
Hymenolepiasis	*Hymenolepis nana, H. diminuta*	Insect	Rodents	Sporadic	Mild
Inermicapsifera infections	*Inermicapsifera mada-gascarensis, I. cubensis*	Insect	Rodents	Sporadic	Mild
Raillietina infections	*Raillietina* spp.	Insect	Birds, rodents	Rare	Mild
Bertiella infection	*Bertiella studeri*	Mite	– – –	Sporadic	Mild
Taeniasis, cysticercosis	*Taenia solium*	Vehicle	Swine	Sporadic	Serious
	T. saginatum	Vehicle	Cattle	Common	Mild
Hydatid disease	*Echinococcus granulosus*	Vehicle	Dog, sheep, cattle, horse, swine	Sporadic	Serious
	E. multilocularis	Vehicle	Dog, fox, rodents	Sporadic	Serious
Coenurosis	*Multiceps* spp.	Vehicle	Dog, sheep, rabbit	Sporadic	Serious

INFECTION	AGENT	MODE OF TRANS- MISSION	COMMON NONHUMAN VERTEBRATE HOSTS	PREVALENCE IN MAN	SERIOUSNESS OF INFECTION IN MAN
ACANTHOCEPHALID INFECTIONS					
Thorny-headed worm infection	*Macracanthorhyn- chus hirudinaceus*	Insects	Swine	Rare	Serious
	Moniliformia dubius	Insects	Rodents, toads, lizards	Rare	Serious
ARTHROPOD INFESTATIONS					
Mosquito bites	Mosquitos	– – –	Vertebrates	Common	Mild
Fly bites	Biting flies	– – –	Vertebrates	Common	Mild
Myiasis	*Dermatobia hominis,* other flies	– – –	Vertebrates	Sporadic	Serious
Tunga penetrans infestations	*Tunga penetrans*	– – –	Mammals	Common	Serious
Flea bites	Fleas	– – –	Dog, cat, rodents	Common	Usually mild
Bug bites	*Cimex* spp., *Triatoma* spp., etc.	– – –	Vertebrates	Common	Usually mild
Mite bites	Mites	– – –	Mammals, birds	Common	Usually mild
Tick bites	Two- and three-host ticks	– – –	Mammals	Common	Usually mild
Tick paralysis	(?)	– – –	Mammals	Rare	Serious
Pentastomiasis	*Linguatula* spp.	Vehicle	Dog, cattle, other vertebrates	Sporadic	Usually mild
	Armillifer armil- latus and others	– –	Snakes, monkeys	Common	Usually mild
Scabies	*Sarcoptes scabiei,* and other mites	Contact	Horse	Sporadic	Sometimes serious

Bibliography

1. Altman, P. L., and Dittmer, D. S.: Biology Data Book. Federation of American Societies of Experimental Biology, Bethesda, Md., 1964.
2. Andrewes, C. H., and Pereira, H. G.: Viruses of Vertebrates. 2nd ed. Baílliène, Tindall and Cassell, London, 1967.
3. Armed Forces Institute of Pathology: Diseases of Non-human Primates (Syllabus). American Registry of Pathology, Washington, D.C., 1968.
4. Barnes, R. D.: Small marsupials as experimental animals. Lab. Animal Care, 18:251–257, 1968.
5. Bendixen, H. J.: Leukemia in Animals and Man. S. Karger, Basel, 1968.
6. Benirschke, K. (Ed.): Comparative Mammalian Cytogenetics. Springer-Verlag, New York, 1969.
7. Benirschke, K.: Models for cytogenetics and embryology. Fed. Proc., 28(No. 1):170–178, 1969.
8. Bernhard, W.: Fine structural lesions induced by viruses. In CIBA Foundation Symposium on Cellular Injury, Boston 1964.
9. Beveridge, W. I. B.: The Art of Scientific Investigation. 3rd ed. Random House, New York, 1957.
10. Beveridge, W. I. B. (Ed.): Using Primates in Medical Research. II. Recent Comparative Research. S. Karger, Basel, 1969.
11. Biester, H. E., and Schwarte, L. H.: Diseases of Poultry. 5th ed. Iowa State University Press, Ames, Iowa, 1965.
12. Black, M. M., and Wagner, B. M.: Dynamic Pathology. The C. V. Mosby Co., St. Louis, 1964.
13. Blood, D. C., and Henderson, J. R.: Veterinary Medicine. 2nd ed. Williams & Wilkins Co., Baltimore, 1963.
14. Brody, J. A., Henle, W., and Koprowski, H. (Eds.): Chronic Infections, Neuropathic Agents and Other Slow Viruses. Current Topics in Microbiology and Immunology. Springer-Verlag, New York, 1967.
15. Brook Lodge Workshop on Spontaneous Diabetes in Laboratory Animals. Diabetologia, Vol. 3 (No. 2), 1967.
16. Bruner, D. W., and Gillespie, J. H.: Hagan's Infectious Diseases of Domestic Animals. 5th ed. Cornell University Press, Ithaca, N.Y., 1966.
17. Burstone, M. S.: Enzyme Histochemistry. Academic Press, New York, 1962.
18. Bustad, L. K., and Crowder, C.: Animals on the Verge of Discovery. Lab. Animal Care, 18(No. 2): 229–304, 1968.
19. Bustad, L. K., and McClellan, R. O.: Swine in Biomedical Research. Pacific Northwest Laboratory, Batelle Northwest Memorial Laboratory, Richland, Wash., 1966.
20. Chadwick, J. S.: Serological responses of insects. Fed. Proc., 26:1675–1679, 1967.
21. Cheng, T. C.: The Biology of Animal Parasites. W. B. Saunders Co., Philadelphia, 1964.
22. Clarke, E. G. C., and Clarke, M. L.: Garner's Veterinary Toxicology. Williams & Wilkins Co., Baltimore, 1967.
23. Clarkson, T. B.: Atherosclerosis: spontaneous and induced. Advances Lipid Res., 1:211–252, 1963.
24. Conalty, M. L. (Ed.): Husbandry of Laboratory Animals. Academic Press, New York, 1967.
25. Cornelius, C. E.: Animal models—a neglected medical resource. New Eng. J. Med., 281(No. 17): 934–944, 1969.
26. Cornelius, C. E., and Kaneko, J. J.: Clinical Biochemistry of Domestic Animals. Academic Press, New York, 1963.
27. Cotchin, E., and Roe, F. J. C.: Pathology of Laboratory Rats and Mice. F. A. Davis, Philadelphia, 1967.
28. Craig, J. M.: Models for obstetrical and gynecological disease. Fed. Proc., 28(No. 1):206–210, 1969.
29. Dalling, T.: International Encyclopedia of Veterinary Medicine. W. Green & Son, Ltd., Edinburgh, 1966.
30. Dalton, A. J., and Hagenav, F. (Eds.): Tumors Induced by Viruses: Ultrastructural Studies. Academic Press, New York, 1962.
31. Davidson, E. H.: Gene Activity in Early Development. Academic Press, New York, 1968.
32. Davis, B. D., Dulbecco, R., Eisen, H. N., Ginsberg, H. S., and Wood, W. B.: Microbiology. Hoeber Medical Division (Harper & Row), New York, Evanston and London, 1968.
33. de Duve, C., and Wattiaux, R.: Function of Lysosomes. Annual Review of Physiology, Annual Reviews, Inc., Palo Alto, Calif., 1966.
34. Dixon, F. J., and Kunkel, H. G. (Eds.): Advances in immunology. Academic Press, New York, 1969.
35. Doyle, R. E., Garb, S., Davis, L. E., Meyer, D. K., and Clayton, F. W.: Domesticated farm animals in medical research. Ann. N.Y. Acad. Sci., 147:129–204, 1968
36. Dubos, R. J., and Hirsch, J. G.: Bacterial and Mycotic Infections of Man. 4th ed. J. B. Lippincott Co., Philadelphia, 1965.
37. Emmel, V. M., and Cowdry, E. V.: Laboratory Technique in Biology and Medicine. 4th ed. Williams & Wilkins Co., Baltimore, 1964.
38. Fawcett, D. W.: The Cell: Its Organelles and Inclusions. An Atlas of Fine Structure. W. B. Saunders Co., Philadelphia, 1966.
39. Fenner, F.: The Biology of Animal Viruses Vols. I and II. Academic Press, New York, 1968.
40. Fenner, F., and Ratcliffe, F. N.: Myxomatosis. Cambridge University Press, London, 1965.
41. Fiennes, R.: The Zoonoses of Primates. Cornell University Press, Ithaca, N.Y., 1967.

Bibliography

42. Frenkel, J. K.: Choice of animal models for the study of disease processes in man. Fed. Proc., 28(No. 1):160–161, 1969.
43. Frenkel, J. K.: Models for infectious diseases. Fed. Proc., 28(No. 1):179–190, 1969.
44. Gajdusek, D. C., Gibbs, C. J., and Alpers, M. (Eds.): Slow, Latent, and Temperate Virus Infections. National Institute of Neurologic Disease and Blindness, Monograph #2, Bethesda, Md., 1965.
45. Gay, W. I.: Methods in Animal Experimentation. Academic Press, New York. Vol. I, 1964; Vol. II, 1965; Vol. III, 1968.
46. Goldsmith, E. I., and Moor-Jankowski, J. (Eds.): Experimental medicine and surgery in primates. Ann. N.Y. Acad. Sci., 162:324, 1969.
47. Good, R. A., Finstad, J., Cain, W. A., Fish, A., Perey, D. Y., and Gatti, R. A.: Models of Immunological Diseases and Disorders. Fed Proc., 28(No. 1):191–205, 1969.
48. Good, R. A., and Gabrielsen, A. E.: The Thymus in Immunobiology. Hoeber Medical Division (Harper & Row), New York, 1964.
49. Gottlieb, D., and Shaw, P. D.: Antibiotics. Vol. I. Mechanism of Action. Springer-Verlag, New York, 1967.
50. Gray, P. G.: The Encyclopedia of the Biological Sciences. Reinhold Publishing Corp., New York, 1961.
51. Green, E. L. (Ed.): Biology of the Laboratory Mouse. 2nd ed. McGraw-Hill Book Co., New York, 1966.
52. Gresham, G. A., and Jennings, A. R.: An Introduction to Comparative Pathology. Academic Press, New York, 1962.
53. Gross, L.: Oncogenic Viruses. 2nd ed. Pergamon Press, Long Island City, N.Y., 1970.
54. Gruneberg, H.: The Genetics of the Mouse. 2nd ed. N. I. J. Hoff, The Hague, 1952.
55. Gruneberg, H.: The Pathology of Development. John Wiley & Sons, Inc., New York, 1963.
56. Gunsalus, I. C., and Stanier, R. Y.: Bacteria. A Treatise on Structure and Function. Vol. V. Heredity. Academic Press, New York, 1964.
57. Gurr, E.: Rational Use of Dyes in Biology and General Staining Methods. Williams & Wilkins Co., Baltimore, 1965.
58. Hafez, E. S. E.: The Behavior of Domestic Animals. Williams & Wilkins Co., Baltimore, 1962.
59. Harris, H.: Hybrid Cells from Mouse and Man. A Study of Genetic Regulation. Proc. Royal Soc., Series B, Vol. 166, No. 1004, 1966.
60. Harris, R. J. C.: Problems of Laboratory Animal Disease. Academic Press, New York, 1962.
61. Hartman, P. E., and Suskind, S. R.: Gene Action. Prentice-Hall, Inc., Englewood Cliffs, N.J. 1965.
62. Hayflick, L. (Ed.): The Mycoplasmatales and the L Phase of Bacteria. Appleton-Century-Crofts, New York, 1969.
63. Holdenreid, R. (Ed.): Viruses of Laboratory Rodents. Monograph #20, National Cancer Institute, Washington, D.C., 1966.
64. Horsfall, F. L., and Tamm, I.: Viral and Rickettsial Diseases of Man. 4th ed. J. B. Lippincott Co., Philadelphia, 1965.
65. Hsu, T. C., and Benirschke, K.: An Atlas of Mammalian Chromosomes. Springer-Verlag, New York, 1967.
66. Hull, T. G.: Diseases Transmitted from Animals to Man. 5th ed. Charles C Thomas, Springfield, Ill., 1963.
66a. Hunter, G. W., Frye, W. W., and Swartzwelder, J. C.: A Manual of Tropical Medicine. 4th ed. W. B. Saunders Co., Philadelphia, 1966.
67. Hutt, F. B.: Animal Genetics. 5th ed. Charles C Thomas, Springfield, Ill., 1963.
68. Innes, J. R. M., and Saunders, L. Z.: Comparative Neuropathology. Academic Press, New York, 1962.
69. Innes, J. R. M., and Steen, O.: Splayleg in rabbits. Lab. Invest., 6:171–186, 1957.
70. Jablonski, S.: Illustrated Dictionary of Eponymic Syndromes and Diseases. W. B. Saunders Co., Philadelphia, 1969.
71. Jarcho, S.: Human Paleopathology. Yale University Press, New Haven. Conn., 1966.
72. Jones, T. C.: Mammalian and Avian Models of Disease in Man. Fed. Proc., 28(No. 1):162–169, 1969.
73. Jubb, K. V. F., and Kennedy, P. C.: Animal Pathology. Academic Press, New York, 1963.
74. King, D. W.: Ultrastructural Aspects of Disease. Hoeber Medical Division (Harper & Row), New York, 1966.
75. King, R. C.: A Dictionary of Genetics. Oxford University Press, New York, 1968.
76. Kitchen, H.: Comparative biology: animal models of human hematologic disease – a review. Pediat. Res., 2:215, 1968.
77. Kraft, L. M., and Moore, A. E.: Papular skin lesions of mice caused by a transmissible agent. Z. Versuchstierk, 1:66–73, 1961.
78. Kral, F., and Schwartzman, R. M.: Veterinary and comparative dermatology. J. B. Lippincott Co., Philadelphia, 1964.
79. Lane-Petter, W.: Animals for Research. Academic Press, New York, 1963.
80. Lane-Petter, W., Worden, A. N., Hill, B. F., Paterson, J. F., and Vezerf, H. G. (Eds.): The UFAW Handbook on Care and Management of Laboratory Animals. E. & S. Livingstone, Edinburgh, 1967.
81. Leader, R. W.: Discovery and exploitation of animal model diseases. Fed. Proc., 28:1804–1809, 1969.
82. Leader, R. W., Gorham, J. R., and Wagner, B. M.: Connective tissue diseases of animals other than man. In B. M. Wagner (Ed.): The Connective Tissue. Williams & Wilkins Co., Baltimore, 1967.
83. Levine, N. D.: Protozoan Parasites of Domestic Animals and of Man. Burgess Publishing Co., Minneapolis, 1961.
84. Lindsey, J. R. (Ed.): Genetics in Laboratory Animal Medicine. National Academy of Science Publication 1724, Washington, D.C., 1969.
85. Lindsey, J. R. (Ed.): Animal Models for Biomedical Research. II. National Academy of Science Publication 1736, Washington, D.C., 1969.

Bibliography

86. Luckey, T. D.: Germfree Life and Gnotobiology. Academic Press, New York, 1963.
87. Lumb, W. V.: Small Animal Anesthesia. Lea & Febiger, Philadelphia, 1963.
88. Lynch, C. J.: The so-called Swiss mouse. Lab. Anim. Care, 19(No. 2):214–220, 1969.
89. Matheson, R.: Medical Entomology. 2nd ed. Comstock Publishing Associates, Ithaca, N.Y., 1944.
90. Mazur, A., and Harrow, B.: Biochemistry: A Brief Course. W. B. Saunders Co., Philadelphia, 1968.
91. Medway, W., Prier, J. E., and Wilkinson, J. S.: Textbook of Veterinary Clinical Pathology. Williams & Wilkins Co., Baltimore, 1969.
92. Merchant, I. A., and Packer, R. A.: Veterinary Bacteriology and Virology. Iowa State University Press, Ames, Iowa, 1961.
93. Miescher, P. A., and Muller-Eberhard, H. J.: Textbook of Immunopathology. Vols. I and II. Grune & Stratton, Inc., New York, 1968.
94. Mihich, E. (Ed.): Immunity, Cancer, and Chemotherapy. Academic Press, New York, 1967.
95. Miller, E. V., Ben, M., and Cass, J. S.: Comparative anesthesia in laboratory animals. Fed. Proc., 28:1373, 1969.
96. Miller, M. E., Christiansen, G. C., and Evans, H. E.: Anatomy of the Dog. W. B. Saunders Co., Philadelphia, 1964.
97. Miller, W. C., and West, G. P.: Encyclopedia of Animal Care (formerly Black's Veterinary Dictionary). 8th ed. Williams & Wilkins Co., Baltimore, 1967.
98. Moore, M. A. S., and Owen, J. J. T.: Experimental studies on the development of the bursa of Fabricius. Develop. Biol., 14:40–51, 1966.
99. Morgan, B. B., and Hawkins, P. A.: Veterinary Helminthology. Burgess Publishing Co., Minneapolis, 1949.
100. Morgan, B. B., and Hawkins, P. A.: Veterinary Protozoology. 2nd ed. Burgess Publishing Co., Minneapolis, 1955.
101. Morris, D.: The Naked Ape. McGraw-Hill Book Co., New York, 1968.
102. Moulton, J. E.: Tumors in Domestic Animals. University of California Press, Berkeley, 1961.
103. Napier, J. R., and Napier, P. H.: A Handbook of Living Primates. Academic Press, New York, 1967.
104. National Academy of Sciences: Scientific and Technical Societies of the United States. National Academy of Sciences, Washington, D.C., 1968.
105. National Academy of Sciences: Animal Models for Biomedical Research. Publication 1594, Washington, D.C., 1968.
106. National Institutes of Health: Viral Etiology of Congenital Malformations. (Workshop.) Bethesda, Md., 1968.
107. Nies, A. S., and Melmon, K. L.: Kinins and arthritis. Bull. Rheum. Dis., 19:512–517, 1968.
108. Nossal, G. J. V.: Antibodies and Immunity. Basic Books, Inc., New York, 1969.
109. Olsen, O. W.: Animal Parasites – Their Biology and Life Cycles. 2nd ed. Burgess Publishing Co., Minneapolis, 1967.
110. Parker, E. P.: Mammals of the World. Vols. I, II, and III. Johns Hopkins Press, Baltimore, 1964.
111. Pennak, R. W.: Collegiate Dictionary of Zoology. Ronald Press, New York, 1964.
112. Petrak, M. L. (Ed.): Diseases of Cage and Aviary Birds. Lea & Febiger, Philadelphia, 1969.
113. Pickles, V. R.: Prostaglandin. Nature, 224:221–225, 1969.
114. Prier, J. E. (Ed.): Basic Medical Virology. Williams & Wilkins Co., Baltimore, 1966.
115. Rebell, G., Taplin, D., and Blank, H.: Dermatophytes: Their Recognition and Identification. Dermatology Foundation of Miami, Miami, Fla., 1964.
116. Reichenbach-Klinke, H., and Elkin, E.: Diseases of Lower Vertebrates. Academic Press, New York, 1965.
117. Reid, M. E.: The Guinea Pig in Research. Human Factors Research Bureau, Inc., Miami, Fla., 1958.
118. Report of the Commission on Enzymes of the International Union of Biochemistry. Pergamon Press, Long Island City, N.Y., 1961.
119. Ribelin, W. E., and McCoy, J. R.: The Pathology of Laboratory Animals. Charles C Thomas, Springfield, Ill., 1965.
120. Rich, M. A. (Ed.): Experimental leukemia. Appleton-Century-Crofts, New York, 1968.
121. Rieger, R., Michaelis, A., and Green, M. M.: A Glossary of Genetics and Cytogenetics. Springer-Verlag, New York, 1968.
122. Roberts, J. C., Jr., and Straus, R.: Comparative Atherosclerosis. Hoeber Medical Division (Harper & Row), New York, 1965.
123. Robinson, R.: Genetic studies of the rabbit. Bibliographica Genetica, 17:229–558, 1958.
124. Rogers, A. W.: Techniques of Autoradiography. American Elsevier Publishing Co., New York, 1967.
125. Rook, A. J., and Walton, G. S.: Comparative Physiology of the Skin. F. A. Davis Co., Philadelphia, 1965.
126. Rosenblum, L. A., and Cooper, R. W.: The Squirrel Monkey. Academic Press, New York, 1968.
127. Rous, P.: Viruses and tumor causation – an appraisal of present knowledge. Nature, 207:457–463, 1965.
128. Ruch, T. C.: Diseases of Laboratory Primates. W. B. Saunders Co., Philadelphia, 1959.
129. Samter, M., and Alexander, H. L.: Immunological Diseases. 2nd ed. Little, Brown & Co., Boston, 1965.
130. Sartorelli, A. C., and Creasey, W. A.: Cancer Chemotherapy. Annual Review of Pharmacology, 1969. Annual Reviews, Inc., Palo Alto, Calif., 1969.
131. Saunders, L. Z.: Myositis in guinea pigs. J. Nat. Cancer Inst., 20:899–904, 1958.
132. Scarpelli, D. C.: A survey of some spontaneous and experimental disease processes of lower vertebrates and invertebrates. Fed. Proc., 28:1825–1833, 1969.
133. Schalm, O. W.: Veterinary Hematology. 2nd ed. Lea & Febiger, Philadelphia, 1965.
134. Schrier, A. M. (Ed.): Laboratory Primate Newsletter. Brown University, Providence, R. I.,
135. Schultz, J., and Gerhardt, P.: Dialysis culture of microorganisms: design, theory, and results. Bact. Rev., 33:1–47, 1969.
136. Schwabe, C. W.: Veterinary Medicine and Human Health. 2nd ed. Williams & Wilkins Co., Baltimore, 1969.

Bibliography

137. Shellenberger, T. E.: Biological studies utilizing Japanese quail. Lab. Animal Care, *18*:244–250, 1968.
138. Simmons, M. L., and Brick, J. O.: The Laboratory Mouse: Selection and Management. Prentice-Hall, Inc., Englewood Cliffs, N.J., 1970.
139. Simpson, G. G.: Primate taxonomy and recent studies of nonhuman primates. Ann. N.Y. Acad. Sci., *102*:497–514, 1962.
140. Sisson, S., and Grossman, J. D.: The Anatomy of Domestic Animals. 4th ed. W. B. Saunders Co., Philadelphia, 1953.
141. Sloss, L. L., and Nobles, L. H.: Earth History: An Illustrated Syllabus in Historical Geology. Northwestern University Press, Evanston, Ill., 1964.
142. Smith, H. A., and Jones, T. C.: Veterinary Pathology. 3rd ed. Lea & Febiger, Philadelphia, 1966.
143. Smith, R. T., Good, R. A., and Miescher, P. A.: Ontogeny of Immunity. University of Florida Press, Gainsville, Fla., 1967.
144. Sodeman, W. A., and Sodeman, W. A., Jr.: Pathologic Physiology: Mechanisms of Disease. 4th ed. W. B. Saunders Co., 1967.
145. Soulsby, E. J.: Textbook of Veterinary Clinical Parasitology. F. A. Davis Co., Philadelphia, 1965.
146. Staats, J.: Standardized nomenclature for inbred strains of mice: fourth listing. Cancer Res., 28(No. 3):391–420, 1968.
147. Stanbury, J. B., Wyngaarden, J. B., and Fredrickson, D. S.: The Metabolic Basis of Inherited Disease. 2nd ed. McGraw-Hill Book Co., Inc., New York, 1966.
148. Steinhaus, E. A. (Ed.): Insect Pathology, An Advanced Treatise. Vol. 2. Academic Press, New York, 1963.
149. Steinhaus, E. A.: Invertebrates and their diseases as models for the study of disease processes in man. Fed. Proc., 28:1810–1814, 1969.
150. Stewart, H. L., Snell, K. C., Dunham, L. J., and Schlyen, S. M.: Transplantable and Transmissible tumors of animals. Atlas of Tumor Pathology, Section XII, Fascicle 40. Armed Forces Institute of Pathology, Washington, D.C., 1959.
151. Storer, T. I., and Usinger, R. L.: General Zoology, McGraw-Hill Book Co., Inc., New York, 1957.
152. Thompson, R. H. S., and King, E. J.: Biochemical Disorders in Human Disease. 2nd ed. Academic Press, New York, 1964.
153. Thompson, S. W.: Selected Histochemical and Histopathological Methods. Charles C Thomas, Springfield, Ill., 1966.
154. Thomson, A. L.: A New Dictionary of Birds. Thomas Nelson & Sons, Camden, N.J., 1964.
155. Valeria, D. A., Miller, R. L., Innes, J. R. M., Pallotta, A. J., and Guttmacher, R. M.: *Macaca mulatta*, Management of a Laboratory Breeding Colony. Academic Press, New York, 1969.
156. Van der Hoeden, J.: Zoonoses. American Elsevier Publishing Co., New York, 1964.
157. Van Nostrand's Scientific Encyclopedia. D. Van Nostrand Co., Inc., Princeton, N.J., 1968.
158. Verplanck, W. S.: A glossary of some terms in the objective science of behavior. Psychol. Rev., Vol. 64, No. 6, Part 2 (Suppl.), 1957.
159. Weinman, D., and Ristic, M.: Infectious Blood Diseases of Man and Animals. Vol. I. Academic Press, New York, 1968.
160. Weir, D. M.: Handbook of Experimental Immunology. F. A. Davis Co., Philadelphia, 1967.
161. Whitlock, J. H.: Diagnosis of Veterinary Parasitisms. Lea & Febiger, Philadelphia, 1960.
162. Wintrobe, M. M.: Clinical Hematology. 5th ed. Lea & Febiger, Philadelphia, 1965.
163. Wolstenholme, G. E. W. (Ed.): Antilymphocyte Serum. CIBA Foundation Study Group No. 29, Little, Brown & Co., Boston, 1967.
164. Wood, H. N., and Braun, A. C.: The transformation and recovery of the crown gall tumor cell. Fed. Proc., 28:1815–1819, 1969.
165. Zweifach, B. W., Grant, L., and McCluskey, R. T.: The Inflammatory Process. Academic Press, New York, 1965.

238